Brain Development
and Epilepsy

Brain Development and Epilepsy

Edited by
PHILIP A. SCHWARTZKROIN
SOLOMON L. MOSHÉ
JEFFREY L. NOEBELS
JOHN W. SWANN

New York   Oxford
OXFORD UNIVERSITY PRESS
1995

Oxford University Press

Oxford   New York
Athens   Auckland   Bangkok   Bombay
Calcutta   Cape Town   Dar es Salaam   Delhi
Florence   Hong Kong   Istanbul   Karachi
Kuala Lumpur   Madras   Madrid   Melbourne
Mexico City   Nairobi   Paris   Singapore
Taipei   Tokyo   Toronto

and associated companies in
Berlin   Ibadan

Copyright © 1995 by Oxford University Press, Inc.

Published by Oxford University Press, Inc.,
200 Madison Avenue, New York, New York 10016

Library of Congress Cataloging-in-Publication Data
Brain development and epilepsy / edited by Philip A. Schwartzkroin . . . [et al.].
      p.   cm.   Includes bibliographical references and index.
   ISBN 0-19-507846-2
   1. Epilepsy in children—Pathogenesis.   2. Developmental
neurology.   I. Schwartzkroin, P. A. (Philip A.)
   [DNLM: 1. Epilepsy—etiology.   2. Central Nervous System-
-embryology.   3. Epilepsy—in infancy & childhood.
WL 385 B814 1995]   RJ496.E6B68   1995
618.92′853071—dc20 DNLM/DLC   94-42513

9 8 7 6 5 4 3 2 1

Printed in the United States of America
on acid-free paper

Preface

Identifying the causes of epilepsy in the immature nervous system is a formidable task that requires commitment from both clinical investigators and basic scientists. Childhood seizure disorders are among the most common epileptic syndromes and are sometimes intractable to conventional treatments. The clinical characterization of these epilepsies and the development of rational therapies have been the subject of serious debate. While we have learned much from studying epilepsy in the mature central nervous system, both clinical experiences and experimental observations suggest that many unique questions, complex issues, and new challenges must be confronted to reach an understanding of epileptogenesis in the immature nervous system.

In recent years, developmental neurobiologists have made significant progress in recognizing the processes that determine normal organization and function of the central nervous system. Although this research provides the necessary basis for examining the factors that contribute to the age-dependent expression of seizures, there has been surprisingly little communication between developmental neurobiologists and the clinicians who deal directly with pediatric epilepsy patients. Few attempts have been made to apply the emerging concepts in developmental neurobiology to an understanding of the origins of the epilepsies of childhood.

In an attempt to meet this need, a conference on "Brain Development and Epilepsy" was arranged to bring together representatives from the pediatric neurology and developmental neurobiology communities. The conference, held in Houston in March 1992, and sponsored by the Methodist Hospital System, Baylor College of Medicine, and the Blue Bird Circle Foundation (with generous support from the American Epilepsy Society, CIBA/Geigy, Parke Davis, Marion Merrell-Dow, and Abbott), was an exciting demonstration of the fruitfulness of this type of interaction. The current volume is an attempt to crystallize some of the discussion that was initiated at that conference.

This volume does not consist of symposium proceedings. Rather, we asked the authors to provide an integrated overview of specific research areas that seem critical to an understanding of the pediatric epilepsies. The chapters attempt to integrate material from basic experimental research with issues of clinical importance. Authors draw on data from their own laboratories for illustration and also summarize relevant data from a wide range of sources. In posing relevant questions and describing experimental approaches, they illustrate how the wealth of knowledge accumulated in basic developmental neurobiology may focus our attempts to understand the epilepsies in the developing brain.

In considering the contents of this volume, the reader may wish to keep in mind several key questions. The first set of questions revolves around the issue of what causes seizures and epilepsy in the immature brain. The two processes—electrogenesis of single seizures and the development of epileptic syndromes—may not be related in a simple way. What are the factors that render the infant susceptible to single seizures, and what are the biological bases for the most intractable epilepsy syndromes? Although identifiable pathologic processes are associated with some seizures, there is often no apparent underlying cause. How important are genetic factors in determining seizure susceptibility, and what role do epigenetic influences play? Which abnormalities (if any) result from disruptions in normal developmental programs—and which programs are critical to the development of normal excitability? The second set of questions focuses on the concept of a "critical period" during which the brain is particularly seizure-prone. Is there a critical period for epileptogenesis early in life, and if so, what are the factors that define seizure "prone-ness" during that period? Are environmental insults to the brain during that period of any special consequence? If there is such a critical period in human development, when is it, and how can we relate the time-dependent phenomena described in animal models to those in children? The third major set of questions concerns the consequences of seizures that occur in the immature brain. Is there an age-dependency of seizure-induced detrimental effects on brain development? Why do certain epileptic syndromes abate after several years? Why do seizures of apparently similar intensity have different sequelae, even within a specific age group? Related to these questions are issues concerning the existence of unique mechanisms of plasticity in the developing nervous system, the relationship between structural damage and functional abnormality, and the appropriateness of early intervention to prevent a permanent epileptic condition.

This book has three sections. The first three chapters provide a descriptive introduction to the various epileptic syndromes and seizure types. These chapters also provide an overview of experimental epilepsy research that is focused on various model systems thought to be relevant to seizures of the immature nervous system. Chapter 1 provides a clinician's view of childhood seizure disorders, describing the phenomena that we hope to better understand and treat, and posing general questions for the basic science investigator. Chapters 2 and 3 focus more sharply on developmental aspects of partial and absence seizures, respectively. Animal models are evaluated with respect to what they have told us about the basic mechanisms that underlie such seizure activity. The next four chapters deal with developmental neurobiological concepts. Chapters 4 and 5 explore basic issues of neuronal proliferation and migration, with special focus on how these very early developmental processes are critical in shaping the brain. The authors discuss pathologies that are often associated with epileptic syndromes in the developing human nervous system and that may reflect errors in these developmental events (programs). Chapters 6 and 7 describe the evolution and ontogeny of the membrane ion channels that determine the excitability of individual neurons. This overview of voltage- and ligand-gated channels sets the stage for subsequent analysis of seizure propensity in the immature brain. The final four chapters attempt to integrate features of the developing nervous system that have obvious importance for epileptogenesis, such as the formation and remodeling of synaptic networks (Chapter 8), functional and morphological plasticity (Chapter 9), consequences of seizure activity for further brain development (Chapter 10), and the basis for rational development of age-specific drug therapies (Chapter 11).

While the views and data presented in these chapters address the issues just posed, the reader should be aware that there are few clear answers in this complex field. Thus, these chapters also illustrate important problems for future studies: How does one go beyond the point of simple correlation (e.g., between structural abnormality and electrophysiologic hyperexcitability) to define cause-and-effect relationships? Do seizures in early life alter the normal course of brain development, and if so, how? Do seizure-related changes in the developing brain worsen an already abnormal condition, or do these changes reflect attempts to compensate for preexisting abnormalities? Are the processes of neuronal differentiation, growth, and connectivity in the developing nervous system the same as those seen following injury? Analyses of these questions leads one to think about the future of research in this area and, in particular, to ask whether—or how—an understanding of basic developmental principles will enable us to better treat the intractable epileptic syndromes of childhood. Can we develop new anticonvulsant drugs based on our growing knowledge of the molecular biology of receptors and channels? Will we be able to intervene during abnormal brain development using basic science technology to prevent the clinical expression of epilepsy?

Recent studies have yielded an overwhelming wealth of data relevant to an understanding of the pediatric epilepsies. While our technologies continue to advance in sophistication, the real limitations may be conceptual. We are only now beginning to put together some of the important pieces of the puzzle. By bringing together clinicians and basic scientists, conceptual frameworks can be developed that allow us to integrate the available information into more meaningful models. We hope this volume will be a catalyst for further progress toward such integration, and thereby provide some help to those interested in basic developmental and clinical issues relevant to the pediatric epilepsies.

Seattle   P. A. S.
New York   S. L. M.
Houston   J. L. N.
August 1994   J. W. S.

Contents

Contributors

VERNE S. CAVINESS, JR.
Department of Neurology
Massachusetts General Hospital
Boston, MA

OLIVIER DULAC
Service de Neuropediatrie
Hôpital Saint-Vincent-de-Paul
Paris, FRANCE

JOHN M. FREEMAN
Pediatric Epilepsy Center
Departments of Pediatrics and
    Neurology
Johns Hopkins Medical Institutions
Baltimore, MD

MARY E. HATTEN
Laboratory of Developmental
    Neurobiology
The Rockefeller University
New York, NY

PETER KELLAWAY
Department of Neurology, Section of
    Neurophysiology; Division of
    Neuroscience; and the Epilepsy
    Research Center
Baylor College of Medicine
Houston, TX

KEVIN M. KELLY
Department of Neurology
University of Michigan Medical School
Ann Arbor, MI

ROBERT L. MACDONALD
Departments of Neurology and
    Physiology
University of Michigan Medical School
Ann Arbor, MI

SUSAN K. MCCONNELL
Department of Biological Sciences
Stanford University
Stanford, CA

SOLOMON L. MOSHÉ
Departments of Neurology,
    Neuroscience, and Pediatrics
Albert Einstein College of Medicine
Bronx, NY

JEFFREY L. NOEBELS
Department of Neurology, Section of
    Neurophysiology; Division of
    Neuroscience; and Department of
    Molecular Genetics
Blue Bird Circle Developmental
    Neurogenetics Laboratory
Baylor College of Medicine
Houston, TX

DOMINICK P. PURPURA
Dean
Albert Einstein College of Medicine
Bronx, NY

RAMAN SANKAR
Departments of Neurology and
    Pediatrics
UCLA School of Medicine
Sepulveda VA Medical Center
Los Angeles, CA

PHILIP A. SCHWARTZKROIN
Departments of Neurological Surgery
    and Physiology/Biophysics
University of Washington School of
    Medicine
Seattle, WA

SHLOMO SHINNAR
Montefiore Epilepsy Management
    Center
Departments of Neurology and
    Pediatrics
Albert Einstein College of Medicine
Bronx, NY

ELLEN S. SPERBER
Departments of Neurology and
    Neuroscience
Albert Einstein College of Medicine
Bronx, NY

NICHOLAS C. SPITZER
Department of Biology and Center for
    Molecular Genetics
University of California, San Diego
La Jolla, CA

JOHN W. SWANN
The Gordon and Mary Cain Pediatric
    Neurology Research Foundation
    Laboratories
Department of Pediatrics and Division
    of Neuroscience
Baylor College of Medicine
Houston, TX

TAKAO TAKAHASHI
Department of Neurology
Massachusetts General Hospital
Boston, MA
Department of Pediatrics
Keio University School of Medicine
Tokyo, JAPAN

BRUCE L TEMPEL
Seattle VA Medical Center, GRECC
Departments of Medicine and
    Pharmacology
University of Washington School
    of Medicine
Seattle, WA

BARRY R. THARP
Departments of Pediatrics and
    Neurology
Blue Bird Circle Pediatric Neurology
    Clinic
Baylor College of Medicine
Houston, TX

CHRISTOPHER A. WALSH
Department of Neurology
Beth Israel Hospital
Harvard Medical School
Boston, MA

CLAUDE G. WASTERLAIN
Department of Neurology
UCLA School of Medicine
Sepulveda VA Medical Center
Los Angeles, CA

Brain Development
and Epilepsy

Introduction

PETER KELLAWAY

In the Beginning: Insights through the EEG

Although Richard Caton demonstrated spontaneous electrical activity in the brains of animals as early as 1875, and Hans Berger recorded the human electroencephalogram (EEG) in 1928, it was not until the early 1930s that studies of brain development and epileptogenesis were undertaken. In 1932 Berger reported that the frequency of the electrical activity of the human brain increased steadily with increasing age from one month through childhood. Descriptive studies of the maturation of the human electroencephalogram appeared in quick succession, confirming and enlarging Berger's observation (Bernhard and Skoglund, 1939; Davis and Davis, 1936; Durup and Fessard, 1936; Lindsley, 1939; Loomis et al., 1936; Smith, 1938a,b,c). In his early studies Berger (1933) found that epilepsy was associated with hypersynchronous bursts of electrocortical activity, but this association was not widely recognized until the demonstration by Gibbs, Gibbs, and Lennox (1937) that the electroencephalograms of epileptics showed paroxysms of high-voltage electrocortical activity during clinical seizures.

At the experimental level, Marinesco and his associates (1936) were among the first to demonstrate a relationship between the degree of morphological maturation and the degree of electrical development in neocortex. In 1940 Pentzik showed that the development of the bioelectric activity of the cortex parallels the course of neuronal and axonal maturation. Subsequently, it was shown that both spontaneous and evoked EEG activity in the cerebral cortex appear only after a certain critical period of development has been attained (Jasper et al., 1937). Working on the guinea pig, Flexner and his associates (Flexner, 1952; Flexner et al., 1950) found that this onset of electrical activity in the frontal lobe coincided with the appearance of all five cellular layers in the cortex, the appearance of Nissl substance in the neurons, and the endpoint of nuclear maturation.

One of the important early experimental findings relating to epileptogenesis in immature cortex was that strychnine spikes cannot be evoked in the cortex before the onset of spontaneous electrical activity (Bishop, 1950; Flexner et al., 1950; Garcia-Austt, 1954). The triphasic waveform characteristic of the strychnine spike in the mature brain is evident in the rabbit from the first postnatal day (Bishop, 1950) but has an extremely long duration and occurs only at long intervals. During the first postnatal month, the duration of the spike shortens in accord with an exponential curve, the most rapid change occurring coincidentally with the early phase of axonal and dendritic maturation of the cortex. The ability of the cortex to produce repetitive discharges was found to be considerably less than in the adult brain. Similarly, the ability of the immature cortex to respond to a fast train of sensory stimuli was low (Ellingson, 1960; Grossman, 1954). Perhaps the most prescient comment on the relationship of this finding to human epilepsy was made by Bishop in 1950: "That in the early postnatal period strychnine spikes of the rabbit are of very infrequent occurrence and thereafter increase markedly in frequency during cortical maturation, may also have significance in evaluating the expectancy of spikes in the EEGs of infants with convulsive disorder. Perhaps if recording paroxysmal spikes is of diagnostic importance, the lengths of records in infants should be materially increased."

Studies of human neonates with seizures have demonstrated that interictal EEG spikes are few and far between; indeed, they are virtually nonexistent in the routine EEG before a gestational age of 35–36 weeks. Similarly, electrical seizure activity is rarely seen before this stage of development, and when present it occurs in an all-or-none manner—that is, without the presence of interictal discharges (Kellaway and Mizrahi, 1987). An early study by Grossman (1955) showed that the tendency of afterdischarge to spread over the cortex from its point of origin was also dependent upon the degree of cerebral maturation. He found that the mature form of afterdischarge—consisting of trains of high-voltage spikes—cannot be elicited in the kitten, and that the repetition rate of slow spike-and-wave discharges is dependent upon the functional maturity of cortex. The complexity of the epileptiform activity has been found to increase with increasing gestational age, the spike component becoming more pronounced until it is the predominant feature of the discharge. This developmental progression occurs with several different methods of inducing epileptiform activity (Mares, 1973; Yamauchi et al., 1976; Zouhar et al., 1980). A related observation was that at a stage of development at which electrical stimulation fails to induce seizures, ictal activity can be induced chemically with pentylenetetrazol (Grossman, 1955; Mares et al., 1980; Purpura, 1964).

Finer-Grained Analysis: Contributions from Single-Cell Studies

The early 1960s was a time when recently developed techniques of intracellular recording and electron microscopy were first applied to the study of the developmental neurobiology of epilepsy. Some of the seminal studies were summarized in proceedings of the first conference on the subject held in Houston in 1963 (Kellaway and Petersén, 1964). In that volume, Crain (1964) reported that neonatal mouse brain cultures could be used to obtain correlative information regarding normal structure and function at a stage of development unattainable in situ. He showed that complex electrical seizure-like discharges could be initiated in neonatal cerebral cortex cultures after only 14 days in vitro. Studies of the maturation of the evoked cortical response (Goldring et al., 1964) and of the postnatal functional development of the corpus callosum of the cat (Grafstein, 1964) were also described in an attempt to elucidate the genesis and elaboration of focal and generalized epileptic activity.

A key contribution of the 1963 Houston meeting was Purpura's summary of his laboratory's work on the relationship of seizure susceptibility to morphologic and physiologic properties of immature cortex (Purpura, 1964). These studies demonstrated the remarkable analytic power of the experimental ontogenetic method for determining structure–function correlations. Using light and electron microscopy and intracellular recording, his laboratory demonstrated that many of the electrographic features of seizure activity of the immature brain reflect the distinctive morphology of neurons and their synaptic relations. Among the many insights arising from this work was the appreciation that "experimentally-produced alterations in morphogenetic patterns can exert profound effects on excitability characteristics of immature neuronal organizations." For example, Purpura and colleagues found that a net increase in excitatory synaptic drive occurs in response to trauma of the immature cortex. This was a consequence, in part, of a rapid and extensive proliferation of axon collaterals in injured tissue—an observation echoed in recent studies of "sprouting" in epileptic tissue.

Evidence that a similar disruption of the stability of the immature cortex may result from deafferentation, sensory deprivation, or aberration of sensory (visual) input was also reported at the 1964 conference (Smith and Kellaway, 1964) and elaborated 20 years later at a second Houston meeting held in 1984 (Kellaway and Noebels, 1989). In the human infant, retinal damage or visual deprivation occurring at a critical time of development may be followed by the appearance of focal occipital spike discharges in the EEG (Kellaway, 1989). Changes in ionic gradients and their regulation also became recognized as important factors in the epileptogenicity of immature cortex. Hypocalcemia was at one time the most common cause of epileptic seizures in the newborn term infant (Kellaway and Hrachovy, 1983); yet in premature infants with a conceptional age of less than 36 weeks, hypocalcemia does not result in electrical or clinical seizures, and the threshold rises again in older children (Kellaway and Prakash, 1974). A similar window of enhanced excitability to low calcium levels has now been described in in vitro slice preparations (Roper et al., 1993).

At the second Houston conference, new experimental techniques and approaches to brain development and epilepsy were also described (Kellaway and Noebels, 1989). For example, the application of the in vitro slice technique to developmental epilepsy research was discussed alongside in vivo studies on seizure processes in the immature brain. In vivo studies of developing animals provided new insights into the mechanisms of seizure control as a function of age and into the propensity of the immature brain to experience status epilepticus. Highly effective tools for studying the role of genetics in epileptic processes were also introduced.

The contributions to this book demonstrate the considerable advances that have been made since the second Houston meeting. The presentations at the third Houston conference in 1992, as elaborated here, emphasize the complexity of the processes underlying epilepsy in the immature brain. Clearly, the basic discoveries that are emerging from contemporary developmental neurobiology will form critical cornerstones for our understanding of those processes. Each advance seems to reveal new problems to be studied, and each points to the challenging avenues of study that lie ahead.

References

Berger, H. (1932) Über das elektrenkephalogramm des Menschen. *Arch. Psychol. Nervenkr. 98:*231–354.

Berger, H. (1933) Über das elektrenkephalogramm des Menschen. *Arch. Psychol. Nervenkr. 100:*301–320.

Bernhard, C. G., and Skoglund, C. R. (1939) On the alpha frequency of human brain potentials as a function of age. *Skand. Arch. Physiol. 82:*178–184.

Bishop, E. F. (1950) The strychnine spike as a physiological indicator of cortical maturity in the postnatal rabbit. *Electroencephalogr. Clin. Neurophysiol. 2:*309–315.

Crain, S. M. (1964) Development of bioelectric activity during growth of neonatal mouse cerebral cortex in tissue culture. In P. Kellaway and I. Petersén (eds.), *Neurological and Electroencephalographic Correlative Studies in Infancy.* New York: Grune and Stratton, pp. 12–26.

Davis, H., and Davis, P. A. (1936) Action potentials of the brain in normal persons and in normal states of cerebral activity. *Arch. Neurol. Psychiatr. 36:*1214–1224.

Durup, G., and Fessard, A. (1936) L'Électroencéphalogramme de l'homme, observations psychophysiologique relatives à l'action des stimuli visuels et auditifs. *Année Psychol. 36:*1–35.

Ellingson, R. J. (1960) Cortical electrical responses to visual stimulation in the human infant. *Electroencephalogr. Clin. Neurophysiol. 12:*663–677.

Flexner, L. B. (1952) Physiologic development of the cortex of the brain and its relationship to its morphology, chemical constitution, and enzyme systems. In S. Cobb (ed.), *The Biology of Mental Health and Disease.* New York: Paul B. Hoeber, pp. 180–192.

Flexner, L. B., Tyler, D. B., and Gallant, L. J. (1950) Biochemical and physiological differentiation during morphogenesis: X. Onset of electrical activity in developing cerebral cortex of fetal guinea pig. *J. Neurophysiol. 6:*427–430.

Garcia-Austt, E., Jr. (1954) Development of electrical activity in cerebral hemispheres of the chick embryo. *Proc. Soc. Exp. Biol. Med. 86:*348–352.

Gibbs, F. A., Gibbs, E. L., and Lennox, W. G. (1937) Epilepsy: A paroxysmal cerebral dysrhythmia. *Brain 60:*377–388.

Goldring, S., Sugaya, E., and O'Leary, J. L. (1964) Maturation of evoked cortical responses in animal and man. In P. Kellaway and I. Petersén (eds.), *Neurological and Electroencephalographic Correlative Studies in Infancy.* New York: Grune and Stratton, pp. 68–77.

Grafstein, B. (1964) Postnatal development of the corpus callosum in the cat: Myelination of a fibre tract in the central nervous system. In P. Kellaway and I. Petersén (eds.), *Neurological and Electroencephalographic Correlative Studies in Infancy.* New York: Grune and Stratton, pp. 52–67.

Grossman, C. (1954) Characteristics and significance of seizure discharges. *Electroencephalogr. Clin. Neurophysiol. 3* (Suppl. 4):249–252.

Grossman, C. (1955) Electro-ontogenesis of cerebral activity. *Arch. Neurol. Psychiatr. 74:*186–200.

Jasper, H. H., Bridgman, C. S., and Carmichael, L. (1937) An ontogenic study of cerebral electrical potentials in the guinea pig. *J. Exp. Psychol. 21:*63–71.

Kellaway, P. (1989) Introduction to plasticity and sensitive periods. In P. Kellaway and J. L. Noebels (eds.), *Problems and Concepts in Developmental Neurophysiology.* Baltimore: Johns Hopkins University Press, pp. 3–28.

Kellaway, P., and Hrachovy, R. A. (1983) Status epilepticus in newborns: A perspective on neonatal seizures. In A. V. Delgado-Escueta (ed.), *Advances in Neurology, Vol. 34: Status Epilepticus.* New York, Raven Press, pp. 93–99.

Kellaway, P., and Mizrahi, E. M. (1987) Neonatal seizures. In H. Lüders, and R. P. Lesser (eds.), *Epilepsy: Electroclinical Syndromes.* New York: Springer-Verlag, pp. 13–47.

Kellaway, P., and Noebels, J. L. (eds.) (1989) *Problems and Concepts in Developmental Neurophysiology.* Baltimore: Johns Hopkins University Press.

Kellaway, P., and Petersén, I. (eds.) (1964) *Neurological and Electroencephalographic Correlative Studies in Infancy.* New York: Grune and Stratton.

Kellaway, P., and Prakash, M. (1974) Hypocalcemia and seizures in the newborn. *Electroencephalogr. Clin. Neurophysiol. 37:*419–420.

Lindsley, D. B. (1939) A longitudinal study of the occipital alpha rhythm in normal children: Frequency and amplitude standards. *J. Gen. Psychol. 55:*197–213.

Loomis, A. L., Harvey, E. N., and Hobart, G. (1936) Electrical potentials of the human brain. *J. Exp. Psychol. 19:*249–279.

Mares, P. (1973) Symmetrical epileptogenic foci in cerebral cortex of immature rat. *Epilepsia 14:*427–435.

Mares, P., Zouhar, A., and Brozek, G. (1980) The electrocorticographic pattern of generalized seizures in rats during ontogenesis. *Physiol. Bohemoslovaca 29:* 193–200.

Marinesco, G., Sager, O., and Kreindler, A. (1936) Etudes electroencephalographiques du chat et du cobay nouveau-nés. *Bull. Acad. Natl. Méd. (Paris) 115:*873–876.

Pentzik, A. S. (1940) Ontogenesis of bioelectric activities and cellular structure of the cortex in rabbits. *Brain Inst. Moscow 5:*273.

Purpura, D. P. (1964) Relationship of seizure susceptibility to morphologic and physiologic properties of normal and abnormal immature cortex. In P. Kellaway and I. Petersén (eds.), *Neurological and Electroencephalographic Correlative Studies in Infancy.* New York: Grune and Stratton, pp. 117–157.

Roper, S. N., Obenaus, A., and Dudek, F. E. (1993) Increased propensity for non-synaptic epileptiform activity in immature rat hippocampus and dentate gyrus. *J. Neurophysiol. 70:*857–862.

Smith, J. M. B., and Kellaway, P. (1964) The natural history and clinical correlates of occipital foci in children. In P. Kellaway and I. Petersén (eds.), *Neurological and Electroencephalographic Correlative Studies in Infancy.* New York: Grune and Stratton, pp. 230–249.

Smith, J. R. (1938a) The electroencephalogram during normal infancy and childhood: I. Rhythmic activities present in the neonate and their subsequent development. *J. Gen. Psychol. 53:*431–453.

Smith, J. R. (1938b) The electroencephalogram during normal infancy and childhood: II. Nature of the growth of the alpha wave. *J. Gen. Psychol. 53:*455–469.

Smith, J. R. (1938c) The electroencephalogram during normal infancy and childhood: III. Preliminary observations on the pattern sequence during sleep. *J. Gen. Psychol. 53:*471–482.

Yamauchi, T., Hirabayashi, Y., Mohri, Y., and Katoaka, N. (1976) Ontogenic studies of seizure patterns and seizure activities induced by cortical focus. *Folia Psych. Neurol. Jpn. 30:*241–252.

Zouhar, A., Mares, P., and Brozek, G. (1980) Electrocorticographic activity elicited by metrazol during ontogenesis in rats. *Arch. Int. Pharmacodyn. 248:*280–288.

1

A Clinician's Look at the Developmental Neurobiology of Epilepsy

JOHN M. FREEMAN

Epilepsy in childhood is <u>not</u> the same as epilepsy in adults. While it has many similarities to the adult disorders, there are vast differences in cause, manifestations, precipitating factors, and often in outcome. There are even age-related, and stage-of-development differences between the various childhood epilepsies. While adult seizure types are characterized by their site of onset and the direction and rapidity of the electrical spread, in many types of seizures in children (such as infantile spasms and the Lennox-Gastaut syndrome) the nature or location of the onset is poorly defined, and the seizure types are age-dependent. These differences between adult and childhood epilepsies raise difficult, sometimes critical questions. For exam-ple, why are the seizures of the newborn so different from those later in infancy? Why are infantile spasms solely a disease of infancy, and how do they cause mental retardation? Why does the preponderance of epilepsy start in childhood? Why is it often outgrown?

Perhaps one of the most important questions in childhood epilepsy has to do with the components of threshold. What is "seizure threshold" and how does it interact with the development of the nervous system? What role does it play in the high incidence of seizures in children? In the effects of fever in precipitating "febrile seizures"? In the ability of children to outgrow these and other seizure types?

Studying the maturation of the developing nervous system and its role in changing the seizure threshold is critical to understanding epilepsy in childhood. Understanding the effects of seizures on development, and of development and plasticity on seizures, may lead to new therapeutic approaches to the childhood epilepsies and to better seizure control. Such understanding may also lead to new insights about the processes involved in adult epilepsy.

Understanding Childhood Epilepsies

From a clinician's perspective, *a* **seizure** *is a sudden electrical discharge in the brain that results in an alteration in sensation, behavior, or consciousness.* **Epilepsy** *is a disorder of recurrent seizures.* Seizures are not of themselves a disease but rather are the response of the central nervous system to a variety of perturbations of its inherent stability. The response of the brain to these perturbations and the type of seizures that may result depend on the type and location of the perturbation and on many intrinsic mechanisms that serve to maintain the stability.

The state and stage of cortical development are factors that clearly influence the brain's response to perturbations, and determine its threshold for seizures. In addition, seizures in infants and in children are often different in form, cause, response to treatment, and outcome from seizures in adults. This diversity of childhood epilepsies may provide clues about brain development, how the brain works at its various stages of development, and how and why it occasionally misfires. Current studies are only beginning to document that the immature brain is not merely a miniature version of the adult brain but is both qualitatively and quantitatively different. These many differences affect the threshold and propagation as well as the clinical manifestations of the seizures.

The purpose of this chapter is to utilize clinical questions about epilepsy, and particularly about the varied epilepsy syndromes in infants and children, to stimulate basic developmental neuroscientists in their research, and to help epileptologists working with adults become more aware of the important interactions between brain development and clinical manifestations of seizure disorders. Such questions include:

> What are the biological components that make up an individual's seizure threshold? Is the threshold for electroencephalographic seizures different from the threshold for clinical seizures?

> How does brain development influence seizure threshold? Why are cortical seizures uncommon in the newborn? Why do seizures most commonly start during infancy and childhood?

> What are the mechanisms by which brain development alters the electrical spread and the clinical manifestations of seizures in infancy and childhood, resulting in the many childhood epileptic syndromes?

> Why do most children outgrow their seizures? What are the differences between those individuals who have only a single seizure and those who have many seizures and between those who eventually outgrow their seizures and those who continue to have difficult-to-control epilepsy?

Society and the Brain: An Analogy

One way to begin to develop an understanding about clinical epilepsy is through the use of an analogy, a comparison between the brain, with its many cells and communities of cells, and society, with its many individuals and communities. Perhaps thinking about perturbations of various types and sizes in society—the accidents, fights, demonstrations, and riots that episodically occur—can help us in thinking about the disruptions in the brain that may cause seizures. Using such an analogy, we might ask questions about the factors that allow an abnormal cell, or group of cells, to recruit sufficient members of its cellular "community" to act synchronously so as to produce various types of seizures or seizure syndromes.

Social Landscapes and Thresholds

Within our varied social communities—rural, urban, etc.—individuals interact in varying but characteristic ways. The individual and population characteristics of these microenvironments, and the nature of interactions within these communities, are based partially on genetic factors, partially on socioeconomic factors, partially on the physical structure of the environment, and so on. These many factors determine how a community will respond to a disturbance. Local environments may selectively foster isolation or community interactions, independence or interdependence. Levels of education, employment, dissatisfaction, poverty, and oppression also influence the threshold of the community for disruption. Some of these factors lower the threshold; others raise the tolerance (resistance) to disruption.

How do we begin to describe the components of differing local environments? What features are important in determining the frequency, character, and qualities of interactions? What are the factors that determine each community's susceptibility to disturbance? Clearly, multiple factors and interactions can be involved in the varieties of disturbance that occur within society.

Brain Regions and Thresholds

Similar questions can be asked about the brain. When an epileptic focus in the brain discharges, why are surrounding cells recruited, or why not? What determines whether sufficient cells are recruited to result in an EEG spike, a seizure discharge, a clinical focal seizure, or a generalized seizure? An appreciation of the multiple components involved in the brain's threshold would allow us to begin to understand these perturbations and the factors that control their magnitude or lead to seizures and epilepsy.

Threshold is defined as the minimal stimulus which is necessary to elicit a response. With respect to "seizure threshold," we can analyze a number of components, such as the threshold for a single cell to fire; the threshold for sufficient cells to fire synchronously to produce a change on the EEG (an electrographic seizure); or the threshold for recruitment of sufficient cells to fire synchronously *and* alter behavior or function—that is, a clinical seizure. Critical questions about seizure threshold include:

> What are the physiological characteristics of a specific brain region (e.g., the frontal cortex) that makes it more easily excitable, more "epilepto-genic" than other brain regions (e.g., the parietal or occipital cortex)?
>
> Are low thresholds for seizures due to the anatomic or cytoarchitectonic differences such as differences in the interconnections between cells (i.e., the localization, types, or ratios of the various synapses)?
>
> Is threshold related to the neurotransmitters which predominate in that specific region or to the local ratio of excitation to inhibition?
>
> Is threshold a function of intrinsic properties of cells in the region (e.g., the distribution and/or characteristics of ion channels)?
>
> Is threshold related to the patterns of local neuronal circuitry (e.g., re-current collaterals) or to influences exerted by distant projection systems?

Since each of these factors clearly differs between lobes and probably even among the varying regions within each lobe, does it make sense to study the electrical properties of a few cells in a small portion of the hippocampus as an example of the diverse forms of epilepsy?

Biologic Factors Affecting the Brain's Threshold for Seizures

We currently have little understanding of the many complex interactions that influence clinical seizure threshold. Among the factors that appear to con-tribute are genetic factors, environmental factors, stresses, and, perhaps most important, age or stages of development.

Genetics

There is likely to be a genetic contribution to every individual's seizure threshold—that is, his or her seizure "prone-ness." This conclusion arises from the clinical observation that under apparently identical provocative and/or environmental conditions, some individuals will have a seizure but others will not. Some individuals may have such a low threshold that they seize spontaneously. Others have a low threshold to seizures but require an additional exogenous stimulus—fever, trauma, stress, lack of sleep—to cross that threshold. Some forms of epilepsy, such as juvenile myoclonic epilepsy (JME) and benign epilepsy of infancy, are clearly genetic and their genes have been localized (Greenber and Delgado-Escueta, 1993). Other sei-zure types, such as febrile seizures, partial complex seizures, and some ab-sence seizures, are not inherited in toto, but have greater or lesser genetic components to their threshold (Treiman, 1993). Mouse models that mimic human absence seizures have been developed (Buchhalter, 1993). These mouse mutants involve different genes, and the seizures arise through differing mechanisms.

These experimental observations support the view that many different genes (and their alleles) may affect the multiple components of threshold. How and where they cause their structural, chemical, physiologic, and age-specific effect(s) are currently unknown, but a number of possible mechanisms have been discussed (Ryan et al., 1991; Shinnar and Moshé, 1991; Treiman, 1993). For example, could these genetic abnormalities determine the structure of ion channels? A large number of subunits of membrane channels have been identified, and a single cell may elaborate several different subunits (Guy and Conti, 1990; Neher, 1992; see Tempel, Chapter 7). Clearly, genetic influences could affect the type and combination of channel components, and therefore the permeability of the membrane channels. Alternatively, genetic influences could be affecting the types and distribution of transmitter receptors and/or the efficiency of membrane pump(s). We know that genetic influences can determine these and many other factors. We don't know yet how or when mutations in most of these systems result in seizure disorders.

Environmental Factors

Many environmental factors can influence seizure threshold. For example, fever can alter the threshold (and lead to a seizure) at any age but is the determining factor for febrile seizures in young children whose genetic and developmental thresholds are sufficiently low (Degen et al., 1991). Excitement and fatigue, as well as concentrations of glucose, calcium, and magnesium, all can play a role in an individual's threshold (Avioli et al., 1991; VanLandingham and Lothman, 1991). Any person who has a tendency to have seizures, whether genetic or symptomatic, is more likely to have a seizure when exposed to such stimuli as fever or stress. How homeostatic balance is maintained in the face of these multiple environmental factors is a major question in understanding seizures in infants and children, as well as in adults.

Age

Age itself is a very important factor affecting threshold for seizures. Newborns have a high cortical threshold for seizures. Although the newborn's cortex has relatively little inhibition, lateral connections between cortical neurons are underdeveloped, synaptic potentials are labile, and cells are unable to fire repetitively for prolonged periods (Moshé, 1987). The newborn's cortical neuron is less able to respond to electrical stimulation, less able to recruit surrounding cells, and thereby less able to generate and maintain a cortical seizure. As the newborn cortex matures anatomically and physiologically, its threshold appears to decrease. The infant and the toddler have increasing susceptibility to febrile seizures and to seizures from other causes. Is this lower threshold the reason that most seizures and most epilepsies begin in childhood?

Over the next few years of a child's development, the threshold appears to increase and gradually approaches adult levels. Thus within a year or two of exhibiting the lowest threshold for febrile seizures, the child's tendency for recurrence of febrile seizures decreases and febrile seizures are "outgrown." The tendency toward nonfebrile seizures also decreases over the first two decades of life, with the most rapid decrease beginning during the second half of the first decade (Annegers et al., 1979; Bancaud et al., 1974; Jasper, 1969).

Clinicians have long discussed the concept of threshold to seizures—the effects of age, genetics, and environmental factors (such as fever, sleeplessness, excitement, medications) on seizure propensity. What do we mean, however, in terms of the physiology of the individual cells and their interactions with their micro- and macroenvironments? Are these age-related differences in seizure susceptibility different from the genetic factors that influence threshold? Are they caused by differences in membrane properties or in receptor protein subunits? Are there concomitant changes in synapse structure and number as a result of synaptic development and pruning? Are they the result of changes in the imbalance of excitatory and inhibitory synapses or transmitters (Bourgeois et al., 1983)? Given that anticonvulsant drugs alter threshold by interacting with different subunits of membrane channels and receptors, it seems likely that a drug will have different effects at different stages of development. Further, it seems feasible that age-specific drugs can be designed which raise threshold by interacting with specific sites that are peculiar to the immature brain (see Dulac, Macdonald, and Kelly, Chapter 11). Can these drugs be designed to be so specific as to alter threshold without altering general levels of cortical function?

Perhaps one of our problems is that we have been looking for *the* factor, or *the* drug without realizing that there are many different epilepsies, and within each of the epilepsy phenotypes there are numerous potential causes of the synchronous firing. Since different medications have different, perhaps multiple effects, it should not be surprising that some individuals with a given seizure manifestation will respond to one medication, whereas others will not. We will discuss this further when we discuss absence seizures.

Focal (Local) Disturbances and Precipitating Causes

Street-corner orators often harangue passers-by on behalf of one or another cause. Few pay attention; most walk on. A small crowd may gather, listen briefly, and on occasion respond, even cheering or marching, but usually dispersing quickly. Only on the rarest of occasions does the speaker incite the crowd to lose its self-control, to demonstrate—even to riot. Why does the crowd occasionally gather? Is the speaker speaking more effectively? Is the threshold of the crowd different? Are the passers-by more interested? Is a demonstration or a riot the result of the charisma of the speaker? The threshold of the crowd? Or the interactions of the two?

Many individuals have a focal abnormality in the brain. This may be a demonstrable anatomic abnormality such as a tumor, an arteriovenous malformation, a scar, a cyst, or an infarct. Many people with such lesions never have seizures and the abnormality appears as an incidental finding on a scan or at autopsy. Others, with similar anatomic or pathologic lesions, may have one or several seizures. Some individuals with anatomic lesions have frequent spikes on their interictal EEG but rarely have seizures. For still others, epilepsy may be a severe problem. The interactions of structural abnormalities with the surrounding brain and the resultant seizures raise a number of important basic questions:

> Why do some structural abnormalities recruit sufficient surrounding cells to become manifest as spikes on the interictal EEG while others do not? Why are the spikes present at some times but not at others?
>
> Why do these focal disturbances sometimes recruit sufficient neighboring cells to become focal seizures, and why do these focal seizures only occasionally spread to become generalized seizures?
>
> Why do most seizures stop spontaneously after only a short period of time?

Because of the importance of cell-to-cell interactions—and cell-to-environment interactions—in seizure genesis, it is critical to focus our research on cell *populations* as well as on the physiology of individual neurons. For example, in studying underlying mechanisms of synchronization as well as desynchronization, it is necessary to examine the interactions of cortical and subcortical systems; to understand the nature of seizure spread and generalization we must study the roles of the thalamus, substantia nigra, and other "deep" structures. Studies of gene expression in mice producing similar spike-and-wave phenotypes (see Noebels and Tharp, Chapter 3) and of age-specific anticonvulsant drug effects (see Dulac, Macdonald, and Kelly, Chapter 11) on oscillating systems can help us generate questions—and answers—about the effects of age, development, and medications on the clinical manifestations of seizure syndromes of childhood.

Seizures and Epilepsy in Children

As defined previously, a *seizure* is a sudden alteration of electrical activity in the brain of sufficient magnitude to alter motor or sensory function, behavior, or consciousness. *Epilepsy* is a chronic disorder characterized by recurrent seizures. An *epileptic syndrome* is a constellation of seizures, EEG patterns, family histories, and age-specific characteristics sufficient to produce a reproducible and recognizable seizure pattern with a predictable outcome.

Seizures may be of two types: *provoked,* by an acute local or systemic disturbance which alters brain function (acute symptomatic seizures), or *unprovoked,* occurring, or recurring, without an obvious precipitating factor. These definitions of provoked and unprovoked seizures are less useful than they first appear. If a child's seizures are due to a specific brain lesion (a tumor, cyst, etc.), are they provoked by that lesion? If so, why do they occur only at certain times? Is the provocation the original damage, or are the seizures due to additional precipitating factors such as lack of sleep, stress, or excitement? Why do some children with specific damage have seizures while others do not? Why do some eventually have their seizures controlled? Why do some outgrow their seizures? Perhaps our thinking would be clearer if we thought of the lesions or the brain damage as *predisposing* rather than provoking factors.

Classification of Seizures

A simplified version of the International Classification of Seizures (Commission on Classification and Terminology of the International League against Epilepsy, 1985, 1989) is shown in Table 1-1. Seizures are classified into two broad categories: partial and generalized.

Partial seizures (also termed *focal* and *local* seizures) have their onset and initial manifestation limited to one part of a hemisphere. When consciousness is maintained, these seizures are termed *simple partial.* When consciousness is impaired or lost, they are termed *complex partial* seizures. Partial seizures may spread to adjacent areas or throughout the cortex. This spread is termed *secondary generalization.* Either type of seizure may secondarily generalize.

Generalized seizures involve both hemispheres from the onset. The clinical manifestation of generalized seizures involves the cerebral cortex, thalamus, and brainstem structures including reticular formation and substantia nigra. Generalized seizures may take many forms. The major groupings

TABLE 1-1.   International Classification of Seizures

New Terms	Old Terms
Partial seizures	Focal seizures
Simple partial (consciousness not impaired)	
Motor symptoms	Focal motor
Sensory symptoms	Focal sensory
Complex partial (consciousness impaired)	Psychomotor temporal lobe
Generalized seizures (convulsive or nonconvulsive)	
Absence	Petit mal
Myoclonic	Minor motor
Atonic	
Tonic-clonic	Grand mal

within generalized seizures are *tonic-clonic* (grand mal), *myoclonic,* and *absence* (staring spells).

Although defining the clinical and EEG manifestations, these definitions do not assist in understanding the basic mechanisms involved in a seizure. For example, it seems counterintuitive to think that generalized seizures could be starting all over the cortex simultaneously. If they start at one location and very rapidly spread throughout the cortex, why are we unable to document the site of origin? Could the site of origin be deep within the brain, (e.g., within the thalamus, the reticular activating system, or the brainstem)? Could the electrical activity spread be rapidly upward from these sites through cortical activating systems, or downward to (and through) postural systems? Is a generalized tonic-clonic seizure caused by the rapid synchronization of cortical firing, whereas the infantile spasms and drop spells of the Lennox-Gastaut syndrome are caused by inhibition of postural tone and cortical desynchronization (Gastaut et al., 1963; Ottino et al., 1971; Vertes, 1981)?

Seizures may also be classified by their cause. First, seizures may be *symptomatic*—of known cause—for example, posttraumatic or caused by a tumor, a vascular abnormality, an infarction, or a developmental abnormality. Second, seizures may be *cryptogenic*—of undiscovered cause—for example, a child may have seizures associated with neurologic problems or mental retardation, but the cause of the seizures (while probably related to these abnormalities) is not clear. Third (and most common), seizures may be *idiopathic*—we do not know the cause and we have no evidence of an underlying neurologic abnormality—that is, the individual is otherwise normal. With better imaging techniques, we are uncovering structural lesions in increasing numbers of individuals with what were formerly called cryptogenic and idiopathic seizures. Whether and how these structural abnormalities constitute a "cause" of the epilepsy in most cases is unclear (Guerrini et al., 1992; Prayson et al., 1993).

Classification of the Epilepsies and Epileptic Syndromes

Another approach is to classify the *epilepsies,* rather than the types of seizures. The epilepsies are again divided into partial and generalized, but each is separated by cause into idiopathic (with age-related onset) and symptomatic (of nonspecific and known etiologies).

The various *epilepsy syndromes* (see Table 1-2) are virtually all age-related and occur during childhood. This fact alone must be telling us something about the young brain at various stages of its development—its response to stimuli, its threshold, its interconnections, its susceptibility to excitation, and its state of inhibition at each stage (McDonald and Johnston, 1990; Vining, 1990). These epilepsy syndromes offer a unique opportunity to explore the response of the developing nervous system to various perturbations and to begin to understand the effects of seizures on central nervous system development, as well as the effects of development on the seizure

TABLE 1-2.　Common Epilepsy Syndromes

Neonatal seizures
　Benign neonatal seizures

Infantile spasms

Lennox-Gastaut syndrome

Benign focal epilepsies
　Benign rolandic seizures
　Benign occipital seizures

Juvenile absence epilepsy (petit mal)

Juvenile myoclonic epilepsy (Janz)

Progressive unilateral encephalopathy of childhood (Rasmussen's encephalopathy)

---

manifestations. Among the questions that may be important to address in studying epilepsy syndromes are:

> Why are some epilepsies convulsive, with tonic and clonic movements, whereas others are nonconvulsive, with only alterations of consciousness?
>
> What do such differences tell us about which brain regions are primarily involved?
>
> What are the developmental factors governing spread and seizure manifestations?

We will review the epilepsy syndromes of childhood by age or stage of onset.

Prenatal Seizures

Seizures are extremely uncommon in utero. Pyridoxine dependency, with its tonic-clonic seizures, is the only seizure type frequently recognized by mothers in utero (Bejsovec et al., 1967). Even with massive destructive lesions of the brain, seizures are infrequently recognized in utero. Further, infants with these lesions rarely seize in the early days of life unless there is an additional insult, such as a hypoxic episode (Volpe, 1987a). Is this paucity of intrauterine seizures because the immature fetus has seizures which are so subtle that they cannot be recognized by the mother (see below)? Does the normal hypoxic environment of the uterus prevent seizures? If so, why are pyridoxine deficiency seizures easily recognized?

Neonatal Seizures

The neonatal period is usually defined as the first month of life, but there is no clear demarcation of this period (other than its onset at birth). The newborn offers the clinician the first opportunity to see and study seizures in the human. Seizures in the neonate are rarely idiopathic, but rather are virtually *always* symptomatic of a central nervous system disturbance (Volpe, 1987b). Some are due to chemical imbalances (e.g., calcium, magnesium, glucose, amino acid disorders, or vitamin deficiencies such as pyridoxine); others are due to developmental abnormalities, trauma, bleeding, or hypoxia. Genetic and benign forms of neonatal seizures have been described (Quattlebaum, 1979; Ryan et al., 1991). Whatever the cause, the clinical manifestations of neonatal seizures are rarely similar to the tonic-clonic seizures seen in older children or adults. The more immature the newborn, the less likely the infant is to have "typical" generalized seizures. Thus a classification of seizures in the newborn (Table 1-3) has little resemblance to the International classification of seizures (Table 1-1).

The newborn's brain is anatomically and physiologically quite different from that of the older child and the adult (Bourgeois et al., 1983; Schwartz-kroin, 1984). Neurons are immature, with different voltage-dependent and transmitter-gated characteristics than in the adult cortex. Increasing myelination after birth may also lead to more effective communication between cells (Pujol et al., 1993). A concomitant decrease in ephaptic transmission may play a role in changing cortical excitability (Hablitz and Heinemann, 1989). As the cortex matures, dendrites are elaborating and then dying back (Moshé, 1987). In the rat there is a "critical period" for seizure susceptibility at the second and third postnatal weeks. Garant et al. conclude their review (Bourgeois et al., 1983) with the statement, "We must avoid conceiving of the immature brain as just a smaller or simpler precursor of the adult brain . . . the maturational processes will affect the initiation, propagation and suppression of seizures as well as their consequences for the brain."

These dramatic age-dependent differences alter the maturing brain's response to acute symptomatic insults and affect its repertoire of seizures (Sperber et al., 1992). Seizures differ between premature and full-term infants (Volpe, 1987b). *Subtle seizures,* the most common form of seizures in the neonate, are even more common and more "subtle" in the premature infant than in the full-term. The seizures are often seen as sudden but subtle changes in the infant's behavioral state. Are these changes really seizures in the usual sense of "excitatory cortical electrical discharges"? Careful video-EEG monitoring has shown that subtle seizures may or may not have EEG accompaniments. Most subtle seizures are now thought to be due to cortical

TABLE 1-3. Neonatal Seizure Classification, in Order of Decreasing Frequency

Subtle
  Motor: swimming, rowing, pedaling
  Apnea: lip-smacking, sucking
  Eyes: deviation, blinking

Generalized tonic

Multifocal clonic

Focal clonic

Myoclonic

From Volpe, 1987b.

release of normally inhibited, subcortical, primitive reflexes, producing reflex movements such as sucking or bicycle-pedaling (Schulte, 1966). When neonatal seizures *are* due to a local cortical lesion, they are likely to be seen as brief, focal clonic movements (Levy et al., 1985). More widespread cortical insults are usually reflected as multifocal clonic seizures with shifting sides and locations, or as tonic stiffenings. Only rarely are neonatal seizures generalized as tonic-clonic.

Infantile Spasms

Infantile spasms (West's syndrome) is an age-related epilepsy syndrome (Holmes, 1992). The seizures have a specific characteristic pattern: a sudden flexion of the body, arms extended, knees flexed, head down. This position is held for a second or two then relaxed—only to be repeated in a few seconds. Infantile spasms occur in series of 5, 10, or 20 spells, each with little or no postictal period. Infantile spasms are the only seizures that occur in such a series. They are most likely to occur as the child is in transition between sleep and wakefulness. Rarely, the seizures may involve only one side of the body, or they may cause extension of the body rather than flexion. These infantile spasms are age-limited, usually starting between 4 and 7 months of age, and rarely starting earlier than 2 months or after 1 year. Untreated, as the cortex matures (by 3–4 years of age), the clinical manifestations and the EEG of infantile spasms gradually evolve into the multiple seizure types of the Lennox-Gastaut syndrome (see below) (Donat, 1992; Palm et al., 1988). Infantile spasms are almost uniformly associated with a characteristic EEG pattern of high-voltage multifocal spikes, often interspersed with a burst-suppression pattern, known as "hypsarrythmia" (Fig. 1-1), which is also age-dependent (Blume, 1988; Kellaway et al., 1979). It is a picture of electroencephalographic chaos.

Infantile spasms may be the major cause of postnatally acquired mental retardation. With the onset of the spasms, the infant usually progressively loses both motor and intellectual milestones. The vast majority of these children are ultimately significantly retarded. Thus infantile spasms may be one of the few epilepsies where the seizures (or their electrical accompaniment) appear to be the cause of (or at least result in) permanent intellectual dysfunction.

Although the clinical characteristics of this age-related epilepsy syndrome are rather uniform, infantile spasms have many etiologies (van Bogaert et al., 1993; Vinters et al., 1993), including metabolic abnormalities of calcium and glucose, aminoacidurias, and genetically based problems such as tuberous sclerosis. In two-thirds of children with infantile spasms, the spasms are considered symptomatic of underlying brain damage; one-third of the children are thought to be normal prior to the onset of spells (Riikonen, 1982). However, as imaging technology has improved, we have begun to find more subtle focal or multifocal cortical abnormalities in the subpopulation previously thought to be idiopathic (Chiron et al., 1993; Chugani et

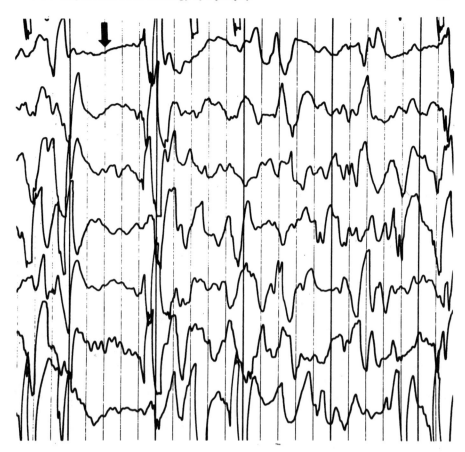

Figure 1-1. Hypsarrthymic EEG pattern. Electroencephalogram shows the chaotic spikes, polyspikes, and slow waves of hypsarrhythmia. Brief voltage suppression (arrow) is usually seen in association with infantile spasms. Time scale = 1-second bars on EEG paper.

al., 1993; van Bogaert et al., 1993). These abnormalities are predominantly in the parietooccipital region. Resection of such cortical abnormalities may result in cessation of the infantile spasms (or other focal seizures) and improvement in mental function (Chugani et al., 1990, 1993).

There is growing evidence that the final common pathway for these seizures lies in the pontine reticular activating system, with its effects on REM sleep and on body tone (Fukuyama et al., 1979; Hrachovy et al., 1981). The pathophysiology of the repetitive nature of the series of spells and the nature of their relation to drowsiness remain ill-defined. The devastating nature of this condition on intellect and the mechanism by which the retardation is produced greatly challenge pediatric epileptology and neuroscience.

The syndrome of infantile spasms raises several basic questions about childhood epilepsy and brain development:

How and why does such etiologic heterogeneity produce such stereotypical seizures? Why are these stereotypical seizures age-dependent? Why do some focal lesions (e.g., porencephalies, dysmigration abnormalities, or unilateral megalencephaly) often cause infantile spasms, while other focal abnormalities (e.g., Sturge-Weber disease) do not?

By what mechanisms and pathways do focal abnormalities produce these generalized seizures and why are they so closely linked to age? Are the cortical alerting mechanisms and their upward-projecting pathways from pontine and midbrain structures important to the normal development of cortical neurons (e.g., do they play a role in the maintenance or the pruning of neuronal interconnections) (Aicardi, 1989; Vertes, 1981)?

How and why do these spells result in intellectual deterioration and permanent mental retardation, whereas most other seizure types do not?

Why are ACTH and prednisone often effective in terminating the spasms and normalizing the EEG? Do they also alter intellectual outcome?

Lennox-Gastaut Syndrome

As children with infantile spasms grow older, with or without treatment, the infantile spasms stop. The now usually substantially retarded child's seizures evolve into the Lennox-Gastaut syndrome (LGS; Donat, 1992; Gastaut et al., 1966). This syndrome usually consists of a combination of focal and/or multifocal generalized tonic, tonic-clonic, myoclonic, atonic, and absence seizures. The hallmark of this syndrome is the sudden flexion spasms, often known as myoclonic, atonic, or akinetic seizures. The child's limited function is further substantially curtailed by the unpredictability of a sudden crash to the ground, with injury to the face or head. The children walk with helmets and face guards; they are rarely far from their protectors.

In addition to evolving from infantile spasms, the Lennox-Gastaut syndrome may result from many other causes, known and unknown, and may even arise in a previously well child or adolescent. In many ways the Lennox-Gastaut syndrome resembles the infantile spasms syndrome, but without the series of seizures; it appears to be a similar epilepsy syndrome superimposed on a more developed nervous system. The EEG in the Lennox-Gastaut syndrome is also extremely abnormal. There are slow spike waves, or polyspike and waves, often runs of multiple spikes seen in sleep. The background is also very abnormal, slow and disorganized (Fig. 1-2). Both the tonic seizures and the characteristic EEG are most often seen during non-REM sleep.

Once the Lennox-Gastaut syndrome begins, intellectual development seems to be halted, or it progresses at a far slower pace than the child's previous rate. There is rarely, however, the rapid intellectual and motor regression seen with infantile spasms.

The Lennox-Gastaut syndrome raises several questions:

What is the relationship of the retardation and the markedly abnormal EEG? Since some individuals have the electrical abnormalities but manifest

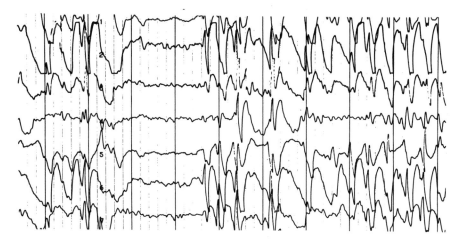

Figure 1-2. Lennox-Gastaut EEG pattern. Electroencephalogram showing the characteristic low spike waves, or polyspike and waves, with runs of multiple spikes often seen in sleep. The background is also very abnormal, slow and disorganized. Time scale = 1-second bars on EEG paper.

neither the seizures nor the retardation, are the electrical abnormalities, the seizures, and the retardation causally linked (Goluden et al., 1991; Huttenlocher and Hapke, 1990)?

What is the relationship of this syndrome to the syndrome of infantile spasms? Are there similar pathophysiologies, pathways of seizure propagation, and electrophysiological mechanisms that result in mental retardation? Are there surgically curable abnormalities in the LGS?

Do the slow spike wave and the hypersynchrony of LGS and of the syndrome of infantile spasms represent an excess of inhibition or a paucity of excitation? Could these influences be modified? Would such modifications alter the associated mental retardation?

How does one begin to understand the neurophysiology or the neurochemistry of either syndrome when there are no animal models?

Does nervous system maturation determine the differences between infantile spasms and Lennox-Gastaut syndrome? Would an understanding of the age-specific characteristics of the central nervous system at these two stages of development help in more effective differential treatment for these syndromes?

Answers to these questions will provide important leads to our clinical understanding, prevention, and treatment of these unfortunate children.

Febrile Seizures

Febrile seizures occur in 3–4 percent of all children and are the paradigm of an age-related threshold disorder (Berg et al., 1990; Freeman and Vining, 1992). There also appears to be a genetic component to the threshold for these seizures (Degen et al., 1991). As discussed previously, the brain's threshold for seizures is initially high at birth, appears to be lowest in the second half of the first year of life, and then increases gradually over the remainder of the first decade and into the second decade. This change in threshold has been deduced from the child's susceptibility to febrile seizures. Febrile seizures are uncommon before about 6 months of life, are most frequent between 6 months and 2 years of age, and progressively decrease in incidence over the next 2–4 years. This change in incidence (and, presumably, threshold) is a paralleled by the age-related incidence of new idiopathic epilepsy and the onset of single seizures (Hauser and Hesdorffer, 1990).

Febrile seizures appear to be the result of interactions of three independent variables, each of which affects threshold. One variable is the child's age, which affects cortical maturity; the second is the individual's genetically determined seizure predisposition; and the third is the intensity of the precipitating agent—in febrile seizures, the amplitude and rate of rise of the fever.

There are several important questions concerning febrile seizures:

> What are the anatomic, physiologic, and molecular or chemical bases of each of these variables? How are they genetically determined and modified by age?

> What are the cellular physiologic features and cell population dynamics which constitute "threshold" for such seizures?

> Are there approaches that could lead to their modification without affecting normal cellular functions?

> Why can a recurrence of febrile seizures be prevented by adequate dosage of some anticonvulsants (e.g., phenobarbital and sodium valproate), but not by others (carbamazepine and phenytoin)? Does this clinical finding tell us something about the neurophysiologic differences between febrile and afebrile (i.e., idiopathic) seizures? Is it giving us an important clue about how these anticonvulsants work to prevent seizures, or about the pathophysiology of these two different seizure types?

Febrile seizures offer us an opportunity to look at the effect of isolated seizures on brain function. Many investigators maintain that seizures require treatment because of their possible adverse effects on the brain, which include kindling, learning problems, structural damage, even death (Shewmon and Erwin, 1988; Siebelink et al., 1988). However, multiple studies of children with febrile seizures have determined that a child with febrile seizures is no more likely to die, to become retarded, or to have learning problems than a child without febrile seizures (Freeman and Vining, 1992; Shinnar, 1993). A child who has had a single febrile seizure has approximately a 30 percent chance of having a second febrile seizure and, depending on the complexity of the seizure (its length, laterality, family history of epilepsy, etc.), has a 2–10 percent chance of subsequently developing nonfebrile seizures. In short, it appears that there are virtually no consequences to febrile seizures other than parental anxiety. There are, however, consequences to treatment with medication, including toxic, allergic, intellectual, and behavioral effects of anticonvulsants (Bourgeois, 1991).

Developing an appropriate rationale for treating or not treating febrile seizures has also helped us develop decision-making paradigms relevant to nonfebrile seizures (Freeman and Vining, 1992). When making such a decision, the physician and the parent must assess the chances of a recurrent seizure, as well as the physical and emotional consequences of such an event. The probability of an adverse occurrence without treatment, and the value assigned to that consequence, must then be compared to the value assigned to the probability of adverse consequences of the treatment and the value assigned to that outcome. This paradigm thus becomes a traditional risk- or cost-benefit analysis. For example, the chance that a child will have a second febrile seizure is approximately 30 percent. Since there are virtually no consequences of that second seizure except the parental anxiety, the "negative value" of that anxiety must be compared to the values attached to the chance of side effects of treatment (such as learning and behavioral problems with phenobarbital or liver disease with valproate) and the consequences of these side effects. It must also be remembered that the risk of further seizures is never zero, even with treatment. When such an analysis is made, it is apparent that a febrile seizure rarely warrants treatment to prevent recurrence.

As the psychosocial consequences of seizures and epilepsy and its consequences on the individual and family are given greater attention, and as outcomes in research play an increasing role in decision-making, febrile seizures provide an excellent decision-making model.

Rasmussen's Syndrome

Rasmussen's syndrome, once called Rasmussen's encephalitis, is an interesting and unusual epilepsy syndrome of childhood (Oguni et al., 1991; Rasmussen, 1958; Vining et al., 1993). The seizures of this epilepsy syndrome usually start between the ages of 3 and 10 years in a previously healthy child. The initial seizure is commonly severe and generalized, without any preceding insult or infection. Shortly thereafter the child begins to have increasingly frequent focal seizures whose clinical manifestations depend on where in the cortex the process begins. The focus is initially very restricted in its manifestations and virtually never multifocal. Gradually, over days, weeks, or months, the focus becomes more intense, eventually leading to epilepsy partialis continua (constant, continual, very focal seizures of one area of the brain, rarely spreading to adjacent areas) in more than half the children. Rasmussen's syndrome is the most common, if not the only cause of epilepsy partialis continua in childhood.

The disease process gradually involves adjacent areas of the cortex, seeming to expand in concentric circles and eventually involving the entire ipsilateral cortex. Even at this stage, while the seizures remain focal or unilateral, careful observation indicates that unlike the typical Jacksonian spread of some unilateral motor seizures, the seizures of Rasmussen's syndrome spread as serial, adjacent, intense, focal seizures. For example, as an intense seizure in the corner of the mouth slows and quiets, then the seizure in the hand (or shoulder) will begin; the foot may start as the arm quiets. The seizures virtually never generalize. The intensity and focality of these seizures have been likened to the seizures in an animal model of GABA withdrawal.

The pathologic hallmarks of Rasmussen's encephalopathy are perivascular inflammation, astrocytosis and gliosis, and neuronal dropout—a picture reminiscent of a prior or ongoing viral encephalitis. Thus Rasmussen originally coined the name "chronic progressive encephalitis" for the entity which has subsequently become known in the literature as "Rasmussen's encephalitis." However, despite years of intense and creative virology, no trace of a viral process has been documented (Asher and Gajdusek, 1991).

In Rasmussen's encephalopathy, these intense cortical focal seizures are eventually associated with damage to the adjacent motor cortex, resulting in a slowly progressive hemiplegia. When the left temporal lobe is involved, progressive loss of language functions is inevitable. In such cases, early removal of the affected language area may improve transfer of language, ultimately resulting in better speech function in the opposite hemisphere (Brandt et al., 1990). We have seen such transfer occur as late as 10 years of age. The slowly progressive intellectual deterioration associated with Rasmussen's syndrome usually results in moderate mental retardation. The intractability of the process and the resistance of the seizures to antiepileptic medications have led some epilepsy centers to surgically remove the locally affected portions of the brain. However, the seizures inevitably return in the remaining ipsilateral cortex (Piatt et al., 1988). Only hemispherectomy (removal of the total hemisphere or of the whole ipsilateral cortex) results in "cure" of the seizures and relief from the adverse effects of medication. This observation has led investigators (Freeman and Vining, 1991; Villemure et al., 1991) to advocate earlier surgical removal of the affected hemisphere. Improvement in the child's mental function has repeatedly followed this hemispherectomy.

One can therefore ask:

What processes could cause such intense, exquisitely focal seizures?

How and why does such intense seizure activity remain so localized? Why doesn't the seizure generalize? Does this restriction of activity tell us anything about the role of inhibition?

Why and how does the epileptic activity, and the associated cortical pathology, gradually involve adjacent tissue, but never involve the opposite side? Given that this intense electrical activity never results in seizures in the opposite side, what does this tell us about "kindling" in the developing human brain?

How does such a focal process cause intellectual deterioration? Does intense focal or unilateral electrical activity interfere with processing in the contralateral cortex? If these seizures occur at a time of learning and brain development, are the effects permanent? Is one good hemisphere better than two hemispheres, when one hemisphere is severely dysfunctional?

What, if anything, do these electrical effects on function in the opposite hemisphere indicate about the possible subtle effects of other types of epilepsy on intellectual function? Does the abnormal EEG so commonly seen in the individual with infrequent seizures (or even completely controlled idiopathic seizures) play any role in the subtle learning and intellectual problems so common in individuals with epilepsy? If so, when appropriate drugs are available should we treat epilepsy until the electric abnormalities are no longer present on the EEG?

The Treatment of Epilepsy

Anticonvulsant Medications

We have made considerable progress in developing a rationale for the design of new drugs capable of blocking seizure activity (Porter, 1989; Rogawski and Porter, 1990; see Dulac, Macdonald, and Kelly, Chapter 11), but since the underlying mechanisms of seizures in immature brain are likely to be different from those in mature brain, drugs designed to block mature CNS processes may be of little value for the immature epilepsy syndromes. Further, since there clearly are many different factors operating in age-dependent epilepsy syndromes, these new compounds will be of greater efficacy in some, but ineffective in other syndromes. Thus even when such compounds are available, we will still rely in large measure on trial and error to find the new compound most effective for a specific epilepsy syndrome or for specific seizures in a given age group.

If we understood the basic mechanisms underlying the age-dependency of seizure threshold—the genetic factors influencing the susceptibility to seizures, the mechanisms by which local lesions and environmental factors interact to change that threshold—then perhaps we would have a more rational approach to the design of drugs. As drugs are developed and as their relative therapeutic indices and mechanisms of action are determined we will be able to use that information to develop hypotheses about the etiology of the syndromes. Then, in turn, we can design compounds to correct or cure each specific syndrome.

Surgery

Surgery has classically been the last resort for the patient with intractable epilepsy. With the appearance of new "designer" drugs, can epilepsy ever be considered intractable? If a child's seizures are well controlled—even completely controlled—with medication, is it better for that child to take medication for the remainder of life than to have an identifiable lesion removed? With brain mapping using grid technology, as well as new imaging technology and functional imaging, we are increasingly able to identify both "eloquent" areas of the brain and foci initiating seizures. Together with patients and their families, we need to consider when the ongoing monetary and psychosocial costs of medication are greater, and when less, than the risks and benefits of surgical removal of an epileptic focus.

Clearly with these advances the "old" risk-benefit ratios are changing. Successful epilepsy surgery is no longer limited to anterior temporal lobectomies and clear cortical lesions.

Diet

There is one other approach to intractable epilepsy in children which deserves mention, if only because it may provide clues not only to new treatment, but also to understanding of basic mechanisms. The ketogenic diet, one of the oldest forms of treatment for epilepsy, when properly used remains one of the most effective treatments for intractable seizures in childhood (Kinsman et al., 1992; Schwartz et al., 1989). The ketogenic diet was based on the observation that seizures are often reduced during fasting. Ketosis is initiated by starvation and then maintained by a carefully calculated diet based on the individual's minimal caloric needs. One gram per kilogram of protein is used for growth, and virtually all remaining calories are taken as fat; sugar is minimized. Minimal errors in diet calculation or "cheating" by eating a few extra nuts or a lollipop may result in a seizure. This diet, while difficult for the child and the family to maintain, appears to be an excellent alternative to the continued seizures and medication toxicity affecting these children.

Some 50 percent of children whose seizures cannot be controlled with combinations of medications will be controlled with the diet. An additional 25 percent of such children will be significantly benefited by either seizure reduction or medication reduction if the family continues this stringent diet for at least one year. Even more remarkable is the fact that when the child with previously intractable seizures has been seizure-free for two years, the diet can be slowly discontinued and the seizures do not return. These children are eventually seizure-free on no anticonvulsant medication. It would appear that in this population of children with intractable seizures, the ketogenic diet has "cured" the child's epilepsy.

Children on the diet are often felt by parents to be brighter and more alert and to exhibit fewer behavior problems than previously. While some of this improvement is due to reduction or freedom from the side effects of medication, part also seems to be due to freedom from the clinical and subclinical seizures and perhaps the abnormal electrical activity.

How does starvation control seizures? How does this high fat–low sugar diet maintain seizure control? If indeed the diet cures epilepsy, how is this "cure" possible?

Conclusion

Epilepsy is not only one condition. There are many different seizure types and patterns, now termed "the epilepsies." When the epilepsies are categorized by the age of onset, the characteristics of the seizures, and also the characteristics of the EEGs, they are termed "epilepsy syndromes." Our review of a few of the various epilepsy syndromes of childhood strongly suggests that the processes underlying these conditions reflect the interactions of the many components which impact and constitute threshold. These components include the following:

1. The anatomic and physiologic changes in membrane and channel structure and in receptor and transmitter balance which occur with age and cortical maturation.

2. The genetically determined alterations in the molecular structure of the cell membrane (e.g., channels and receptors).

3. The changing interactions between regional communities of cells within the developing and evolving cortex.

4. The magnitude and characteristics of varied stresses, both those such as trauma, hypoxia, and developmental abnormalities, which damage the developing nervous system, and the more transient precipitants such as fever or excitement, which temporarily alter threshold.

Thus as neuroscientists study the basic mechanisms underlying seizures and epilepsies, they must come to understand that many different factors, working at many different levels, interact and cause individual cells to "fire repetitively."

Perhaps even more important for understanding epilepsy are the multiple factors affecting communication within large populations of cells. These factors may cause populations of cells to be recruited to fire synchronously, resulting in a spike on the EEG or in the laboratory preparation. It is the simultaneous firing of even larger populations of cells which, in vivo, produce the alterations in behavior or function that are termed "seizures."

Epilepsy in children is not the same as epilepsy in adults. There is much to be learned from understanding the challenges and the questions posed while studying the varied epilepsy syndromes of childhood. Understanding the maturation of the developing nervous system and its interaction with changing seizure threshold might explain why and how most children "outgrow" their epilepsy, and what we might do to foster the process. Understanding the effects of seizures themselves on development, and the effects of development and plasticity on seizures, could allow us to prevent the devastating outcomes which affect many children.

Acknowledgments

I would like to express my appreciation to the many individuals who have contributed ideas and who have read, criticized, and edited this paper. Among them are Drs. Santiago Arroyo, Marvin Cornblath, Solomon Moshé, Russell T. Richardson, Philip A. Schwartzkroin, and Eileen P. G. Vining.

References

Aicardi, J. (1989) The outcome of childhood epilepsy: Benign and malignant. American Epilepsy Society Meeting, Boston, MA.

Annegers, J. F., Hauser, W. A., Elveback, L. R. (1979) Remission of seizures and relapse in patients with epilepsy. *Epilepsia 20:*729–737.

Asher, D. M., and Gajdusek, D. C. (1991) Virologic studies in chronic encephalitis. In F. Andermann (ed.), *Chronic Encephalitis and Epilepsy.* Boston: Butterworth-Heineman, pp. 147–158.

Avioli, M., Drapeau, C., Louvel, J., Pumain, R., Olivier, A., and Villemure, J.-G. (1991) Epileptiform activity induced by low extracellular magnesium in the human cortex maintained in vitro. *Ann. Neurol. 30:*589–596.

Bancaud, J., Yailairach, J., Morel, P., et al. (1974) "Generalized" epileptic seizures elicited by electrical stimulation of the frontal lobe in man. *Electroencephalogr. Clin. Neurophysiol. 37:*275–282.

Bejsovec, M., Kulenda, Z., and Ponca, E. (1967) Familial intrauterine convulsions in pyridoxine dependency. *Arch. Dis. Child. 42:*201–207.

Berg, A. T., Shinnar, S., Hauser, W. A., and Leventhal, J. M. (1990) Predictors of recurrent febrile seizures: A metaanalytic review. *J. Pediatr. 116:*329–337.

Blume, W. T. (1988) The EEG of the Lennox-Gastaut syndrome. In E. Niedermeyer and R. Degen (eds.), *The Lennox-Gastaut Syndrome.* New York: Alan R. Liss, pp. 159–176.

Bourgeois, B. F. D. (1991) Relationships between anticonvulsant drugs and learning disabilities. *Semin. Neurol. 11:*14–19.

Bourgeois, B. F. D., Prensky, A. L., Palkes, H. S., Talent, B. K., and Busch, S. G. (1983) Intelligence in epilepsy: A prospective study in children. *Ann. Neurol. 14:*438–444.

Brandt, J., Vining, E. P. G., Stark, R. E., Ansel, B. M., and Freeman, J. M. (1990) Hemispherectomy for intractable epilepsy in childhood: Preliminary report on neuropsychological and psychosocial sequelae. *J. Epilepsy 3* (Suppl.):261–270.

Buchhalter, J. R., (1993) Animal models of inherited epilepsy. *Epilepsia 34* (Suppl. 3): S31–S41.

Chiron, C., Dulac, O., Bulteau, C., et al. (1993) Study of regional cerebral blood flow in West syndrome. *Epilepsia 34:*707–715.

Chugani, H. T., Shewmon, D. A., Shields, W. D., et al. (1993) Surgery for intractable infantile spasms: Neuroimaging perspectives. *Epilepsia 34:*764–771.

Chugani, H. T., Shields, W. D., Shewmon, D. A., Olson, D. M., Phelps, M. E., and Peacock, W. J. (1990) Infantile spasms: I. PET identifies focal cortical dysgenesis in cryptogenic cases for surgical treatment. *Ann. Neurol. 27:*406–413.

Commission on Classification and Terminology of the International League against Epilepsy. (1985) Proposal for classification of epilepsies and epileptic syndromes. *Epilepsia 26:*268–278.

Commission on Classification and Terminology of the International League against Epilepsy. (1989) Proposal for revised classification of epilepsies and epileptic syndromes. *Epilepsia 30:*389–399.

Degen, R., Degen, H. E., and Hans, K. A. (1991) A contribution to the genetics of febrile seizures: Waking and sleep EEG in siblings. *Epilepsia 32:*515–522.

Donat, J. F. (1992) The age-dependent epileptic encephalopathies. *J. Child. Neurol.* 7:7–21.

Freeman, J. M., and Vining E. P. G. (1991) Hemispherectomy: The ultimate focal resection. In H. Lüders (ed.), *Epilepsy Surgery*. New York: Raven Press, pp. 111–118.

Freeman, J. M., and Vining E. P. G. (1992). Decision making and the child with febrile seizures. *Pediatr. Rev. 13:*298–304.

Fukuyama, Y., Shionaga, A., and Iida, Y. (1979) Polygraphic study during whole night sleep in infantile spasms. *Eur. Neurol. 18:*302–311.

Gastaut, H., Roger, J., Ouahchi, S., Timsit, M., and Broughton, R. (1963) An electro-clinical study of generalized epileptic seizures of tonic expression. *Epilepsia 4:*15–44.

Gastaut, H., Roger, J., Soulayrol, R., Tassinari, C. A., Régis, H., and Dravet, C. (1966) Childhood epileptic encephalopathy with diffuse slow spike-waves (otherwise known as "Petit mal variant") or Lennox syndrome. *Epilepsia* 7:139–179.

Goluden, K. J., Shinnar, S., Koller, H., Katz, M., and Richardson, S. A. (1991) Epilepsy in children with mental retardation: A cohort study. *Epilepsia 32:*690–697.

Greenber, D. A., and Delgado-Escueta, A. V. (1993) The chromosome 6p epilepsy locus: Exploring mode of inheritance and heterogeneity through linkage analysis. *Epilepsia 34* (Suppl. 3):S12–S18.

Guerrini, R., Dravet, C., Raybaud, C., et al. (1992) Epilepsy and focal gyral anomalies detected by MRI: Electroclinico-morphological correlations and follow-up. *Dev. Med. Child. Neurol. 34:*706–718.

Guy, H. R., and Conti, F. (1990) Pursuing the structure and function of voltage-gated channels. *TINS 13:*201–206.

Hablitz, J. J., and Heinemann, U. (1989) Alterations in the microenvironment during spreading depression associated with epileptiform activity in the immature cortex. *Dev. Brain Res. 46:*243–252.

Hauser, W. A., and Hesdorffer, D. C. (1990) Incidence and prevalence. In W. A. Hauser and D. C. Hesdorffer (eds.), *Epilepsy: Frequency, Causes and Consequences*. New York: Demos, pp. 1–51.

Holmes, G. L., (1992) Severe seizures in infancy and early childhood. *Int. Pediatr.* 7:237–254.

Hrachovy, R. A., Frost, J. D., and Kellaway, P. (1981) Sleep characteristics in infantile spasms. *Neurology 31:*688–694.

Huttenlocher, P. R., and Hapke, R. J. (1990) A follow-up study of intractable seizures in childhood. *Ann. Neurol. 28:*699–705.

Jasper, H. H. (1969) Introduction. In H. Gastaut, H. Jasper, J. Bancaud, and A. Waltregny (eds.), *The Physiopathogenesis of the Epilepsies*. Springfield, Ill.: Charles C Thomas, pp. 201–208.

Kellaway P, Hrachovy, R. A., Frost, J. D., Jr., and Zion, T. (1979) Precise characterization and quantification of infantile spasms. *Ann. Neurol. 6:*214–218.

Kinsman, S. L., Vining, E. P. G., Quaskey, S. A., Mellits, E. D., and Freeman,

J. M. (1992) Efficacy of the ketogenic diet for intractable seizure disorders: Review of 58 cases. *Epilepsia 33:*1132–1136.

Levy, S. R., Abroms, I. F., Marshall, P. C., and Rosquete, E. E. (1985) Seizures and cerebral infarction in the full-term newborn. *Ann. Neurol. 17:*366–390.

McDonald, J. W., and Johnston, M. V. (1990) Physiological and pathophysiological roles of excitatory amino acids during central nervous system development. *Brain Res. Rev. 15:*41–70.

Moshé S. L. (1987) Epileptogenesis and the immature brain. *Epilepsia 28* (Suppl. 1): S3–S15.

Neher, E. (1992) Ion channels for communication between and within cells. *Science 256:*498–502.

Oguni, H., Andermann, F., and Rasmussen, T. B. (1991) The natural history of the syndrome of chronic encephalitis and epilepsy: A study of the MNI series of forty-eight cases. In F. Andermann (ed.), *Chronic Encephalitis and Epilepsy.* Boston: Butterworth-Heinemann, pp. 7–36.

Ottino, C. A., Meglio, M., Rossi, G. F., and Tercero, E. (1971). An experimental study of the structures mediating bilateral synchrony of epileptic discharges of cortical origin. *Epilepsia 12:*299–311.

Palm, D. G., Brandt, M., and Korinthenberg, R. (1988) West syndrome and Lennox-Gastaut syndrome in children with porencephalic cysts: Long-term follow-up after neurosurgical treatment. In E. Niedermeyer and R. Degen (eds.), *The Lennox-Gastaut Syndrome.* New York: Alan R. Liss, pp. 419–426.

Piatt, J. H., Hwang P. A., Armstrong, D. C., Becker, L. E., and Hoffman, H. J. (1988) Chronic focal encephalitis (Rasmusssen syndrome): Six cases. *Epilepsia 29:*268–279.

Porter, R. J. (1989) Mechanisms of action of new antiepileptic drugs. *Epilepsia 30* (Suppl. 1):S29–S34.

Prayson, R. A., Estes, M. L., and Morris, H. H. (1993) Coexistence of neoplasia and cortical dysplasia in patients presenting with seizures. *Epilepsia 34:*609–615.

Pujol, J., Vendrell, P., Junqué, C., Martí-Vilalta, J. L., and Capdevila, A. (1993) When does human brain development end? Evidence of corpus callosum growth up to adulthood. *Ann. Neurol. 34:*71–75.

Quattlebaum, T. G. (1979) Benign familial convulsions in the neonatal period and early infancy. *J. Pediatr. 95:*257–259.

Rasmussen, T. (1958) Focal seizures due to chronic localized encephalitis. *Neurology 8:*435–445.

Riikonen, R. (1982) A long-term follow-up study of 214 children with the syndrome of infantile spasms. *Neuropediatrics 13:*14–23.

Rogawski, M. A., and Porter, R. J. (1990) Antiepileptic drugs: Pharmacological mechanisms and clinical efficacy with consideration of promising developmental stage compounds. *Pharmacol. Rev. 42:*223–286.

Ryan, S. G., Wiznitzer, M., and Hollman, C. (1991) Benign familial neonatal convulsions: Evidence for clinical and genetic heterogeneity. *Ann. Neurol. 29:*469–473.

Schulte, F. J. (1966) Neonatal convulsions and their relation to epilepsy in early childhood. *Dev. Med. Child. Neurol. 8:*381–392.

Schwartz, R. H., Eaton, J., Bower, B. D., and Aynsley-Green, A. (1989) Ketogenic diets in the treatment of epilepsy: Short-term clinical effects. *Dev. Med. Child. Neurol. 31:*145–151.

Schwartzkroin, P. A. (1984) Epileptogenesis in the immature CNS. In P. A. Schwartzkroin and H. V. Wheal (eds.), *Electrophysiology of Epilepsy*. New York: Academic Press, pp. 389–412.

Shewmon, D. A., and Erwin, R. J. (1988) The effect of focal interictal spikes on perception and reaction time: I. General considerations. *Electroencephalogr. Clin. Neurophysiol. 69:*9–337.

Shinnar, S. (1993) Treatment decisions in childhood seizures. In W. E. Dodson and J. M. Pellock (eds.), *Pediatric Epilepsy: Diagnosis and Therapy*. New York: Demos, pp. 215–221.

Shinnar, S., and Moshé, S. L. (1991) Age specificity of seizure expression in genetic epilepsies. In V. E. Anderson (ed.), *Genetic Strategies in Epilepsy Research* (Epilepsy Research Suppl. 4). Amsterdam: Elsevier.

Siebelink, B. M., Bakker, D. J., Binnie, C. D., and Kasteleijn-Nolst Trenité, D. G. A. (1988) Psychological effects of subclinical epileptiform EEG discharges in children: II. General intelligence tests. *Epilepsy Res. 2:*117–121.

Sperber, E. F., Haas, K. Z., and Moshé, S. L. (1992) Developmental aspects of status epilepticus. *Int. Pediatr. 7:*213–222.

Treiman, L. J. (1993) Genetics of epilepsy: An overview. *Epilepsia 34* (Suppl. 3): S1–S11.

Van Bogaert, P., Adamsbaum, C., Robain, O., Diebler, C., and Dulac, O. (1993) Value of magnetic resonance imaging in West syndrome of unknown etiology. *Epilepsia 34:*701–706.

VanLandingham, K. E., and Lothman, E. W. (1991) Self-sustaining limbic status epilepticus: II. Role of hippocampal commisures in metabolic response. *Neurology 41:*1950–1957.

Vertes, R. P. (1981) An analysis of ascending brainstem systems involved in hippocampal synchronization and desynchronization. *J. Neurophysiol. 46:*1140–1159.

Villemure, J.-G., Andermann, F., and Rasmussen, T. B. (1991) Hemispherectomy for the treatment of epilepsy due to chronic encephalitis. In F. Andermann (ed.), *Chronic Encephalitis and Epilepsy*. Boston: Butterworth-Heineman, pp. 235–244.

Vining, E. P. G. (1990) Chaos, balance, and development: Thoughts on selected childhood epilepsy syndromes. *Epilepsia 31* (Suppl. 3):S30–S36.

Vining, E. P. G., Freeman, J. M., Brandt, J., Carson, B. S., and Uematsu, S. (1993) Progressive unilateral encephalopathy of childhood (Rasmussen's syndrome): A reappraisal. *Epilepsia 34:*639–650.

Vinters, H. V., De la Rosa, M. J., and Farrell, M. A. (1993) Neuropathologic study of resected cerebral tissue from patients with infantile spasms. *Epilepsia 34:*772–779.

Volpe, J. J. (1987a) Hypoxic-ischemic encephalopathy: Clinical aspects. In J. J. Volpe (ed.), *Neurology of the Newborn,* 2nd ed. Philadelphia: W. B. Saunders, pp. 236–279.

Volpe, J. J. (1987b) Neonatal seizures. In J. J. Volpe (ed.), *Neurology of the Newborn,* 2nd ed. Philadelphia: W. B. Saunders, pp. 129–157.

2

Partial (Focal) Seizures in Developing Brain

SOLOMON L. MOSHÉ
SHLOMO SHINNAR
JOHN W. SWANN

There are multiple causes of seizures. *Reactive,* or *provoked,* seizures occur in response to changes in the environment or internal state, such as high fever or hypoglycemia (Engel, 1989; Moshé et al., 1990). These seizures are transient events and do not recur if the appropriate trigger factors are avoided. *Epileptic* seizures occur at unpredictable intervals in the absence of any clearly identifiable precipitants. Since epileptic seizures may be the result of structural brain abnormalities, the term *symptomatic,* or *lesional, epilepsy* has been proposed. The brain-associated abnormalities can be severe or so subtle that their identification depends on the resolution of the most advanced technology. At times, even with state-of-the-art technology, no lesions can be found (Roger et al., 1989). The term *idiopathic epilepsy* is used for those seizures not associated with any evidence of central nervous system (CNS) pathology other than the seizure. Genetic factors may have an important role in epilepsy, indirectly through gene-determined occurrence of specific brain anomalies that can induce seizures or indirectly by altering the predisposition of an individual to seizures per se, as is the case with benign rolandic epilepsy (Lerman, 1985; Loiseau et al., 1988).

The incidence of seizures is highest during the first few years of life (Hauser and Kurland, 1975). Seizures are classified as partial or generalized (see Freeman, Chapter 1). This chapter deals with the neurobiology of *partial,* or *focal,* seizures during development, first presenting the clinical phenomenology and then describing animal model systems. Partial seizures are most often the result of focal dysfunction, although at times they may occur in conditions that affect the brain diffusely (Moshé and Shinnar, 1993). As described in this chapter, some early-onset partial seizures have features similar to adult-onset partial seizures. Other types of partial seizures have distinct age-specific characteristics. Acute, provoked seizures secondary to systemic insults such as hypoglycemia, hypoxia, or fever are often focal. Conversely, focal structural lesions in young infants can be associated with age-specific secondarily generalized seizure disorders such as infantile spasms or the Lennox-Gastaut syndrome. In early-onset partial epilepsies, the clinical onset of the seizures is often variable from seizure to seizure, suggesting that the focus may not be firmly fixed. Some age-specific partial epilepsies in older children, such as benign rolandic epilepsy, are genetically determined and may spontaneously remit. The spike foci are often bilateral and may shift sides on the EEG (Figure 2-1).

To understand the ontogenetic features of partial seizures, we will review human and animal studies.

Human Partial Seizures during Infancy, Childhood, and Adolescence

The classification of human seizures relies heavily on clinical (behavioral) semiology (Chapter 1). At all ages, partial seizures are most often associated with focal dysfunction, although not necessarily with identifiable focal structural lesions. However, in children, focal dysfunction can produce multifocal seizures; furthermore, during specific developmental periods, focal dysfunction can result in seizures with bilateral manifestations that can be loosely characterized as "generalized" (e.g., infantile spasms).

Partial Seizures Associated with Focal Dysfunction

The clinical manifestations of partial seizures in early childhood are often similar to those seen in older age groups (Dravet et al., 1989; Duchowny et al., 1992; Pratap and Gururaj, 1989; Watanabe et al., 1987). However, the early features may be subtle and can be easily missed or considered to be "baby" behaviors. Observers are more likely to recognize motor manifestations affecting gross movements such as those seen with seizure generalization. Since infants cannot tell us about any preceding aura, it is difficult to make precise comparisons with adult seizures beyond what we observe on video-EEG recordings. Another feature typical of early partial seizures is variability of the seizure semiology during different bouts; in adults the spread patterns are usually better established, and the seizures appear to be relatively stereotyped.

While the clinical manifestations of seizures originating in the temporal lobe may be similar in early life to those seen in older patients, the patho-

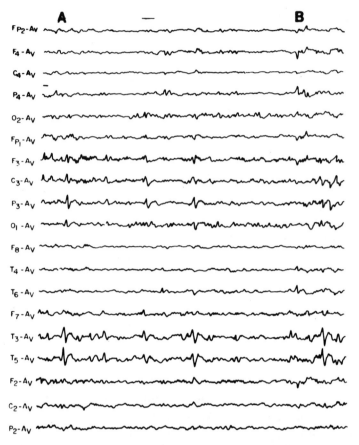

Figure 2-1. The EEG features of benign rolandic epilepsy. Note the presence of bilateral independent centrotemporal spikes. The second spike (B) has a horizontal dipole with a positivity in the frontal areas and a negativity in the centrotemporal region. Upward deflections represent a negativity and downward deflections a positivity for the first electrode in the pair and vice versa. Average reference montage. Right-side electrodes are denoted by even numbers, left-side electrodes by odd numbers.

logical substrate appears to be different. In adults with refractory complex partial seizures, the most common pathological substrate is mesial temporal sclerosis (Wieser et al., 1993). Based on retrospective studies, one of the risk factors for mesial temporal sclerosis has been postulated to be convulsions in early life (Cendes et al., 1993; Falconer, 1971; Falconer et al., 1964). Such isolated, often prolonged convulsions may be followed by a period of remission; seizures then reemerge and are often intractable (French et al., 1993; Wieser et al., 1993). Neuropathology of resected tissue has shown that many of these patients have mesial temporal sclerosis. Based on these studies one might assume that partial seizures in early childhood would also be associated with mesial temporal pathology, but this is not the case (see also Sankar, Wasterlain, and Sperber, Chapter 10). The majority of refractory partial epilepsies of early onset are extratemporal in origin (Nespeca et al., 1990). Extratemporal lesions may produce seizures which result in the slow development of hippocampal sclerosis, a possibility that may account for the dual pathology discovered by Lévesque et al. (1991) (mesial sclerosis, hamartomas, etc.).

Most children with refractory complex partial seizures are developmentally delayed. These behavioral findings together with commonly observed multifocal EEG as well as neuroimaging abnormalities suggest diffuse brain dysfunction (Chugani et al., 1988, 1990, 1992). In contrast, in adults with refractory complex partial seizures and mesial temporal sclerosis, a single focus is usually identified. The patient is of normal intelligence, although specific cognitive deficits may be present. These differences are summarized in Table 2-1.

Given that there are many differences in etiology and prognosis between childhood- and adult-onset seizures, and that a variety of epileptic syndromes tend to either remit (benign rolandic epilepsy, childhood absence) or have their onset in adolescence (juvenile myoclonic epilepsy), it is often assumed that neurologic factors associated with puberty play a role in these changes. While this premise is interesting, a definitive link between seizure onset and remission and puberty has yet to be demonstrated (Annegers et al., 1979; Diamantopoulos and Crumrine, 1986; Shinnar and Moshé, 1991). Epidemiologic studies (Annegers et al., 1979; Diamantopoulos and Crumrine, 1986; Shinnar and Moshé 1991) as well as studies on the remission of childhood seizures and on withdrawing antiepileptic drugs in children (Annegers et al., 1979; Shinnar and Kang, 1988; Shinnar and Moshé, 1991; Shinnar et al., 1985) have failed to find a reproducible pattern of seizure changes that correlates with puberty. Studies of the long-term prognosis of partial seizures suggest that the probability of attaining remission may be a function of the age of onset and the duration of the seizure disorder without a special role for puberty (Annegers et al., 1979; Shinnar and Moshé, 1991; Sofianov, 1982). However, these studies are all limited by an inadequate definition of

TABLE 2-1. Refractory Partial Seizures in Children and Adults: Association with Structural Abnormalities

	Children	Adults
Lesions	+ +	+
Developmental abnormality	+ + +	+
Stroke	+ +	+
Vascular abnormality	+	+
Tumor	+	+ +
Mesial temporal sclerosis	?	+ + +

puberty. Few investigators have used quantitative measures such as the Tanner scale and none have used endocrine markers of puberty. At this time it remains unclear whether there is a special etiological role for puberty or whether the second decade of life simply marks a gradual transition between childhood- and adult-onset seizure disorders.

Partial Seizures without Known Pathology

Benign Rolandic Epilepsy

Benign rolandic epilepsy is the best described benign focal epilepsy of childhood (Lerman, 1985; Loiseau et al., 1988). Onset is between 4 and 10 years of age. Seizures tend to occur at night and can be generalized tonic-clonic or partial. When partial, the seizures often involve the mouth and face. The EEG shows characteristic centrotemporal stereotyped spikes, which increase in frequency during drowsiness and sleep (Blom et al., 1975; Lerman, 1985). The EEG abnormalities may shift from side to side or may be bilateral (Fig. 2-1). Although the EEG does show focal spikes, neuroimaging studies are uniformly normal. The clinical seizures remit in early adolescence and the EEG abnormality disappears a few years later (Blom and Heijbel, 1982; Blom et al., 1975; Kellaway, 1981; Lerman, 1985; Loiseau et al., 1988; Trojaborg, 1966).

Benign rolandic epilepsy is thought to be an autosomal dominant disorder with reduced penetrance (Heijbel et al., 1975; Lerman, 1985; Metrakos and Metrakos, 1970). Studies of siblings suggest that 30 percent will have the EEG abnormality (Heijbel et al., 1975; Lerman, 1985; Metrakos and Metrakos, 1970). Only a fraction of those with the EEG abnormality will have clinical epilepsy. The factors that determine whether the EEG trait will be expressed, and whether seizures will also be expressed, are unknown. Prolonged EEG recordings from children with benign rolandic epilepsy reveal that up to 30 percent will also have at least occasional bursts of generalized spike and wave, which is the characteristic signature abnormality of the primary generalized epilepsies (Blom et al., 1975; Lerman, 1985; Metrakos and Metrakos, 1970); however, clinical absence seizures are uncommon. This finding emphasizes the variable expression of the disorder in childhood, though the precise relationship between the benign rolandic epilepsy and primary generalized seizures is not well understood.

Other Benign Focal Epilepsies of Childhood

Other benign focal epilepsies of childhood are less well understood than benign rolandic epilepsy and have a far more variable prognosis (Delgado-Escueta and Enrile-Bacsal, 1984). Population studies of the occurrence of spike foci in children of different ages suggest that spike foci in childhood are not always associated with seizures (Kellaway, 1981; Lairy and Harrison, 1968; Trojabor, 1966). The semiology, frequency, and probability of ultimate remission of the seizures vary with the localization of the spike focus.

Partial Seizures Associated with Bilateral or Diffuse Dysfunction

Neonatal Seizures

During the neonatal period seizures have distinct characteristics based on the behavioral repertoire of neonates. While generalized tonic-clonic seizures do occur, particularly in the full-term infant, in the premature infant more subtle forms of seizures are far more common (see Freeman, Chapter 1). The semiology of the seizures can be focal or generalized regardless of whether the region of dysfunction is focal or diffuse. In the premature infant, seizures often mimic the normal behavioral repertoire of babies of that age. Such behaviors may be brainstem- rather than cortically-mediated (Hrachovy and Frost, 1989; Kellaway et al., 1983). Older patients suffering the same degree of brain dysfunction may not survive; if they do, seizures may not be a prominent consequence. These observations suggest that the immature brain is more likely than the adult brain to respond to intense environmental stressors such as hypoxia-ischemia or bleeding with seizures (Tuchman and Moshé, 1990).

Febrile Seizures

Febrile seizures are an excellent example of the complex interplay among environmental, developmental, and genetic influences occurring in childhood seizures (see Freeman, Chapter 1). The majority of febrile seizures are generalized tonic-clonic convulsions consistent with the genetic nature of the disorder and the systemic insult (fever). However, up to 16 percent of otherwise normal children with normal neurologic examinations and normal development will present with focal febrile seizures (Berg et al., 1990, 1992; Nelson and Ellenberg, 1976, 1978).

Bilateral Motor Seizures Associated with Focal or Multifocal Pathology

Infantile Spasms

This syndrome is an example of an age-specific response of the CNS to a variety of focal or global-systemic lesions. It can also occur in association with a variety of genetic metabolic disorders. While infantile spasms are a form of myoclonic seizures which are bilateral (see Freeman, Chapter 1), there are reports of focal lesions associated with infantile spasms and hypsarrhythmia Fig. 2-2; Alvarez et al,. 1987; Hrachovy and Frost, 1989; Meencke, 1988). The hypsarrhythmic pattern may represent the spread of the epileptic activity and recruitment of multiple brain sites, which produces an age-specific seizure pattern. The rapid synchronization may be due to the relative immaturity of other brain sites that participate in the control or containment of focal epileptic discharges later in life. Such brain sites may include structures of the brainstem (Alvarez et al., 1987; Hrachovy and Frost, 1989). After the hypsarrhythmic pattern resolves, patients may continue to

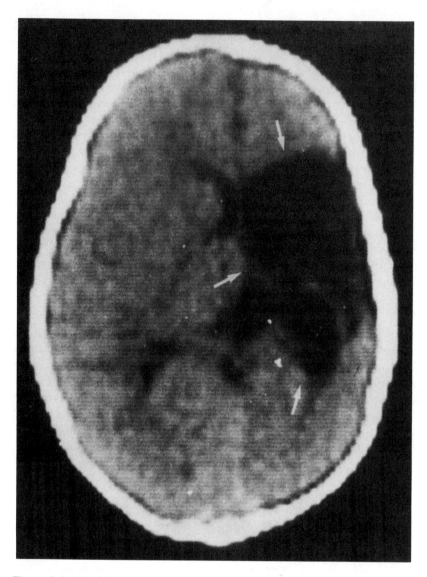

Figure 2-2. (A) CT scan demonstrating wedge-shaped hypodense lesion (arrows) suggestive of an old infarct in the right middle cerebral artery distribution in a 6-month-old infant. (B) Sleep EEG from the same patient demonstrating hypsarrhythmia. There is voltage attenuation and virtually complete absence of sleep spindles in the right hemisphere. Bipolar montage. Right-side electrodes are denoted by even numbers, left side electrodes by odd numbers. (Reproduced with permission from Alavarez et al., 1987.)

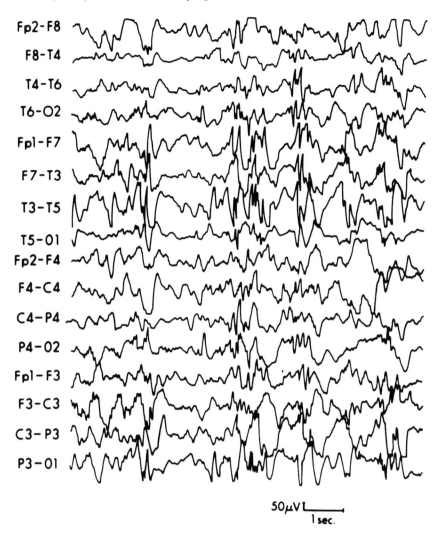

Fp2-F8
F8-T4
T4-T6
T6-O2
Fp1-F7
F7-T3
T3-T5
T5-O1
Fp2-F4
F4-C4
C4-P4
P4-O2
Fp1-F3
F3-C3
C3-P3
P3-O1

50μV

1 sec.

Figure 2-2. (Continued)

have focal seizures. Recently, subtle focal abnormalities have been demonstrated on PET scanning and corticography and some of these children have significantly improved following surgical resections (Chugani et al., 1988). These focal lesions seem to involve the parietooccipital structures rather than the temporal lobes (Chugani et al., 1992). The surgical treatment requires large resections that are almost hemispherectomies. Based on these findings, Shewmon and colleagues (Shewmon, Altman, et al., 1990; Shewmon, Shields, et al., 1990) have proposed that, early in life, focal lesions may produce secondary epileptogenesis by altering the epileptic potential of other brain sites, leading to the development of multifocal seizure foci and the clinical expression of infantile spasms or Lennox-Gastaut syndrome.

Summary of the Clinical Data

The susceptibility to seizures changes with age. A window of increased epileptogenicity occurs during the first few years of life (Hauser and Hesdorffer, 1990). Genetically determined syndromes such as febrile seizures and benign rolandic epilepsy have their own windows of augmented seizure susceptibility and remission. The unique behavioral manifestations of the seizures appear to relate to the age of onset of seizures as well as the specific epileptic syndrome. Unique features include the presence of alternating seizures (Gastaut et al., 1974), seizures with migratory foci, multifocal seizures with focal lesions, and rapid secondary generalization with possible prominent involvement of brainstem structures.

To understand the clinical syndromes, it is important to obtain a clearer insight into how development influences epileptogenicity. For this purpose, these developmental influences have been studied in animal models of epilepsy in which the investigator has better control of many contributing factors.

Animal Models of Focal Seizures

Correlative ontogenetic studies require an understanding of the differences in the developmental process among various mammals (reviewed in Dobbing and Sands, 1979; Moshé and Cornblath, 1993). For example, mice and rats are born before the main period of neuroblast differentiation; synaptogenesis and myelination are largely postnatal events. In human brain neuroblasts are almost completely differentiated and have completed their proliferation before birth, but myelination occurs postnatally.

Gottlieb, Keydor, and Epstein (1977) compared the age-related stages of brain growth in humans and rodents and suggested that the developmental status of the full-term human brain may be roughly equivalent to the rodent brain at 5 to 8 days of age. Thirty-five-day-old rats are considered pubescent animals (Moshé and Cornblath, 1993). Recent experimental evidence suggests that postnatal age-related changes in seizures susceptibility are not linear; instead, as seems to be the case clinically, there are developmentally discrete periods of altered seizure susceptibility and expression. The first such period in the rat is the first postnatal week, during which the immature brain is less prone to develop electrographic seizures than at any other age (see below). During the rat's second and third postnatal weeks (ages roughly corresponding to human infants and young children; Gottlieb et al., 1977), there is an increased susceptibility to focal seizures. This increased epileptogenicity has been described in in vitro slices of hippocampus and neocortex subjected to various conditions that increase neuronal excitability (Hablitz, 1987; Hablitz and Heinemann, 1987; Schwartzkroin, 1984; Swann and Brady, 1984). Similar data have been obtained in whole-animal experiments including studies on neocortical focal epileptogenesis (Mares, 1973), electrically induced neocortical afterdischarges (Mares et al., 1980), amygdala kindling (Moshé, 1981), hippocampal kindling (Haas et al., 1990; Michelson et al., 1989), and hippocampal electrical stimulations (Velísek and Mares, 1991). The concordance of these observations suggests that the increased susceptibility to seizures during weeks 2 and 3 of life is not restricted to a single structure or to a specific model but probably represents a widespread phenomenon. Another window of altered epileptogenicity may exist during periadolescence. Evidence from amygdala-kindling studies (Moshé, 1981; Moshé et al., 1981) and studies of kainic acid–induced seizures (Albala et al., 1984) indicates that 30- to 35-day-old rats may be more resistant to the development of secondarily generalized seizures than younger or older rats (Table 2-2).

First Postnatal Week

In Vivo Studies

More than 20 years ago, during in vivo neurophysiologic studies of the ontogeny of seizures in kittens, Purpura and colleagues observed that the immature neocortex and hippocampus were less prone to develop electrographic seizures than the mature cortex (Purpura, 1964, 1969). The kitten neocortex was considered to be electrophysiologically "stable" and less susceptible to seizures than the cortex of mature animals (Prince and Gutnick, 1972). Electric stimulations elicited broad action potentials, and repetitive discharging was infrequent. Similar data have been obtained in rats. Michelson and colleagues (Michelson and Lothman, 1991, 1992; Michelson et al., 1989; Michelson and Wong, 1991) found that urethane-anesthetized or freely moving 7-day-old rats have the highest threshold for the hippocampal afterdischarges (ADs). Velísek and his associates also found elevated (compared to other age groups) hippocampal AD thresholds in 7-day-old rats; at times currents as high as 2,000 μA are needed to elicit hippocampal ADs (unpublished observations). Seven-day-old rats have long refractory periods following electrical hippocampal stimulations compared to rats in the second or third postnatal week (Velísek and Mares, 1991).

TABLE 2-2. Features of Developmental Seizures of Focal Onset in Rats

	Focal Epileptogenicity	*Secondary Generalization*
First week	Decreased	Limited
Second–third week	Increased	Enhanced
Periadolescence	Increased	Diminished

Note: Age-related epileptogenicity is relative to adult animals.

In Vitro Studies

Recent in vitro intracellular recordings from slices from hippocampus and neocortex taken during the first postnatal week are consistent with many of these earlier findings. Intracellular recordings have shown that action potentials routinely have slower rising and falling phases (Kriegstein et al., 1987; Schwartzkroin and Kunkel, 1982; Schwartzkroin et al., 1982). Often no seizure-like discharges occur (Hablitz, 1987; Hablitz and Heinemann, 1987). When ADs are elicited, they are far less synchronized than those recorded from tissue taken from rats 2–3 weeks of age (Kriegstein et al., 1987; Schwartzkroin and Kunkel, 1982; Schwartzkroin et al., 1982; Swann and Brady, 1984).

Second and Third Postnatal Weeks

In Vivo Studies

Kindling is one of the best models of epilepsy in which to study how seizures propagate from a focus and progressively recruit many additional brain structures; this spread culminates in the emergence of generalized seizures (Goddard et al., 1969). Kindling, once induced, permanently changes the susceptibility of the brain to seizures (Goddard et al., 1969). Occasionally, spontaneous seizures occur as well (Pinel and Rovner, 1978; Wada and Osawa, 1976; Wada et al., 1974).

The behavioral manifestations of kindled seizures induced by stimulating limbic structures have been described for various ages starting with 7-day-old rats (Baram et al., 1993; Moshé and Cornblath, 1993). Progression through the various seizure stages in young animals is different from kindled seizure stages in prepubescent and adult rats (Table 2-3). Stages 0–2 represent local events, stage 3 the involvement of the hemisphere ipsilateral to the stimulation site, stages 4–5 bilateral (generalized) seizures, while stages 6 and 7 (Haas et al., 1990; Sperber et al., 1990) may reflect spread to the brainstem (Browning, 1985; Burnham, 1985; Gale, 1989). Compared to older rats, pups spend proportionally less time in the early stages of kindling (stages 0–2), which are associated with focal seizures (Moshé, 1981). Instead there is an early appearance of bilateral, although often asynchronous seizures, indicating a tendency for seizure generalization. The ability of immature rats to exhibit bilateral asymmetric seizures, in contrast to adult rats, may reflect a lack of complete myelination of the corpus callosum (Agrawal and Davison, 1973; Carey, 1982; Davison, 1970; DeMeyer, 1967). Pups do not often experience stage 5 seizures, which are characterized by falling. Instead, they experience many stage 3–4 seizures intermixed with isolated stage 5 seizures followed by the explosive onset of stage 6 and stage 7 seizures (Haas et al., 1990; Sperber et al., 1990). Another differentiating feature is the ease with which stage 6 and stage 7 seizures occur in rat pups, indicating perhaps rapid spread to brainstem structures (Haas, 1990). Sponta-

TABLE 2-3. Developmental Features of Kindling in Rats

Kindling Stage	Pups (less than 18 days)	Pubescents (30–35 days)	Adults (older than 60 days)
0	Behavioral arrest	Behavioral arrest	Behavioral arrest
1	Facial movements	Chewing	Chewing
2	Rhythmic head movements or turning of body to stimulated site	Head nodding	Head nodding
3	Unilateral forelimb clonus and ± hindlimb clonus; "wet dog" shakes	Contralateral forelimb clonus	Contralateral forelimb clonus
3.5	Alternating forelimb clonus		
4	Bilateral forelimb clonus or rotatory movements of tonically extended forelimbs; rearing not consistent	Bilateral symmetrical forelimb clonus with rearing	Bilateral symmetrical forelimb clonus with rearing
5	Bilateral forelimb clonus with rearing and falling*	Bilateral forelimb clonus with rearing and falling	Bilateral forelimb clonus with rearing and falling
6	Wild running and jumping with or without vocalizations	No available studies	Wild running and jumping with vocalizations
7	Tonus	No available studies	Tonus
8	Spontaneous seizures		Spontaneous seizures

*This stage may be absent in rat pups (see text).
Modified from Moshé and Cornblath, 1993 (with permission).

neous seizures occur more readily in pups compared to adults (Baram et al., 1993; Haas et al., 1992).

Amygdala or hippocampal kindling can be produced in 15-day-old pups using frequent stimulations, say, every 15 minutes (Lee et al., 1989; Moshé and Albala, 1983; Moshé et al., 1983). In adults, stimulations delivered every 15 minutes either significantly retard or fail to induce kindling (Goddard et al., 1969; Moshé et al., 1983; Peterson et al., 1981; Racine, 1972). Hippocampal stimulation in rat pups results in the same stages and rates of kindling as amygdala stimulation (Haas et al., 1990). This is different from adult kindling in which the amygdala kindles faster than the dorsal hippocampus (Goddard et al., 1969). Thus the immature hippocampus appears to be more susceptible to the development of kindled seizures than the adult hippocampus (Haas et al., 1990; Lee et al., 1989).

There is another difference between adult rats and 15-day-old rat pups, involving the phenomenon of kindling antagonism (Applegate and Burchfiel,

1990; Burchfiel and Applegate, 1989). In adult rats, concurrent kindling of two limbic foci results in the suppression of generalized seizures from one or both sites. Pups do not show kindling antagonism between the amygdala and hippocampus, or between the amygdala on each side (Haas et al., 1990, 1992; Sperber et al., 1990). These data may indicate that, early in life, different brain areas can mutually enhance their epileptogenic potential leading to the development of multifocal epilepsy, a common clinical phenomenon in young children, especially in those with infantile spasms. The data also suggest that during the critical period, the immature CNS is more prone to the development of secondarily generalized seizures that may have their onset from multiple limbic seizure foci. This increase in seizure susceptibility extends beyond the local generation of epileptic discharges and involves the mechanisms that participate in seizure propagation to recruit additional structures that may increase seizure severity.

In Vitro Studies

During the second and third weeks of life, the hippocampal CA_1 region is more prone to the development of epileptiform afterdischarges following repetitive orthodromic stimulation (Schwartzkroin, 1984), in response to lowering extracellular calcium levels (Hamon and Heinemann, 1988), or even spontaneously (Schwartzkroin, 1984) than at any other stage of development. This is also the case in the CA_3 area of the hippocampus. Swann and colleagues (Swann and Brady, 1984; Swann et al., 1991) have shown that applications of $GABA_A$ antagonists such as penicillin, bicuculline, or picrotoxin in slices from this age group induce prolonged seizurelike discharges. In contrast, in slices from adult animals, similar applications of $GABA_A$ antagonists produce short-lived epileptiform bursts, which are like interictal spikes (Fig. 2-3). The electrographic seizures that occur in 2- to 3-week-old rat pups arise from the CA_3 subfield itself and do not depend on activity in dentate or CA_1 pyramidal cells for their occurrence (Chesnut and Swann, 1988; Swann et al., 1987). Hablitz and Heinemann (1987, 1989) reported that neocortical slices obtained from the anterior frontal cortex of animals at this age also exhibit a greater propensity toward the development of ictal discharges following the application of picrotoxin than slices obtained from adult animals.

Periadolescence

In Vivo Studies

Periadolescence can be defined as a developmental stage immediately prior to, during, and immediately after the onset of puberty. In rats it includes animals 30–40 days old (Spear and Brake, 1983). During this period the susceptibility to seizures changes again. The amygdala-induced AD threshold is lowest in 35-day-old rats (Moshé, 1981). This finding may be evidence of

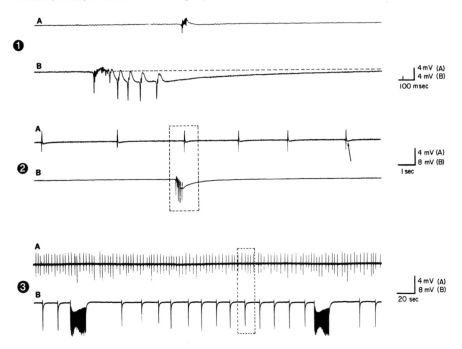

Figure 2-3. Comparison of spontaneous epileptiform discharges recorded extracellularly from the CA$_3$ cell body layer of a slice taken from a mature (traces A) and an 11-day-old rat pup (traces B). Slices were bathed in 1.7 mM penicillin. Recordings at three different time bases are shown. Events in (1) are shown framed by a dashed line in (2). Likewise, traces in (2) are those framed in (3). (Reproduced with permission from [Swann and Brady, 1984].)

increased focal epileptogenicity (Table 2-2), although this age-specific sensitivity has not been studied in detail. On the other hand, there is evidence from both kindling studies and studies using the chemoconvulsant kainic acid indicating that 30- to 35-day-old rats are more resistant to the development of generalized seizures than younger or older animals (Albala et al., 1984; Moshé, 1981; Moshé et al., 1981).

Factors Underlying the Developmental Periods of Differential Susceptibility to Seizures

Experimental studies have suggested that a wide variety of factors can contribute to changes in seizure susceptibility during critical developmental periods. These factors range from age-dependent differences in the development of synaptic inhibition and excitation to ionic microenvironmental imbalances.

Synaptic Inhibition

In Purpura's studies (Purpura, 1964, 1969), the apparent lack of excitability of the neonatal cortex during the first postnatal week was thought to be the product of several neurophysiologic factors, including the relative inexcitability of immature neurons. Subsequent studies demonstrated that there are differences in the developmental patterns of expression of inhibitory postsynaptic potentials (IPSPs) between species and brain regions. It seems clear that in the rat, early in neonatal life, the neocortex has little if any functional inhibition (Luhmann and Prince, 1991). The same appears to be true for hippocampal area CA_1 (Zhang et al., 1991). However, in area CA_3 functional synaptic inhibition is more precocious and appears early in postnatal life (Swann et al., 1989). It seems likely that in areas of brain such as hippocampal area CA_1, the late onset of synaptic inhibition could contribute to enhanced seizure susceptibility. However, in other areas, such as hippocampal CA_3, these inhibitory synapses may play a central role in preventing seizure generation at critical periods in development.

In addition to $GABA_A$ receptor-mediated IPSPs the $GABA_B$ receptors mediate large, prolonged IPSPs in both mature hippocampus and neocortex (Newberry and Nicoll, 1985). The ontogeny of $GABA_B$ IPSPs parallels that of their $GABA_A$ counterpart. In hippocampal area CA_1, late IPSPs and hyperpolarizing responses to baclofen have not been observed during the neonatal period (Brady and Swann, 1984; Janigro and Schwartzkroin, 1988; Schwartzkroin, 1982; Schwartzkroin and Kunkel, 1982; Schwartzkroin et al., 1982). In neocortex, application of baclofen fails to produce any responses in the majority of neocortical neurons studied during the first postnatal week (Luhmann and Prince, 1991). In contrast, immature CA_3 pyramidal cells uniformly respond to bath-applied baclofen with large membrane hyperpolarizations (Brady and Swann, 1984; Janigro and Schwartzkroin, 1988; Swann et al., 1989). Thus it appears that the formation of many local circuit inhibitory synapses progresses during early postnatal life and that inhibitory synapses that generate $GABA_A$- and $GABA_B$-mediated IPSPs form roughly at the same time in a given brain region. However, the timing of the formation of these synapses is different from one area of the brain to another (Swann, Chapter 8).

As mentioned, a late onset of functional synaptic inhibition could conceivably contribute to increased seizure susceptibility in early life. However, most studies in rodents have shown that during the second and third postnatal week, when seizure susceptibility is unusually high, synaptic inhibition is functional. Indeed, at these times application of $GABA_A$ receptor antagonists will produce seizure discharges that are unusually prolonged in nature (Brady and Swann, 1984; Hablitz, 1987; Hablitz and Heinemann, 1987). Studies have implicated excitatory amino acid synaptic transmission in the generation of these protracted events (Brady and Swann, 1984, 1986; Lee and Hablitz, 1991; Swann et al., 1993). Synaptic inhibition in the epileptic cortical or hippocampal focus may be functional at this stage of development.

Synaptic Excitation

There is ample evidence indicating that glutamate-mediated excitatory postsynaptic potentials (EPSPs) undergo dramatic changes during postnatal life. The properties of these early-formed synapses are thought to contribute to enhanced seizure susceptibility (Swann, Chapter 8). EPSPs are unusually prolonged in both neonatal cortex and hippocampus (Burgard and Hablitz, 1993; Kriegstein et al., 1987). Moreover, the biophysical properties of excitatory amino acid receptors change dramatically with brain maturation (Carmignoto and Vicini, 1992; Hestrin, 1992; Schwartzkroin, Chapter 9). This is likely a reflection of developmental alterations in the expression of different subunits for the receptors (Pellegrini-Giampietro et al., 1991). In many brain regions the receptors undergo a transient developmental increase in density (McDonald and Johnston, 1990). This occurs at a time when the animals are most susceptible to seizures. In the hippocampus, local excitatory recurrent collaterals form dense networks of axon arbors which decrease in complexity with maturation (Gomez-Di Cesare et al., unpublished; Swann, Chapter 8). Thus it is possible that the properties of some excitatory synapses that exist only transiently in early postnatal life promote epileptogenesis and contribute to seizure generation.

During the course of electrographic seizures, individual neurons undergo a sustained membrane depolarization. In the immature hippocampus this sustained depolarization appears to be a separate physiologic process from the rhythmic repetitive discharges of seizures; it is synaptically mediated and may play a pivotal role in seizure generation (Swann, Smith, and Brady, 1993). The sustained depolarization appears to be produced exclusively in the proximal portion of the CA_3 pyramidal cell basilar dendrites. As the hippocampus matures, the CA_3 networks appear to be remodeled and seizure susceptibility decreases concomitantly. These recent results indicate that age-dependent alterations in a population of excitatory synapses that are restricted to only a fraction of the dendritic tree may have an overriding influence in determining whether hippocampal seizures occur (Swann, Chapter 8).

The Ionic Microenvironment

The role of extracellular K^+ in the generation of seizures has been the subject of much discussion (Dichter et al., 1972; Prince, 1978; Somjen, 1979; Swann et al., 1989). In mature animals, ion-sensitive microelectrode studies have shown that following an interictal spike in the neocortex or hippocampus, there are substantial increases in extracellular K^+. Repeated interictal spiking within short time intervals can lead to temporal summation of extracellular K^+ accumulation; recovery to baseline levels may take many seconds. The increase in $[K^+]_0$ is thought to lead to membrane depolarization and thereby increase neuronal excitability via a positive feedback process. In this way, changes in $[K^+]_0$ may contribute to the transition from an interictal state (repeated isolated events) to ictal (seizure) episodes (Connors et al., 1982; Hablitz and Heinemann, 1987; Mutani et al., 1984; Swann et al., 1988; Traynelis and Dingledine, 1988).

In the immature CNS during the second to third postnatal week, the extracellular $[K^+]_0$ changes accompanying interictal spikes in the hippocampal CA_3 subfield are much greater than those observed in mature animals, as indicated in Figure 2-4 (Swann et al., 1986). In addition, in the mature brain, $[K^+]_0$ reaches a ceiling level of 10–12 mM during the course of an electrographic seizure. By contrast, in the immature CNS, the K^+ ceiling level is much higher than that seen in the mature brain, with values of 14–20 mM routinely observed (Hablitz and Heinemann, 1989; Swann et al., 1986). The ages when changes in $[K^+]_0$ are unusually large coincide with the period during which the immature hippocampus demonstrates its marked propensity for seizures (Fig. 2-4).

In the CA_3 subfield and neocortex, increases in $[K^+]_0$ follow and do not precede the onset of epileptiform events (Hablitz and Heinemann, 1987; Swann et al., 1986). Therefore, these changes may be the product of the synchronized discharges (Swann et al., 1986) and may contribute to prolonging a seizure-like discharge and aiding in its spread to other brain regions. In hippocampal area CA_3, changes in $[K^+]_0$ vary greatly across the hippocampal laminae. K^+ transients are largest in the proximal position of the basilar dendritic layer (Swann et al., 1986). This is the site where excitatory synapses are thought to produce the sustained depolarizations associated with electrographic seizures (Swann, Smith, and Brady, 1993; Swann, Smith, Brady and Pierson, 1993). It is possible that $[K^+]_0$ changes are at least part, the product of a unique form of excitatory amino acid synaptic transmission that exists in developing hippocampus and contributes importantly to the generation of prolonged seizure discharges. In addition, delayed development of the glia may allow for the accumulation of potassium in the extracellular space, which may lead to general hyperexcitability (Schwartz-kroin, 1984).

Myelination

Incomplete myelination may explain some of the age-specific differences in the expression of the motor seizures and electrographic seizure patterns, as well as the poor interhemispheric synchrony of the ADs (Moshé, 1981). Myelin assembles slowly during the last part of gestation and more rapidly afterward. Myelination occurs first in the phylogenetically older parts of the brain such as the brainstem and later in the corpus callosum and fronto-pontine tracts (Agrawal and Davison, 1973; Davison, 1970; Eayrs and Goodhead, 1959). Characteristic features of bilateral kindled seizures in 15-

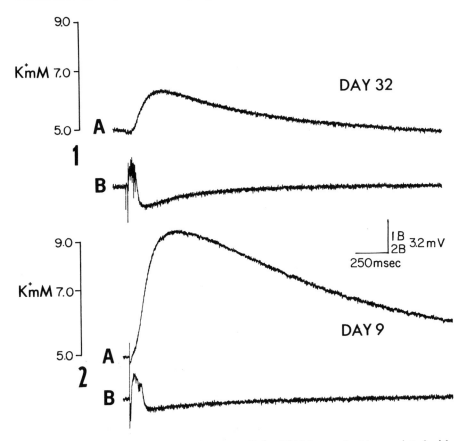

Figure 2-4. Comparison of changes in extracellular [K$^+$] (traces in A) associated with interictal spike discharging recorded in the rat hippocampal CA$_3$ subfield on postnatal days 32 and 9. Recordings were made in the striatum oriens at the edge of the cell body layer. Extracellular fields recorded simultaneously are shown in traces B. (Reproduced with permission from Swann et al., 1986.)

day-old pups suggest a proportionately larger brainstem role and lesser involvement of prefrontal motor regions (Moshé et al., 1990). In fact, 15-day-old pups resemble adult rats with prefrontal lesions (Corcoran et al., 1976). This observation suggests that prefrontal inputs are necessary for the expression of adultlike stage 5 seizure patterns. In humans, immaturity of prefrontal inputs along with the incomplete myelination may account for the age-specific clinical phenomenology of infantile spasms.

Catecholamines and Seizures

Age-related changes in the levels of neurotransmitters influence the patterns of seizure propagation. In humans, dysfunction of central monoaminergic systems has been implicated in the expression of infantile spasms (Hrachovy and Frost, 1989). However, the results are inconclusive. In animals, cate-cholamines and especially norepinephrine play an important role in contain-ing kindled seizures within the focus. Norepinephrine depletion accelerates the development of kindling in adult (Corcoran and Weiss, 1990; McIntyre, 1981; McIntyre et al., 1987) and pubescent rats (Goddard et al., 1969; Mich-elson and Butterbaugh, 1985; Moshæ and Albala, 1983; Peterson et al., 1981). In this respect, norepinephrine-depleted adult rats resemble 15- to 18-day-old rat pups in whom the levels of norepinephrine are lower than in older rats (Moshé et al., 1981). On the other hand, pubescent (35-day-old) rats have lower norepinephrine levels than adults but kindle slower than adults (Moshé et al., 1981). In pubescent rats hormonal influences may play a role, since gonadal steroid hormones can suppress kindling in young rats but not in adults (Holmes and Weber, 1986).   ˙

Substantia Nigra and Seizure Expression

A large number of studies have implicated seizure-modifying circuits which include several subcortical nuclei. One such system may include a GABA-sensitive substantia nigra (SN)–based circuit. The SN and especially the pars reticulata (SNR) may be critically involved in the expression and con-trol of generalized seizures in rats (for review, see Moshé and Sperber, 1990). The potentially crucial role in the adult rat was first suggested by the dra-matic increases in deoxyglucose utilization seen in the SN during kindling (Engel et al., 1978). In 15-day-old rats, however, there is no such deoxyglu-cose accumulation in the SN (Ackermann et al., 1989).

The SN changes are not specific for the kindling model. Deoxyglucose studies have been performed in rats injected with kainic acid or exposed to flurothyl. Immature animals are more susceptible to the development of either kainic acid or flurothyl seizures than are adults (Albala et al., 1984; Sperber and Moshé, 1988). Yet in these models, as in kindling, there is lower glucose utilization (than in the adult) in the SN during seizures even when the rat pup is experiencing severe seizures (Albala et al., 1984; Sperber et al., 1992).

Pharmacologic studies suggest that the nigral effects on seizures are age-specific. Some of the age-related differences in seizure susceptibility may be due to functional differences of the SN GABA receptors. There are age-specific differences in the density of $GABA_A$ and $GABA_B$ nigral receptors. Although in vitro muscimol ($GABA_A$) receptor binding studies of the SN region indicate that there are no differences in the receptor density of the $GABA_A$ low-affinity site as a function of age, there are differences in the density of high-affinity receptors. Specifically, the SN of immature rats shows only 13 percent of the adult level of high-affinity receptors (Wurpel et al., 1988). Furthermore, in vitro $GABA_B$ receptor binding studies reveal that the $GABA_B$ receptor density is higher in the pup SN than in the adult (Fig. 2-5; Garant et al., 1992).

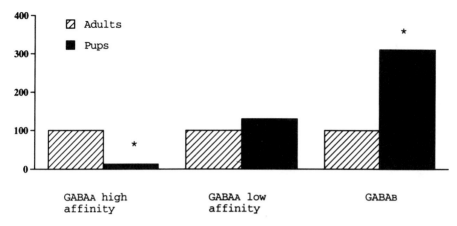

Figure 2-5. Age-specific changes in the expression of nigral GABA receptors. Adult values are considered to be 100 percent. Asterisk denotes significant differences.

Pharmacologic studies have shown that in adults the nigral effects on seizures appear to be mediated by the $GABA_A$ receptor since an agonist (muscimol) and an antagonist (bicuculline) produce opposing effects on seizures (Sperber et al., 1989b). Both high- and low-affinity subtypes of $GABA_A$ receptor may be involved because bicuculline is an antagonist of the low-affinity site, while muscimol acts on both the high- and low-affinity site. The importance of the low-affinity site is also reflected in the results of combined γ-vinyl GABA–bicuculline infusions in which bicuculline abolishes the anticonvulsant effect of GVG (Xu, Sperber, and Moshé, 1991). In adult rats, the nigral $GABA_B$ receptor does not appear to participate in the control of seizures because baclofen infusions have no effect on seizures (Sperber, Wurpel, and Moshé, 1989). The indirect effect of GVG must then be the result of $GABA_A$ receptor activation (Xu, 1991b).

In pups, the nigral GABA-mediated effects on seizures are complex. There are some similarities with the adult effects, as well as marked differences (Sperber et al., 1987; Sperber, Wurpel, and Moshé, 1989; Sperber, Wurpel, and Zhao, et al., 1989; Xu, Garant, et al., 1991; Xu, Sperber, et al., 1991). Bicuculline has a similar proconvulsant effect in the two groups, suggesting that the $GABA_A$ low-affinity receptor acts in the same fashion regardless of the rat's age. On the other hand, in pups, but not in adults, baclofen is capable of suppressing seizures (Sperber, Wurpel, and Moshé, 1989). The $GABA_B$ receptor binding data may explain the age-specific effects of baclofen, anticonvulsant in pups and no effect in adults (Fig. 2-6).

The most marked age-related differences in the nigral effects on seizures involve muscimol, since similar doses of muscimol are anticonvulsant in adults but proconvulsant in 2-week-old pups (Moshé and Garant, 1994). Identical results have been obtained using nigral infusions of THIP (4,5,6,7-tetrahydroisoxazolo[5,4-c]pyridin-3-ol), a selective $GABA_A$ receptor agonist

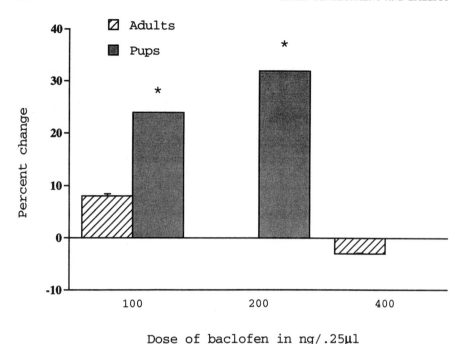

Figure 2-6. Effects of intranigral infusions of baclofen on seizures as a function of age. The percentage change reflects differences in seizure duration from control values. Asterisk denotes significant differences.

(Xu et al., 1992). Because THIP is a relatively specific high-affinity $GABA_A$ receptor agonist (Xu et al., 1992), the proconvulsant effects of both drugs are likely to be mediated by the nigral high-affinity $GABA_A$ receptors. These apparent paradoxical findings may be due to an ontogenetic difference in the action of GABA at nigral $GABA_A$ receptors. Other investigators have observed that GABA agonists can produce both excitatory and inhibitory effects during early development (Chesnut and Swann, 1988; Mueller et al., 1983, 1984). Furthermore, in kittens initial nigral responses to caudate stimulation are either excitatory or inhibitory, while in adults almost all responses are inhibitory (Fisher et al., 1982).

The observed phenomena may be due to site-specific (for the SN) developmental differences in the density, molecular composition, and function of $GABA_A$ receptors. Molecular cloning techniques have confirmed that central $GABA_A$ receptors are a heterogeneous family of related proteins (Angelotti and Macdonald, 1993a, b; Khrestchatisky et al., 1989; Laurie et al., 1992; Levitan, Blair, et al., 1988; Levitan, Schofield, et al., 1988; Schofield et al., 1987, 1990). The heterogeneity of these subunits is also expressed during development (Gambarana et al., 1990). This molecular divergence may be partly responsible for the diverse pharmacologic effects. There may be specific $GABA_A$ isoforms of the $GABA_A$ receptors in nigral neurons associated with proconvulsant or anticonvulsant effects. Moshé and Garant (1995) have proposed that the putative proconvulsant isoform may be expressed in the SN early in life as the predominant isoform of the few available high-affinity sites. With maturation, the increases in nigral $GABA_A$ high-affinity binding sites may reflect the appearance of a putative anticonvulsant isoform which in adults constitutes the majority of the high-affinity sites. In adults, GABAergic drugs that act on the $GABA_A$ high-affinity site may predominantly activate the anticonvulsant site. With larger doses, the proconvulsant site may become involved. This hypothesis could explain why muscimol partially attenuates the GVG effect in the dual infusion studies (Xu, Garant, et al., 1991) and the proconvulsant effects of high doses of muscimol and THIP in adult rats (Fig. 2-7; Moshé and Garant, 1995). In fact, recent in situ hybridization studies indicate that the expression of the $\alpha 1$ subunit of the $GABA_A$ receptor in the SNR is lower in pups than that in adults (Sperber et al., 1991). The expression of the isoforms may vary with age and thus account for the developmentally bound site-specific (nigral) effect of $GABA_A$ receptor agonists on seizures. Further studies on the molecular composition of $GABA_A$ receptors may help elucidate why genetically determined epileptic syndromes occur in certain strains of animals and in some human families. These studies could also lead to possible new pharmacologic strategies to control systems essential for seizure propagation and modification, thus

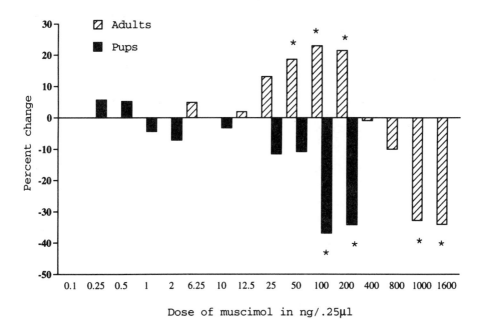

Figure 2-7. Effects of intranigral infusions of muscimol on seizures as a function of dose and age. The percentage change reflects differences in seizure duration from control values. Asterisk denotes significant differences. Note the biphasic effect in adults. In pups, the only significant changes are indicative of proconvulsant effects.

aiding the development of age-appropriate treatments of seizure disorders (see also Chapter 11).

Conclusion

Development alters the susceptibility of the brain to focal seizures. There are periods of either decreased or increased seizure susceptibility depending on the level of maturation of various factors that can influence the expression and the control of seizures. As with seizure susceptibility, the underlying ontogenetic processes are not linear but have characteristic age-specific patterns that may be recapitulated during disease states or during conditions of excessive stimulation. The slow and prolonged postsynaptic events during the first week of life in the rodent can be considered a reflection of the slow, asynchronous, often fragmented seizure discharges observed in newborn human infants (Chapter 1). Some seizures (see-saw) in human infants are similar to kindling stage 3.5 in rat pup (Gastaut et al., 1974). Although the exact human age equivalent is unknown, correlative ontogenetic studies suggest that the period during which age-specific seizure patterns such as infantile spasms are expressed (the first year of life) may be related to the second and third postnatal week in the rat (Gottlieb et al., 1977; Moshé, 1987; Moshé et al., 1992). Thus the study of seizures, epilepsy, and their substrates at different ages may provide important insights about normal brain development in experimental animals and in humans.

Acknowledgments

The work described in this chapter was supported by NIH grants NS-20253 (S.L.M.), NS-26151 (S.S.), and NS-18309 (J.W.S.).

References

Ackermann, R. F., Moshé, S. L., and Albala, B. J. (1989) Restriction of enhanced ^{14}C-2-deoxyglucose utilization to rhinencepahlic structures in immature amygdala-kindled rats. *Exp. Neurol. 104*:73–81.

Agrawal, H. C., and Davison, A. N. (1973) Myelination and amino acid imbalance in the developing brain. In W. Himwich (ed.), *Biochemistry of the Developing Brain*. New York: Marcel Dekker, pp. 143–168.

Albala, B. J., Moshé, S. L., and Okdada, R. (1984) Kainic-acid–induced seizures: A developmental study. *Dev. Brain Res. 13*:139–148.

Alvarez, L. A., Shinnar, S., and Moshé, S. L. (1987) Infantile spasms due to unilateral cerebral infarcts. *Pediatrics 79*:1024–1026.

Angelotti, T. P., and Macdonald, R. L. (1993a) Assembly of $GABA_A$ receptor subunits: α_1, β_1 and $\alpha_1\beta_1\gamma_{25}$ subunits produce unique ion channels with dissimilar single-channel properties. *Neuroscience 13*:1429–1440.

Angelotti, T. P., and Macdonald, R. L. (1993b) Assembly of GABA_A receptor subunits: Analysis of transient single-cell expression utilizing a fluorescent substrate/marker gene technique. *Neuroscience 13:*1418–1428.

Annegers, J. F., Hauser, W. A., and Elveback, L. R. (1979) Remission of seizures and relapse in patients with epilepsy. *Epilepsia 20:*729–737.

Applegate, C. D., and Burchfiel, J. L. (1990) Evidence for a norepinephrine-dependent brain-stem substrate in the development of kindling antagonism. *Epilepsy Res. 6:*23–32.

Baram, T. Z., Hirsch, E., and Schultz, L. (1993) Short-interval amygdala kindling in neonatal rats. *Dev. Brain Res. 73:*79–83.

Berg, A. T., Shinnar, S., Hauser, W. A., Alemany, M., Shapiro, E. D., Salomon, M. E., and Crain, E. F. (1992) Predictors of recurrent febrile seizures: A prospective study of the circumstances surrounding the initial febrile seizure. *N. Engl. J. Med. 327:*1122–1127.

Berg, A. T., Shinnar, S., Hauser, W. A., and Leventhal, J. M. (1990) Predictors of recurrent febrile seizures: A meta-analytic review. *Pediatrics 116:*329–337.

Blom, S., and Heijbel, J. (1982) Benign epilepsy of children with centrotemporal EEG foci: A follow-up study in adulthood of patients initially studied as children. *Epilepsia 23:*629–631.

Blom, S., Hiejbel, J., and Bergfors, P. G. (1975) Benign epilepsy of children with centrotemporal EEG foci–discharge rate during sleep. *Epilepsia 16:*133–140.

Brady, R. J., and Swann, J. W. (1984) Postsynaptic actions of baclofen associated with its antagonism of bicuculline-induced epileptogenesis in hippocampus. *Cell Mol. Neurobiol. 4:*403–408.

Brady, R. J., and Swann, J. W. (1986) Ketamine selectively suppresses synchronized afterdischarges in immature hippocampus. *Neurosci. Lett. 69:*143–149.

Browning, R. A. (1985) Role of the brain-stem reticular formation in tonic-clonic seizures: Lesion and pharmacological studies. *Fed. Proc. 44:*2425–2431.

Burchfiel, J. L., and Applegate, C. D. (1989) Stepwise progression of kindling: Perspectives from the kindling antagonism model. In D. P. Cain and D. Teskey (eds.), *Neuroscience and Biobehavioral Reviews.* New York: Pergamon, pp. 289–308.

Burgard, E. C., and Hablitz, J. J. (1993) Developmental changes in NMDA and non-NMDA receptor-mediated synaptic potentials in rat neocortex. *J. Neurophysiol. 69:*230–240.

Burnham, W. M. (1985) Core mechanisms in generalized convulsions. *Fed. Proc. 44:*2442–2445.

Carey, E. (1982) The biochemistry of fetal brain development and myelination. In C. Jones (ed.), *Biochemical Development of the Fetus and Neonate.* Amsterdam: Elsevier Biomedical Press, pp. 287–336.

Carmignoto, G., and Vicini, S. (1992) Activity-dependent decrease in NMDA receptor responses during development of the visual cortex. *Science, 258:*1007–1011.

Cendes, F., Andermann, F., Gloor, P., Lopes-Cendes, I., Andermann, E., Melanson, D., Jones-Gotman, M., Robitaille, Y., Evans, A., and Peters, T. (1993) Atrophy of mesial structures in patients with temporal lobe epilepsy: Cause or consequence of repeated seizures? *Ann. Neurol. 34:*795–801.

Chesnut, T. J., and Swann, J. W. (1988) Epileptiform activity induced by 4-aminopyridine in immature hippocampus. *Epilepsy Res. 2:*187–195.

Chugani, H. T., Shewmon, D. A., Peacock, W. J., Shields, W. D., Mazziotta, J. C., and Phelps, M. E. (1988) Surgical treatment of intractable neonatal onset seizures: The role of positron emission tomography. *Neurology 38:*1178–1188.

Chugani, H. T., Shewmon, D. A., Sankar, R., Chen, B. C., and Phelps, M. E. (1992) Infantile spasms: II. Lenticular nuclei and brain stem activation on positron emission tomography. *Ann. Neurol. 31:*212–218.

Chugani, H. T., Shields, W. D., Shewmon, D. A., Olson, D. M., Phelps, M. E., and Peacock, W. J. (1990) Infantile spasms: I. PET identifies focal cortical dysgenesis in cryptogenic cases for surgical treatment. *Ann. Neurol. 27:*406–413.

Connors, B. E., Ransom, B. R., Kunis, D. M., and Gutnick, M. J. (1982) Activity-dependent K^+ accumulation in the developing rat optic nerve. *Science 216:*1341–1343.

Corcoran, M. E., Urstad, H., McCaughran, J. A. J., and Wada, J. A. (1976) Frontal lobe and kindling in the rat. In J. A. Wada (eds.), *Kindling.* New York: Raven Press, pp. 215–225.

Corcoran, M. E., and Weiss, G. K. (1990) Noradrenaline and kindling revisited. In J. A. Wada (ed.), *Kindling 4.* New York: Plenum, pp. 141–153.

Davison, A. N. (1970) The biochemistry of the myelin sheath. In A. N. Davison and A. Peters (eds.), *Myelination.* Springfield, Ill.: Charles C Thomas, pp. 80–161.

Delgado-Escueta, A. V., and Enrile-Bascal, F. (1984) Juvenile myoclonic epilepsy of Janz. *Neurology 34:*285–294.

DeMeyer, W. (1967) Ontogenesis of the rat corticospinal tract. *Arch. Neurol. 16:*203–211.

Diamantopoulos, N., and Crumrine, P. K. (1986) The effect of puberty on the course of epilepsy. *Arch. Neurol. 43:*873–876.

Dichter, M. A., Herman, C. J., Hofmeier, G., and Seltzer, M. (1972) Silent cells during interictal discharges and seizures in hippocampal penicillin foci: Evidence for the role of extracellular K^+ in the transition from the interictal state to seizures. *Brain Res. 48:*173–183.

Dobbing, J., and Sands, J. (1979) Comparative aspects of the brain growth spurt. *Early Hum. Dev. 3:*79–83.

Dravet, C., Catani, C., Bureau, M., and Roger, J. (1989) Partial epilepsies in infancy: A study of 40 cases. *Epilepsia 30:*807–812.

Duchowny, M., Lewin, B., Jaykar, P., Resnick, T., Alvarez, L., Morrison, G., and Dean, P. (1992) Temporal lobectomy in early childhood. *Epilepsia 33:*298–303.

Eayrs, J. T., and Goodhead, B. (1959) Postnatal development of the cerebral cortex in the rat. *J. Anat. 93:*385–402.

Engel, J. J. (1989) *Seizures and Epilepsy: Contemporary Neurology Series.* Philadelphia: F. A. Davis.

Engel, J. J., Brown, L. L., and Wolfson, L. (1978) Anatomical correlates of electrical and behavioral events related to amygdaloid kindling. *Ann. Neurol. 3:*538–544.

Falconer, M. (1971) Genetic and related etiological factors in temporal lobe epilepsy: A review. *Epilepsia 12:*13–31.

Falconer, M. A., Serafetinides, E. A., and Corsellis, J. A. N. (1964) Etiology and pathogenesis of temporal lobe epilepsy. *Arch. Neurol. 10:*233–248.

Fisher, R. S., Levine, M. S., Hull, C. D., and Buchwald, N. A. (1982) Postnatal ontogeny of evoked neuronal responses in the substantia nigra of the cat. *Dev. Brain Res. 3:*443–462.

French, J. A., Williamson, P. D., Thadani, V. M., Darcey, T. M., Mattson, R. H.,

Spencer, S. S., and Spencer, D. D. (1993) Characteristics of medial temporal lobe epilepsy: I. Results of history and physical examination. *Ann. Neurol. 34:*774–780.

Gale, K. (1989) GABA in epilepsy: The pharmacologic basis. *Epilepsia 30:*S1–S11.

Gamabarana, G., Pittman, R., and Siegel, R. E. (1990) Differential expression of rat GABA$_A$ receptor subunit mRNAs during development. *J. Neurobiol. 12:*4151–4172.

Garant, D. S., Velísek, L., Sperber, E., and Moshé, S. L. (1992) Why do infants have seizures? *Int. Pediatr. 7:*199–212.

Gastaut, H., Broughton, R. Tassinari, C. A., and Roger, J. (1974) Unilateral epileptic seizures. In P. J. Vinken and G. W. Bruyn (eds.), *Handbook of Clinical Neurology: The Epilepsies.* New York: American Elsevier, pp. 235–245.

Goddard, G. V., McIntyre, D. C., and Leech, C. K. (1969) A permanent change in brain function resulting from daily electrical stimulation. *Exp. Neurol. 25:*295–330.

Gottlieb, A., Keydor, I., and Epstein, H. T. (1977) Rodent brain growth stages: An analytical review. *Biol. Neonate, 32:*166–176.

Haas, K., Sperber, E. F., and Moshé, S. L. (1990) Kindling in developing animals: Expression of severe seizures and enhanced development of bilateral foci. *Dev. Brain Res. 56:*275–280.

Haas, K., Sperber, E. F., and Moshé, S. L. (1992) Kindling in developing animals: Interactions between ipsilateral foci. *Dev. Brain Res. 68:*140–143.

Hablitz, J. J. (1987) Spontaneous ictal-like discharges and sustained potential shifts in the developing rat neocortex. *J. Neurophysiol. 58:*1052–1065.

Hablitz, J. J., and Heinemann, U. (1987) Extracellular K$^+$ and Ca^{2+} changes during epileptiform discharges in the immature rat neocortex. *Brain Res. 433:*299–303.

Hablitz, J. J., and Heinemann, U. (1989) Alterations in the microenvironment during spreading depression associated with epileptiform activity in the immature neocortex. *Dev. Brain Res. 46:*243–252.

Hamon, B., and Heinemann, U. (1988) Developmental changes in neuronal sensitivity to excitatory amino acids in area CA$_1$ of the rat hippocampus. *Brain Res. 466:*286–290.

Hauser, W. A., and Hesdorffer, D. C. (1990) *Epilepsy: Frequency, Causes and Consequences.* New York: Demos, pp. 1–52.

Hauser, W. A., and Kurland, L. T. (1975) The epidemiology of epilepsy in Rochester, Minnesota, 1935–1967. *Epilepsia 16:*1–66.

Heijbel, J., Blom, S., and Rasmuson, M. (1975) Benign epilepsy of childhood with centrotemporal EEG foci: A genetic study. *Epilepsia 16:*285–293.

Hestrin, S. (1992) Developmental regulation of NMDA receptor-mediated synaptic currents at a central synapse. *Nature 357:*686–689.

Holmes, G. L., and Weber, D. A. (1986) Effects of ACTH on seizure susceptibility in the developing brain. *Ann. Neurol. 20:*82–88.

Hrachovy, R. A., and Frost, J. D. (1989) Infantile spasms: A disorder of the developing nervous system. In P. Kellaway and J. L. Noebels (eds.), *Problems and Concepts in Developmental Neurophysiology.* Baltimore: Johns Hopkins University Press, pp. 131–147.

Janigro, D., and Schwartzkroin, P. A. (1988) Effects of GABA and baclofen on pyramidal cells in the developing rabbit hippocampus: an "in vitro" study. *Brain Res. 41:*171–184.

Kellaway, P. (1981) The incidence, significance and natural history of spike foci in children. In C. E. Henry (ed.), *Current Clinical Neurophysiology: Update on EEG and Evoked Potentials.* New York: Elsevier, pp. 151–175.

Kellaway, P., Frost, J. D., and Hrachovy, R. A. (1983) Infantile spasms. In P. L. Morselli, C. E. Pippenger, and J. K. Penry (eds.), *Antiepileptic Drug Therapy in Pediatrics.* New York: Raven Press, pp. 115–136.

Khrestchatisky, M., MacLennan, A. J., Chiang, M. Y., Xu, W., Jackson, M., Brecha, N., Sternini, C., Olsen, R. W., and Tobin, A. J. (1989) A novel alpha subunit in rat brain GABA$_A$ receptors. *Neuron 3:*745–753.

Kriegstein, A. R., Suppes, T., and Prince, D. A. (1987) Cellular and synaptic physiology and epileptogenesis of the developing rat neocortical neurons in vitro. *Dev. Brain Res. 34:*161–171.

Lairy, G. C., and Harrison, A. (1968) Functional aspects of EEG foci in children. In P. Kellaway and I. Petersen (eds.), *Clinical Electrophysiology of Children.* New York: Grune and Stratton, pp. 197–212.

Laurie, D. J., Seeburg, P. H., and Wisden, W. (1992) The distribution of 13 GABA$_A$ receptor subunit mRNAs in the rat brain: II. Olfactory bulb and cerebellum. *J. Neurosci. 12:*1063–1076.

Lee, S., Murata, R., and Matsuura, S. (1989) The developmental study of hippocampal kindling. *Epilepsia 30:*266–270.

Lee, W. L., and Hablitz, J. J. (1991) Excitatory synaptic involvement in epileptiform bursting in the immature rat neocortex. *J. Neurophysiol. 66:*1894–1901.

Lerman, P. (1985) Benign partial epilepsy with centro-temporal spikes. In J. Roger, C. Dravet, M. Bureau, F. E. Dreifuss, and P. Wolf (eds.), *Epileptic Syndromes in Infancy, Childhood and Adolescence.* London: John Libbey Eurotext, pp. 150–158.

Lévesque, M. F., Nakasato, N., Vinters, H., and Babb, T. L. (1991) Surgical treatment of limbic epilepsy associated with extrahippocampal lesions: The problem of dual pathology. *J. Neurosurg. 75:*364–370.

Levitan, E. S., Blair, L. A. C., Dionne, V. E., and Barnard, E. A. (1988) Biophysical and pharmacological properties of cloned GABA$_A$ receptor subunits expressed in *Xenopus* oocytes. *Neuron 1:*773–781.

Levitan, E. S., Schofield, P. R., Burt, D. R., Rhee, L. M., Wisden, W., Kohler, M., Fujita, N., Rodriguez, H., Stephenson, F. A., Darlison, M. G., Barnard, E. A., and Seeburg, P. H. (1988) Structural and functional basis for GABA$_A$ receptor heterogeneity. *Nature 335:*76–79.

Loiseau, P., Duche, B., Cordova, S., Dartigues, J. F., and Cohadon, S. (1988) Prognosis of benign childhood epilepsy with centrotemporal spikes: A follow-up study of 169 patients. *Epilepsia 29:*229–235.

Luhmann, H. J., and Prince, D. A. (1991) Postnatal maturation of the GABAergic system in rat neocortex. *J. Neurophysiol. 65:*247–263.

Mares, J., Mares, P., and Trojan, S. (1980) The ontogenesis of cortical self-sustained after-discharges in rats. *Epilepsia 21:*111–121.

Mares, P., (1973) Ontogenetic development of bioelectrical activity of the epileptogenic focus in rat neocortex. *Neuropadiatrie 4:*434–445.

McDonald, J. W., and Johnston, M. V. (1990) Physiological and pathophysiological roles of excitatory amino acids during central nervous system development. *Dev. Brain Res. 15:*41–70.

McIntyre, D. C. (1981) Catecholamine involvement in amygdala kindling of the rat. In J. A. Wada (ed.), *Kindling 2.* New York: Raven Press, pp. 67–79.

McIntyre, D. C., Rajalla, J., and Edson, N. (1987) Suppression of amygdala kindling with short interstimulus intervals: Effect of norepinephrine depletion. *Exp. Neurol. 95:*391–402.

Meencke, H.-J. (1988) Pathology of childhood epilepsies. *Cleveland Clin. J. Med. 56:*S111–S120.

Metrakos, J. D., and Metrakos, K. (1970) Genetic factors in epilepsy. *Mod. Probl. Pharmacopsychiatr. 4:*71–86.

Michelson, H., and Lothman, E. (1991) An ontogenetic study of kindling using rapidly recurring hippocampal seizures. *Dev. Brain Res. 61:*79–85.

Michelson, H. B., and Butterbaugh, G. G. (1985) Amygdala kindling in juvenile rats following neonatal administration of 6-hydroxydopamine. *Exp. Neurol. 90:*588–593.

Michelson, H. B., and Lothman, E. W. (1992) Ontogeny of epileptogenesis in the rat hippocampus: A study of the influence of GABAergic inhibition. *Dev. Brain Res. 66:*237–243.

Michelson, H. B., Williamson, J. M., and Lothman, E. W. (1989) Ontogeny of kindling: The acquisition of kindled responses at different ages with rapidly recurring hippocampal seizures. *Epilepsia 30:*672.

Michelson, H. B., and Wong, R. K. S. (1991) Excitatory synaptic responses mediated by GABA(A) receptors in the hippocampus. *Science 253:*1420–1423.

Moshé, S. L. (1981) The effects of age on the kindling phenomenon. *Dev. Psychobiol. 14:*75–81.

Moshé, S. L. (1987) Epileptogenesis and the immature brain. *Epilepsia 28* (Suppl.):S3–S15.

Moshé, S. L., and Albala, B. J. (1982) Kindling in developing rats: Persistence of seizures into adulthood. *Dev. Brain Res. 4:*67–71.

Moshé, S. L., and Albala, B. J. (1983) Maturational changes in postictal refractoriness and seizure susceptibility in developing rats. *Ann. Neurol. 13:*552–557.

Moshé, S. L., Albala, B. J., Ackermann, R. F., and Engel. J. J. (1983) Increased seizure susceptibility of the immature brain. *Dev. Brain Res. 7:*81–85.

Moshé, S. L., and Cornblath, M. (1993) Developmental aspects of epileptogenesis. In E. Wyllie (ed.), *The Treatment of Epilepsy: Principles and Practice.* Philadelphia: Lea & Febiger, pp. 99–110.

Moshé, S. L., and Garant, D. S. (1995) Substantia nigra GABA receptors can mediate anticonvulsant or proconvulsant effects. *Epilepsy Res.* (Suppl.) (in press).

Moshé, S. L., Sharpless, N. S., and Kaplan, J. (1981) Kindling in developing rats: Afterdischarge thresholds. *Brain Res. 211:*190–195.

Moshé, S. L., and Shinnar, S. (1993) Early intervention. In J. Engel, Jr. (ed.), *Surgical Treatment of the Epilepsies.* New York: Raven Press, pp. 123–132.

Moshé, S. L., and Sperber, E. F. (1990) Substantia nigra–mediated control of generalized seizures. In G. Gloor, R. Kostopoulos, M. Naquet, and P. Avoli (eds.), *Generalized Epilepsy: Cellular, Molecular and Pharmacological Approaches.* Boston: Birkhauser, pp. 355–367.

Moshé, S. L., Sperber, E. F., and Haas, K. (1990) Pathophysiology of experimental seizures in developing animals. In M. Sillanpaa, S. I. Dam, M. Johannessen, and G. Blennow (eds.), *Pediatric Epilepsy.* Stroud, Hampshire, England: Wrightson Biomedical, pp. 17–30.

Moshé, S. L., Sperber, E. F., Haas, K., Xu, S., and Shinnar, S. (1992) Effects of the maturational process on epileptogenesis. In H. Lüders (ed.), *Epilepsy Surgery.* New York: Raven Press, pp. 741–747.

Mueller, A. L., Chestnut, R. M., and Schwartzkroin, P. A. (1983) Actions of GABA in developing rabbit hippocampus: An in vitro study. *Neuroscience 39:*193–198.

Mueller, A. L., Taube, J. S., and Schwartzkroin, P. A. (1984) Development of hyperpolarizing inhibitory postsynaptic potentials and hyperpolarizing response to gamma-aminobutyric acid in rabbit hippocampus studied in vitro. *J. Neurosci. 4:*860–867.

Mutani, R., Futamachi, K. J., and Prince, D. A. (1984) Potassium activity in immature cortex. *Brain Res. 75:*27–39.

Nelson, K. B., and Ellenberg, J. H. (1976) Predictors of epilepsy in children who have experienced febrile seizures. *N. Engl. J. Med. 295:*1029–1033.

Nelson, K. B., and Ellenberg, J. H. (1978) Prognosis in children with febrile convulsions. *Pediatrics 61:*720–727.

Nespeca, M., Wyllie, E., Lüders, H., Rothner, D., and Hahn, J. E. A. (1990) EEG recording and functional localization studies with subdural electrodes in infants and young children. *J. Epilepsy 3* (Suppl.):107–124.

Newberry, N. R., and Nicoll, R. A. (1985) Comparison of the action of baclofen with gamma-aminobutyric acid on rat hippocampal pyramidal cells in vitro. *J. Physiol. 360:*161–185.

Pellegrini-Giampietro, D. E., Bennett, M. V., and Zukin, R. S. (1991) Differential expression of 3 glutamate receptor genes in developing rat brain: An in situ hybridization study. *Proc. Natl. Acad. Sci. 88:*4157–4161.

Peterson, S. L., Albertson, T. E., and Stark, L. G. (1981) Intertrial intervals and kindled seizures. *Exp. Neurol. 71:*144–153.

Pinel, J. P. J., and Rovner, L. I. (1978) Experimental epileptogenesis: Kindling-induced epilepsy in rats. *Exp. Neurol. 58:*190–202.

Pratap, R. C., and Gururaj, A. K. (1989) Clinical and electroencephalographic features of complex partial seizures in infants. *Acta Neurol. Scand. 79:*123–127.

Prince, D. A. (1978) Neurophysiology of epilepsy. *Ann. Rev. Neurosci. 1:*395–415.

Prince, D. A., and Gutnick, M. J. (1972) Neuronal activities in epileptogenic foci of immature cortex. *Brain Res. 45:*455–468.

Purpura, D. P. (1964) Relationship of seizure susceptibility to morphological and physiologic properties of normal and abnormal immature cortex. In P. Kellaway and I. Petersén (eds.), *Neurologic and Electroencephalographic Correlative Studies in Infancy.* New York: Grune and Stratton, pp. 117–154.

Purpura, D. P. (1969) Stability and seizure susceptibility of immature brain. In H. H. Jaspar, A. A. Ward, and A. Pope (eds.), *Basic Mechanisms of the Epilepsies.* Boston: Little Brown, pp. 481–505.

Racine, R. J. (1972) Modification of seizure activity by electrical stimulation: I. After-discharge threshold. *Electroencephalogr. Clin. Neurophysiol. 32:*269–279.

Roger, J., Driefuss, F. E., Martinez-Lage, M., Munari, C., Porter, R. J., Seino, M., and Wolf, P. (1989) Proposal for revised classification of epilepsies and epileptic syndromes. *Epilepsia 30:*389–399.

Schofield, P. R., Darlison, M. G., Fujita, N., Burt, D. R., Stephenson, R. A., Rodriguez, H., Rhee, L. M., Ramachandran, J., Reale, V., Glencorse, T. A., Seeburg, P. G., and Barnard, E. A. (1987) Sequence and functional expression of the GABA$_A$ receptor shows a ligand-gated receptor superfamily. *Nature 328:*221–227.

Schofield, P. R., Shivers, B. D., and Seeburg, P. (1990) The role of receptor subtype diversity in the CNS. *TINS 13:*8–11.

Schwartzkroin, P. A. (1982) Development of rabbit hippocampus: Physiology. *Dev. Brain Res. 2*:469–486.

Schwartzkroin, P. A. (1984) Epileptogenesis in the immature CNS. In P. A. Schwartzkroin and H. V. Wheal (eds.), *Electrophysiology of Epilepsy.* London: Academic Press, pp. 389–412.

Schwartzkroin, P. A., and Kunkel, D. D. (1982) Electrophysiology and morphology of the developing hippocampus of fetal rabbits. *J. Neurosci. 2*:469–486.

Schwartzkroin, P. A., Kunkel, D. D., and Mathers, L. H. (1982) Development of rabbit hippocampus: Anatomy. *Dev. Brain Res. 2*:452–468.

Shewmon, A., Altman, K., Olson, D. M., and Shields, W. D. (1990) Selective carotid amytal suppression of independent multifocal spikes in children. *Epilepsia 31*:5.

Shewmon, D. A., Shields, W. D., Chugani, H. T., and Peacock, W. J. (1990) Contrasts between pediatric and adult epilepsy surgery: Rationale and strategy for focal resection. *J. Epilepsy 3* (Suppl.):141–155.

Shinnar, S., and Kang, H. (1988) Discontinuing antiepileptic drug therapy in children with epilepsy. In W. A. Hauser (ed.), *Current Trends in Epilepsy.* Landover, Md.: Epilepsy Foundation of America, pp. 43–50.

Shinnar, S., and Moshé, S. L. (1991) Age specificity of seizure expression in genetic epilepsies. In V. E. Anderson, W. A. Hauser, I. E. Leppik, J. L. Noebels, and S. S. Rich (eds.), *Genetic Strategies in Epilepsy Research.* New York: Raven Press, pp. 69–85.

Shinnar, S., Vining, E. P. G., Mellits, E. D., D'Souza, B. J., Holden, K., Baumgardner, R. A., and Freeman, J. M. (1985) Discontinuing antiepileptic medication in children with epilepsy after two years without seizures: A prospective study. *N. Engl. J. Med. 313*:976–980.

Sofianov, N. G. (1982) Clinical evolution and prognosis of childhood epilepsies. *Epilepsia 23*:61–69.

Somjen, G. G. (1979) Extracellular potassium in the mammalian central nervous system. *Ann. Rev. Physiol. 41*:159–177.

Spear, L. P., and Brake, S. C. (1983) Periadolescence: Age-dependent behavior and pharmacological responsivity in rats. *Dev. Psychobiol. 6*:83–109.

Sperber, E. F., Brown, L. L., and Moshé, S. L. (1992) Functional mapping of different seizure states in the immature rat using ^{14}C-2-deoxyglucose. *Epilepsia 33*:44.

Sperber, E. F., Haas, K., and Moshé, S. L. (1990) Mechanisms of kindling in developing animals. In J. A. Wada (eds.), *Kindling 4.* New York: Plenum, pp. 157–167.

Sperber, E. F., and Moshé, S. L. (1988) Age-related differences in seizure susceptibility to flurothyl. *Dev. Brain Res. 39*:295–297.

Sperber, E. F., Pellegrini-Giampietro, D. E., Friedman, L. K., Zukin, R. S., and Moshé, S. L. (1991) Maturational differences in gene expression of GABA-A α1 receptor subunit in rat substantia nigra. *Soc. Neurosci. Abstr. 17*:171.

Sperber, E. F., Wong, B. Y., Wurpel, J. N. D., and Moshé, S. L. (1987) Nigral infusions of muscimol or bicuculline facilitate seizures in developing rats. *Dev. Brain Res. 37*:243–250.

Sperber, E. F., Wurpel, J. N. D., and Moshé, S. L. (1989a) Evidence for the involvement of nigral GABA$_B$ receptors in seizures in rat pups. *Dev. Brain Res. 47*:143–146.

Sperber, E. F., Wurpel, J. N. D., Zhao, D. Y., and Moshé, S. L. (1989b) Evidence for the involvement of nigral GABA$_A$ receptors in seizures of adult rats. *Brain Res. 480*:378–382.

Swann, J. W., and Brady, R. J. (1984) Penicillin-induced epileptogenesis in immature rats CA$_3$ hippocampal pyramidal cells. *Dev. Brain Res. 12*:243–254.

Swann, J. W., Brady, R. J., and Martin, D. L. (1989) Postnatal development of GABA-mediated synaptic inhibition in rat hippocampus. *Neuroscience 28*:551–562.

Swann, J. W., Brady, R. J., Smith, K. L., and Pierson, M. G. (1988) Synaptic mechanisms of focal epileptogenesis in the immature nervous system. In J. W. Swann, and A. Messer (eds.), *Disorders of the Developing Nervous System: Changing View on Their Origins, Diagnoses, and Treatment*. New York: Alan R. Liss, pp. 19–49.

Swann, J. W., Smith, K. L., and Brady, R. L. (1987) Localized synaptic interactions mediate the sustained depolarization of seizure-like discharges in immature hippocampus. *Soc. Neurosci. Abstr. 13*:1156.

Swann, J. W., Smith, K. L., and Brady, R. J. (1986) Extracellular K$^+$ accumulation during penicillin-induced epileptogenesis in the CA$_3$ region of immature rat hippocampus. *Dev. Brain Res. 30*:243–255.

Swann, J. W., Smith, K. L., and Brady, R. J. (1991) Age-dependent alterations in the operations of hippocampal neural networks. *Ann. N.Y. Acad. Sci. 627*:264–276.

Swann, J. W., Smith, K. L., and Brady, R. J. (1993) Localized excitatory synaptic interactions mediate the sustained depolarization of electrographic seizures in developing hippocampus. *J. Neurosci. 13*:4680–4689.

Swann, J. W., Smith, K. L., Brady, R. J., and Pierson, M. G. (1993) Neurophysiological studies of alterations of seizure susceptibility during brain development. In P. A. Schwartzkroin (ed.), *Concepts and Models in Epilepsy Research*. Oxford: Oxford University Press, pp. 209–243.

Traynelis, S. F., and Dingledine, R. (1988) Potassium-induced spontaneous electrographic seizures in the rat hippocampal slice. *J. Neurophysiol. 59*:259–276.

Trojaborg, W. (1966) Focal spike discharges in children, a longitudinal study. *Acta Paediatr. Scand. 55* (Suppl. 168):1–113.

Tuchman, R. F., and Moshé, S. L. (1990) Neonatal seizures. Diagnostic and treatment controversies. In M. Sillanpää, S. I. Johannessen, G. Blennow, and M. Dam (eds.), *Paediatric Epilepsy*. Hampshire, England: Wrightson Biomedical, pp. 57–64.

Velísek, L., and Mares, P. (1991) Increased epileptogenesis in the immature hippocampus. *Exp. Brain Res. Ser. 20*:183–185.

Wada, J. A., and Osawa, T. (1976) Spontaneous recurrent seizure state induced by daily electric amygdaloid stimulation in Senegalese baboons. *Neurology 26*:273–286.

Wada, J. A., Sato, M., and Corcoran, M. E. (1974) Persistent seizure susceptibility and recurrent spontaneous seizures in kindled cats. *Epilepsia 15*:465–478.

Watanabe, K., Yamamoto, N., Negoro, T., Takaesu, E., Aso, K., Furune, S., and Takahashi, I. (1987) Benign complex partial epilepsies in infancy. *Pediatr. Neurol. 3*:208–212.

Wieser, H.-G., Engel, J. J., Williamson, P. D., Babb, T. L., and Gloor, P. (1993) Surgically remediable temporal lobe syndromes. In J. J. Engel (eds.), *Surgical Treatment of the Epilepsies*, 2nd ed. New York: Raven Press, pp. 49–63.

Wurpel, J. N. D., Tempel, A., Sperber, E. F., and Moshé, S. L. (1988) Age-related changes of muscimol binding in the substantia nigra. *Dev. Brain Res. 43:*305–307.

Xu, S. G., Garant, D. S., Sperber, E. F., and Moshé, S. L. (1991) Effects of substantia nigra γ-vinyl-GABA infusions on flurothyl seizures in adult rats. *Brain Res. 566:*108–114.

Xu, S. G., Garant, D. S., Sperber, E. F., and Moshé, S. L. (1992) The proconvulsant effect of nigral infusion of THIP on flurothyl-induced seizures in rat pups. *Dev. Brain Res. 68:*275–277.

Xu, S. G., Sperber, E. F., and Moshé, S. L. (1991) Is the anticonvulsant effect of substantia nigra infusion of gamma-vinyl GABA (GVG) mediated by the GABA$_A$ receptor in rat pups? *Dev. Brain Res. 59:*17–21.

Zhang, L., Spigelman, I., and Carlen, P. L. (1991) Development of GABA-mediated, chloride-dependent inhibition in CA$_1$ pyramidal neurones of immature rat hippocampal slices. *J. Physiol. 444:*25–49.

3

Absence Seizures in Developing Brain

JEFFREY L. NOEBELS
BARRY R. THARP

Nonconvulsive generalized absence seizures represent a major category of epilepsy in the developing brain that is receiving increased attention from both basic and clinical points of view. The excitement is fueled partly by fresh insights into the cellular mechanisms underlying the hypersynchronous spike-wave discharge, an EEG pattern that has served, since its discovery, as the electrocortical signature of this important seizure type (Gibbs et al., 1935). The precise identities of intrinsic neuronal membrane conductances and synaptic connections contributing to rhythmic neuronal oscillations in the neocortex (Connors and Gutnick, 1990) and thalamus (Crunelli et al., 1989; Huguenard and Prince, 1992; Steriade, 1992; Steriade et al., 1993; von Krosigk et al., 1993) are becoming clearer. This information, in turn, is providing the framework for specific hypotheses regarding potential ion channel and receptor defects underlying the electrogenesis of abnormal thalamo-cortical synchronization (Crunelli and Leresche, 1991; Gloor and Fariello, 1988), as well as offering the promise of pinpointing the molecular targets and mechanisms of action of existing antiabsence pharmacologic agents (Coulter et al., 1989; Lytton and Sejnowski, 1992).

In parallel with the basic descriptions of excitability mechanisms for thal-amocortical network oscillations in normal brain, additional research interest in absence epilepsies is being driven by the development over the last decade of experimental gene models of the cortical spike-wave phenotype in animals possessing many of the attributes of the human disorder. These models, based on single-locus mutations (Noebels, 1979) and inbred strains (Marescaux, Vergnes, and Depaulis, 1992), foster the search for naturally occurring lesions underlying spike-wave epileptic phenotypes, allow comparisons of their individual attributes with the human disorders, and facilitate the pursuit of alternative therapeutic strategies.

Finally, a steep increase in the biotechnology of chromosome analysis has propelled an international effort to map and sequence the genes for familial absence seizures in human pedigrees. Generalized absence epilepsies make a logical neurogenetic target, since they were one of the first defined seizure types to be recognized as strongly hereditary in origin (Lennox, 1960). Interestingly, it is the prospect of molecular genetic diagnosis of inherited epilepsies, and with it the promise of formulating rational therapy, that has focused much recent attention on refining the clinical characterization of generalized absence epilepsy phenotypes. The greatest possible diagnostic precision is required, since the search for single-gene disorders by positional cloning depends heavily on accurate ascertainment of cases and the ability to exclude unrelated genetic disorders.

Questions Regarding the Developmental Neurobiology of Absence Epilepsies

Since primary generalized absence epilepsies arise predominantly in children, the developmental aspects of these syndromes play a central role in neurobiologic, genetic, and clinical lines of research and raise testable hypotheses for each. For example, what is the molecular explanation for the fact that the cortical spike-wave seizure pattern of 3 cycles per second (c/s) is rarely observed in children before the second year of life? Does the ontogeny of gene expression for a primary molecular defect (e.g., in a specific subtype of membrane ion channel, receptor, or synaptic connection that endows the network with its oscillating properties) directly account for the appearance of EEG discharges at a specific age? Or does the abnormal firing mode arise secondarily, perhaps years later, in thalamocortical circuits that bear a preexisting error but are destabilized only following the maturation of other modulatory synaptic inputs?

Similar questions can be posed about the loss of abnormal excitability, since in many cases absence seizures disappear in adolescence. How are the seizures outgrown? Is it through the steady maturation of inhibitory synaptic control mechanisms that constitute the brain's normal defense against aberrant synchronization? Does it involve the selective seizure-induced expression of new patterns of gene transcription within the epileptic circuit that directly mask the primary excitability defect in the bursting neurons? The distinction between these two possibilities is not inconsequential, since in the latter case antiepileptic therapy might, in theory, have the unexpected effect of prolonging the duration of the seizure disorder. Interestingly, clinical data are conflicting about the age of onset and long-term prognoses. Some studies have reported a more favorable outcome in children whose seizures began between ages 4 and 8 years (Livingston et al., 1965; Roger, 1974); another found no correlation between long-term prognosis and the age of onset of absence seizures (Sato et al., 1983). Could a critical period of neural plasticity in the developing brain explain why the age of seizure onset has an important bearing on clinical outcome?

Finally, there remains the real issue of how useful the chronological age of seizure onset will prove to be as a phenotypic marker in human gene mapping studies of generalized absence epilepsies; that is, how informative is this trait in correctly sorting and assigning multiple family pedigrees for linkage analysis? Does a difference of 5 or 10 years in the age of onset between two children with otherwise identical seizures actually signify a separate genetic disease, or is the diagnostic overlap between currently recognized absence syndromes still too great to use this parameter as an identifying trait to map and clone specific childhood epilepsy genes? This question might have gone unasked until recent findings showed an inverse correlation between the age of onset of symptoms (and a direct correlation with the severity) and the length of an abnormal DNA insert within a gene in patients affected by unstable genetic mutations. This correlation between clinical penetrance and the expanded length of "triplet repeat" intragenic DNA sequences has been found in a group of inherited diseases all involving the nervous system, the newly termed "dynamic mutations" of Huntington disease, Kennedy disease, fragile X, myotonic dystrophy, and spinocerebellar ataxia (Martin, 1993). These variable-age penetrance mutations provide a set of convincing examples that the clinical expression of a single molecular disease gene can be developmentally regulated over a period spanning several decades, effectively challenging the assumption that different ages of phenotypic expression signify different genetic diseases.

In framing the preceding questions we referred to spike-and-wave seizure expression in the neocortex as if it represented the result of a single epileptogenic process. Despite the reasonably stereotyped morphology of the spike-and-wave EEG discharge pattern, there is substantial evidence that this is not the case; in particular, different kinds of inherited lesions and intervening mechanisms underlying generation of the spike-and-wave pattern appear to vary considerably with regard to their onset and modifiability during development. To the gene hunter, electrophysiologist, and clinician, these differences may ultimately prove to be as informative as the similarities. In the present chapter we will review current clinical, genetic, and electrophysiological evidence for neurobiological heterogeneity in this important class of epilepsy, with special emphasis on its developmental aspects.

Clinical Recognition of Diverse Generalized Absence Seizure Phenotypes

Minor seizures of the absence type were first described several centuries ago. According to Lennox (1960), Esquirol used the term "petit mal" in 1815 to describe these distinctive events. The Swiss neurologist Tissot, however, actually used the word "petits" in 1770 to describe the minor seizures that occurred between the "grand accès" (generalized tonic-clonic seizures) of a 14-year-old girl with epilepsy. In 1854 Delasiauve applied the term "absence" to minor seizures associated with brief, abrupt, and discrete periods of "intellectual collapse." During the early years of the twentieth century the term "petit mal" was used for all minor seizures, including typical complex partial seizures, and "absence" was used for more typical petit mal seizures, the type now associated with the classical 3 c/s spike-and-wave EEG pattern.

Some confusion over terminology was perpetuated by Lennox, who used the term "petit mal triad" to describe the major features of absence seizures: "a stare, a jerk, a fall." He recognized that "pure petit mal" was usually characterized by a stare only, had a strong familial tendency, and occurred in otherwise normal children. The other two symptoms of the triad were associated with brief seizures that he labeled "myoclonic" and "atonic" (astatic) epilepsy, respectively. These latter seizures were more likely to occur in children with brain lesions and mental retardation whose EEG contained atypical, or slow, spike-and-wave discharges (less than 2.5 c/s). Most of these children would now be classified as cases of the Lennox-Gastaut syndrome. This diagnosis encompasses a heterogeneous population of patients with static encephalopathies that result in abnormalities on neurological examination, mental retardation, and several types of seizures, including drop attacks (atonic seizures), atypical absences, and tonic seizures. A family history of seizures is less likely, and the prognosis for full recovery is poor (Chapter 1). Though the medications available in Lennox's time for the treatment of the petit mal triad, primarily the diones and acetazolamide, were effective for children with myoclonic and astatic absences, the success rate was lower for children with the typical or pure petit mal seizure.

In the 1970s and 1980s the International League against Epilepsy (ILAE) published a classification of seizures which has become widely accepted by the neurological community (Dreifuss 1981; Gastaut, 1970). The ILAE committee recommended that "absence" become the preferred term to describe brief nonconvulsive seizures and that the term "petit mal" be avoided. They divided seizures into partial (focal), generalized (seizures in which the first clinical changes suggest initial involvement of both hemispheres and where the ictal EEG patterns are bilateral and widespread in both hemispheres), and unclassifiable. The generalized seizures were in turn defined according to whether they were convulsive or nonconvulsive. The division of absence seizures into typical and atypical was mainly on the basis of the EEG. Typical absences were characterized as regular and symmetrical 2–4 (usually 3) c/s spike-and-wave complexes occurring on a normal EEG background. Atypical absences showed a more heterogeneous, asymmetrical, and irregular (slow spike-and-wave or other paroxysmal activity) discharge occurring on an abnormal background. Clinically, the latter seizures were thought to be more often associated with a significant change in motor tone and a less abrupt onset and/or cessation. Typical absences usually showed an abrupt impairment of consciousness only, with very mild clonic/atonic/tonic components, sometimes with eyelid or perioral myoclonias, automatisms, or autonomic signs.

With the advent of video-EEG monitoring, more detailed clinical descriptions of nonconvulsive seizures have emerged and blurred Lennox's distinction of typical and atypical absences (Penry et al., 1975). Holmes et al. (1987) analyzed the video-EEGs of 926 absence seizures in 54 patients. They divided their patients into typical and atypical groups solely on the basis of the morphology of the EEG paroxysmal activity. As expected, they found that an abnormal EEG background, multiple seizure types, mental retardation, and developmental delay occurred more frequently in the atypical group. Interestingly, however, both types of seizures usually had an abrupt onset and ending, and automatisms were more frequent in the typical group, while changes in tone were seen more often in the atypical group. They concluded that a single clinical feature could not adequately distinguish the two seizure types, and that the clinical spectrum of absence seizures probably represented a continuum rather than distinct subtypes.

Clinical Heterogeneity of Epilepsy Syndromes Featuring Generalized Absence Seizures

In 1981 the ILAE accepted a Classification of Epileptic Syndromes to supplement the classification of seizure types. The ILAE commission defined a syndrome as "an epileptic disorder characterized by a cluster of signs and symptoms customarily occurring together. The signs and symptoms may be strictly clinical . . . or may be findings detected by ancillary studies" (Commission, 1989). This group emphasized that syndromes might represent specific disorders or broader concepts; that syndromes of high specificity might include syndromes of lesser specificity; and that some syndromes may represent specific diseases and other vague entities without a known etiology. The syndrome classification was developed on the basis of two principles. The first separated epilepsies according to whether the seizures were generalized (including the absence epilepsies) or partial, and the second according to the presumed etiology (primary, or idiopathic, epilepsy vs. secondary, or symptomatic, epilepsy). The primary generalized absence epilepsies (listed according to increasing age) included childhood absence epilepsy (CAE), juvenile absence epilepsy (JAE), and juvenile myoclonic epilepsy (JME) (see Fig. 3-1). Epilepsy associated with the Lennox-Gastaut syndrome, West syndrome (infantile spasms with hypsarrhythmia), epilepsy with myoclonic absences (EMA), and myoclonic-astatic epilepsy (MAE) were classified as idiopathic and/or symptomatic generalized epileptic syndromes. The latter disorder has been considered part of the Lennox-Gastaut syndrome since it also features "atypical" absence seizures; however, some authors feel that the strong genetic disposition and normal developmental status prior to seizures define it as a specific entity (Doose, 1992).

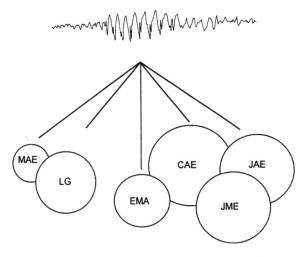

Figure 3-1. Phenotypic heterogeneity of currently recognized human spike-and-wave absence epilepsy syndromes. Partially overlapping syndromes show variations in frequency of EEG discharges, character of clinical seizures, age of onset, severity of associated neurological problems, genetic disposition, and prognosis.

According to this classification, absence seizures are included in a particular syndrome according to the age of onset (e.g., childhood and juvenile), associated clinical epileptic features (e.g., astatic and myoclonic accompaniments to the absence), and nonepileptic clinical and prognostic features (e.g., the Lennox-Gastaut syndrome with its associated static encephalopathy; JME with its generalized tonic-clonic and myoclonic seizures with a poor prognosis for cessation of seizures before adulthood). Absence seizures may be easily provoked by hyperventilation and, less frequently, by photic stimulation, and there is some clinical and biochemical evidence suggesting that these also could represent two distinct syndromes. One group reports that the two are inherited independently, even though both types of activation may occasionally occur in the same individual (Doose and Gerken, 1973). A second study has suggested that central dopaminergic mechanisms are involved in the systems generating the photic-induced discharges, but not in seizure discharges provoked by hyperventilation (Quesney et al., 1980).

The presence of a second seizure type adds to the clinical heterogeneity of absence syndromes. Generalized tonic-clonic seizures occur in approximately 40 percent of children with absence epilepsy. These seizures usually follow the onset of absence seizures by several years and often first appear in adolescence. They may also precede the absences in about 10 percent of cases (Covanis et al., 1992), though in Doose's study of 108 children with absence epilepsy convulsive seizures were reported to be the initial seizure in 46 (Doose et al., 1973). In this same study, convulsive seizures occurred in 39 of the 105 affected relatives of children with absence epilepsy, whereas only 10 affected relatives had absence seizures. Children with both absence and convulsive seizure types are more likely to continue to have both types of seizures in adulthood than those who presented with absence seizures alone (Aicardi, 1986). These clinical data again raise the possibility of multiple epileptogenic mechanisms underlying these absence syndromes.

Developmental Features of Absence Syndromes

The absolute age of onset of absence syndromes may span the extremes of the age range, with onset reported in the first year of life (Cavazzuti et al., 1989) or in adulthood even as late as the ninth decade (Thomas et al., 1992). Nevertheless, the time of seizure onset has played a key role in assigning specific cases to one of the four major absence seizure syndromes: childhood absence epilepsy (CAE), epilepsy with myoclonic absences (EMA), juvenile absence epilepsy (JAE), and juvenile myoclonic epilepsy (JME). In most studies there remains significant overlap between each. Figure 3-2 shows the relative incidence of the absence syndromes during the first 20 years of life. There is some debate as to whether the syndromes of EMA and CAE are really different, although in the myoclonic variety the clinical expression of the absences appears quite distinct, the incidence of mental retardation and mental deterioration is higher, and the seizures are less responsive to therapy. There is also an overlap with the secondary generalized epilepsies, since many children with EMA will manifest progressive slowing of the spike-and-wave discharges for 3 c/s to 2.5 c/s or less, typical of the Lennox-Gastaut syndrome. EMA thus is still a heterogeneous designation and may represent multiple disorders ranging from a more benign form similar to CAE to a more malignant variety, which may be clinically indistinguishable from the Lennox-Gastaut syndrome.

Juvenile absence epilepsy (JAE) appears at about the same age as the absence seizures of juvenile myoclonic epilepsy (JME), which often precede the myoclonic and generalized tonic-clonic epilepsies by several years. The absences are clinically quite similar in these two syndromes, and the EEG, particularly in the early stages, may be indistinguishable. JME is a lifelong disorder, whereas JAE may resolve spontaneously in the late teens. JAE therefore appears to fall on the developmental age spectrum between CAE and JME.

The poor temporal resolution, combined with the qualitative overlap of the clinical and EEG features of these syndromes, makes classification of the individual child difficult at times. The seizures of the childhood and juvenile absence syndromes are virtually identical when witnessed clinically. Several authors have noted that ictal retropulsion is more common in the childhood variety (Wolf and Inouye, 1984) and loss of contact with the environment more severe (Panayiotopoulos et al., 1989), whereas the seizure frequency is less and generalized tonic-clonic seizures are more common in

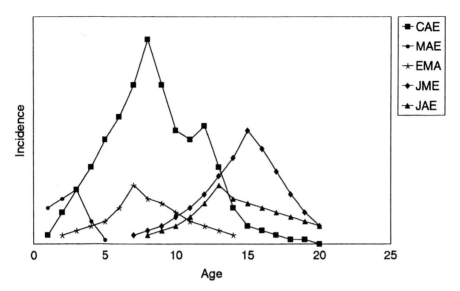

Figure 3-2. Relative incidence of human absence epilepsy syndromes during first two decades of life. The five syndromes show developmental variation in the ages of seizure onset and duration of clinical seizure activity. In temporal order of peak incidence: MAE, myoclonic astatic epilepsy; EMA, epilepsy with myoclonic absences; CAE, childhood absence epilepsy; JAE, juvenile absence epilepsy; JME, juvenile myoclonic epilepsy.

the juvenile syndrome. Subtle EEG differences have also been reported (Gomez and Westmoreland, 1987).

Nonhereditary Absence Syndromes

Further compounding the syndrome classification are absence seizures arising in conjunction with isolated birth defects (Guerrini et al., 1990) and those which occur in individuals with focal epileptogenic processes, particularly those involving the frontal regions (Dalby, 1969; Gordon, 1979). Though focal EEG features are often present interictally and the ictal events are usually not associated with typical spike-and-wave discharges, the similarity with typical absence epilepsy may occasionally be striking, including brief episodes of loss of contact with the environment associated with generalized, frontally dominant spike–and–slow-wave activity. Seizures with similar clinical and electrographic features have been produced in animals by strategically placed focal bihemispheric lesions or application of epileptogenic agents (Fisher and Prince, 1977; Marcus and Watson, 1966) and can be disrupted by section of the corpus callosum (secondary bilateral synchrony). These studies have led to speculation (Gloor, 1979) that at least one category of generalized absence seizures in humans might be caused by a similar interaction of cortical foci.

The proposal is strengthened by the appearance of absence seizures in children with obvious diffuse cortical pathology, such as the Lennox-Gastaut syndrome. The clinical differentiation of these secondary generalized seizures from those that occur in the child with primary generalized absence epilepsy may be impossible without considering other clinical, historical, and radiological features. Patients with what appear to be idiopathic absences accompanied by 3 c/s spike-and-wave activity and good clinical response to valproic acid or ethosuximide may have focal or lateralized features including versive movements, circling behavior, and lateralized (or at times focal) myoclonic jerks. These cases may represent otherwise typical nonconvulsive seizures with mild superimposed hemispheric pathology resulting in an asymmetric clinical expression. Clinical absence seizures can also be caused by toxic and metabolic perturbations, for example, drug withdrawal, renal failure, or high doses of thyroxine (Sundaram et al., 1985) or other medication (Yohai and Barnett, 1989). Rare instances of reflex induction of absences have also been reported, such as those evoked by mental imagery (Bencze et al., 1988).

These overlapping features have led some investigators to question the validity of the syndrome approach to seizure classification and to propose that absence seizures actually represent a spectrum of abnormal brain excitability, with the genetic "typical" absence seizure at one end and the "atypical" absence occurring in the child with significant cerebral pathology at the other. The admixture of these genetic and acquired lesions partly determines the individual clinical "epileptic phenotype" (Berkovic et al., 1987). Studies in animal models are beginning to reveal that seizure-linked plasticity changes may also contribute to the phenotypic complexity of certain spike-wave seizure disorders (see below). Even though the human seizure phenotypes may indeed extend beyond those controlled by various single-gene diseases, it is difficult to dismiss the syndrome approach entirely, since there are easily recognized groups of children that share very similar patterns of clinical and EEG seizure expression, have family histories suggesting significant genetic influences, and show normal neurological and intellectual development with good responses to standard antiepileptic medications.

Human Genetic Studies of Primary Generalized Epilepsy Syndromes

Lennox was well aware of the genetic aspects of the epilepsies, particularly in neurologically and mentally normal children. He found that the concordance of petit mal seizures in identical twins was 75 percent, over 10 times that of dizygotic twins (Lennox, 1960). He also noted the similarity of the pattern of spike-and-wave discharge in twins that shared the epileptic trait, and he reported that about one-third of individuals with "fast spike-wave"—

c/s spike-and-wave complexes—had a family history of epilepsy. Other researchers have since recognized that there is an increased incidence of other seizure types in the near relatives of children with absence seizures, including benign partial epilepsy. Generalized spike–and–slow-wave discharges are also not uncommonly seen in the EEGs of patients with rolandic epilepsy and in their asymptomatic siblings, suggesting a possible genetic link between the expression of partial and generalized epilepsies (Degan and Degan, 1990).

The family studies of Metrakos and Metrakos (1961) showed a striking penetrance of the spike-and-wave trait in relatives of children with petit mal reaching 43 percent in the 4 to 16-year-old group. This led them to propose an autosomal dominant mode of inheritance with age-dependent penetrance. Subsequent studies have shown a lower incidence in first-degree relatives and raise questions about the hypothesis of a single autosomal dominant gene (Doose et al., 1973). It has been speculated that the high incidence of spike-and-wave discharges found by Metrakos and Metrakos in the EEGs of near relatives of the probands reflects an overinterpretation of the normal paroxysmal patterns common in childhood, particularly during drowsiness and hyperventilation. This is given credence by the high incidence of generalized epileptiform discharges in their control subjects (approximately 10 percent) as compared to approximately 1 percent in other studies of normal children. Furthermore, these studies were done at a time when all forms of absence seizure were considered together and before the introduction of the concept of epileptic syndromes, thus including cases with other than the childhood form of absence epilepsy. Individuals with photosensitive seizure disorders were included, and these also probably represent a separate epileptic syndrome (Doose and Gerken, 1973). Doose and Baier (1989) also pointed out that the incidence of generalized spike-and-wave discharges in the relatives of probands with absence epilepsy was related to the age at which the EEG was performed; over 30 percent of those recorded at 2–3 years of age had an abnormal EEG, the incidence dropping to under 4 percent at 12–13 years and even lower in adult asymptomatic relatives.

Juvenile myoclonic epilepsy was the first absence syndrome to be examined by genetic linkage analysis, and two groups have reported that JME maps as a single locus to human chromosome 6p using HLA serotype (Greenberg et al., 1988) and RFLP markers (Durner et al., 1991). Curiously, the actual mode of inheritance (recessive or dominant) remains undefined, and this may be the result of genetic heterogeneity within the 35 families most recently analyzed, despite the adoption of clear clinical and laboratory criteria for case ascertainment in probands and family members (Greenberg and Delgado-Escueta, 1993).

The Italian League against Epilepsy (1993) has collected information on 74 families with multiple cases of idiopathic epilepsy (defined by at least three members affected with a form of idiopathic epilepsy in one or more generations) and found significant concordance of the clinical forms. In families with a proband having childhood absence epilepsy (CAE), 24.4 percent of affected relatives also had CAE, 25.6 percent had febrile seizures, and 36.6 percent had generalized tonic-clonic seizures. In first-degree affected relatives, there was a 42.5 percent concordance for the same seizure type. This study did not find cases of CAE in families in which the proband had benign rolandic epilepsy or juvenile myoclonic epilepsy (JME). These findings differ from those of Janz et al. (1989), who found that absence seizures occurred in 26 percent of first-degree relatives of JME patients. Delgado-Escueta et al. (1990) found that 18 percent of siblings of patients with JME had CAE.

Ancillary Diagnostic Indicators for Classifying Absence Syndrome

Other diagnostic markers will be needed to further clarify subtypes of generalized spike-wave absence epilepsy in human pedigrees for genetic linkage analysis. Dynamic imaging of human brain metabolism has so far proven unhelpful in this regard, and these negative results are mirrored in the few experimental models studied to date. Positron emission tomography (PET) has been used to study cerebral glucose metabolism in patients with absence seizures. The results have been somewhat conflicting, possibly because of the age of the patients in the individual studies and the precise clinical classification of the seizures. In an ictal PET study of children with typical childhood absence epilepsy (Engel et al., 1985), a diffuse increase in cerebral metabolic rate for glucose (CMRGlc) was found, whereas in another study of a more heterogeneous population of older individuals, no change or a decrease in CMRGlc was seen (Ochs et al., 1987). Neither study identified any focal abnormalities related to the seizures. Metabolic studies of a genetic rat model of petit mal–like seizures have shown a diffuse cortical and subcortical increase in CMRGlc, again without any predilection for the brain areas thought to generate the spike-and-wave discharges (Nehlig et al., 1991), and no focal metabolic changes linked to spike-wave discharges were found in either of two mutant mouse models of spike and wave, the *tottering (tg)* and *stargazer (stg)* mice, using the autoradiographic ^{14}C-2-deoxyglucose method (Noebels and Sidman, 1979, and unpublished observations). Despite convincing experimental evidence that thalamic neurons are involved in the generation of rhythmic cortical oscillations, metabolic studies have never shown preferential changes in these regions during spike-and-wave seizures, apart from one study where γ-butyrolactone-induced discharges enhanced by parenteral doses of the convulsant drug penicillin showed abnormal *fos* staining in paraventricular and lateral habenular nuclei (Zhang et al., 1991). In contrast, focal abnormalities in glucose metabolism are common in the Lennox-Gastaut syndrome with atypical absences, and they may reflect areas of abnormal signaling, although it is unlikely that they are specifically correlated with the EEG spike-and-wave discharge.

The lack of specific cellular pathology in the few cases of primary generalized absence studied at autopsy constitutes an additional obstacle to further progress in delineating the absence syndromes. Early clinical depth EEG studies showed widespread involvement of the neocortex, limbic system, and diencephalon without any clear evidence for a reproducible site of initiation in primary generalized epilepsies (Angeleri et al., 1964; Niedermayer et al., 1969; Williams, 1953), and no single region has yet been established where a primary lesion is requisite for the seizures to occur. Individuals with primary generalized epilepsy are typically considered to be free of gross cerebral pathology; their seizures presumably arise from membrane defects that are beyond the resolution of current noninvasive imaging techniques. Meencke, however, has shown subtle increases in the amount of cerebral microdysgenesis in primary generalized epilepsy, consisting primarily of diffuse heterotopias in the frontal lobes of a small number of patients with simple absences, myoclonic absences, and awakening grand mal seizures (Meenke, 1985). Though similar foci of cerebral cortical microdysgenesis may occur in individuals without epilepsy, they may be fewer in number and differently located (Kaufmann and Galaburda, 1989). If these findings can be reproduced by other pathologists and correlated with specific EEG abnormalities, it is possible that some subtypes of generalized epilepsy might be related to subtle dysplastic events in early brain development (see Caviness, Hatten, McConnell, and Takahashi, Chapter 4; Walsh, Chapter 5).

Heterogeneity of Absence Epilepsies as Revealed by Experimental Models

Genetic Heterogeneity

Single-locus neurological mutations in the mouse provide a powerful genetic model system in which to explore the diversity of molecular mechanisms underlying spike-and-wave epilepsy. Cellular lesions identified in these genetically defined epileptic nervous systems can be compared with unaffected coisogenic control littermates identical at every other allele, and the mutant gene sequence, once identified, can be used to search for homologous human genes. A systematic EEG survey of over 110 mapped mouse mutants revealed 5 mutant genes in the mouse, located on separate chromosomes, that display a pattern of spontaneous 6–7 c/s spike-wave discharges accompanied by behavioral arrest, an occasional myoclonic jerk of the head, immediate resumption of normal cortical rhythms without postictal phenomena, and uniform sensitivity to ethosuximide (Fig. 3-3; Noebels, 1992). A sixth absence mutation, transmitted as an autosomal dominant trait with no associated neurological abnormalities, has also now been identified (Qiao, Noebels, and Davisson, unpublished). At three of these loci (*tg, mh,* and *stg*) multiple alleles have been isolated with variable phenotypic features, demonstrating allelic as well as locus heterogeneity of the spike-wave trait. In two of them, *stg* and *tg,* the duration and the frequency of the spike-wave discharges are reliably determined by the specific gene inherited (Qiao and Noebels, 1991).

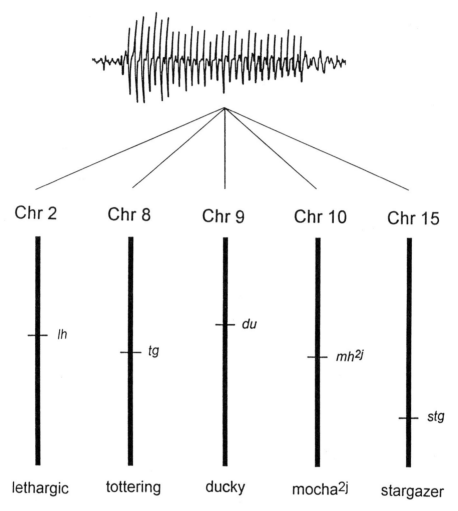

Figure 3-3. Genetic heterogeneity in murine models of spontaneous generalized spike-and-wave absence epilepsy. Five independent recessive mutations, identified by EEG screening of mapped mutant loci, *lethargic* (*lh*); *ducky* (*du*), *tottering* (*tg*), *mocha²ʲ* (*mh²ʲ*), and *stargazer* (*stg*), all show the stereotyped 6 spikes per second cortical discharge accompanied by behavioral arrest and a normal interictal EEG pattern.

These mutants provide the strongest available evidence for genetic heterogeneity of the spike-and-wave trait in the mammalian brain. The mutational analysis shows that single genes causing spike-wave absences do exist and reveals that in mice the epileptic trait can vary in terms of its mode of inheritance. In some gene errors the defect is expressed as a pure seizure phenotype transmitted as a dominant excitability trait; in others (so far, all recessive) the seizures arise in combination with other neurological deficits.

Finally, the clinical severity of the seizure disorder can depend on the specific mutant molecular defect inherited.

Developmental Variability of Seizure Onset

The extreme reproducibility of single-locus mouse mutations allows the developmental onset of seizures to be precisely correlated with the specific gene defect. Two mutants, *tg* and *stg* (Noebels, 1984; Qiao and Noebels, 1993), both show a fully penetrant onset of spontaneous seizure activity within a 2-day temporal window ending on postnatal day 18. At this time seizures are brief, well-defined, and low in frequency (0.5–1 seizure per hour). Within 1 week the spontaneous seizure frequency attains the maximal adult level of seizures (45–120 seizures per hour) in both mutants (Fig. 3-4). Since the third postnatal week remains within the prepubescent stage of murine development, seizure onset in these models corresponds to a childhood, rather than juvenile epilepsy syndrome in human. In comparison, the ontogeny of phenotypically similar, but not identical, absence seizures in inbred rat strains is delayed into the juvenile, if not young adult period. The Wistar rat model developed by Marescaux and coworkers is an inbred strain which has been selectively bred for spontaneous spike-wave discharges, ranging from 7 to 11 spikes per second, accompanied by ethosuximide-sensitive clinical absence seizures. In an ontogenetic study, none of the rats showed seizures at 30 days postnatal, 28 percent of the rats showed spontaneous seizures by 40 days, and 100 percent displayed the trait by 120 days of age (Vergnes et al., 1986). The seizures continued to increase in frequency and duration through 18 months of age. A second highly inbred rat strain, WAG/Rij, showed a somewhat similarly delayed temporal onset; only 18 percent showed an occasional discharge at 75 days postnatal, rising to 100 percent by 140 days (Coenen and Van Luitjelaar, 1987). The gene or genes linked with these inbred disorders have not been isolated, and it is not certain whether the delay is a characteristic of the ontogeny of the specific molecular defects involved or a multigenic interaction with the background genetic strain.

Regardless of which molecular defect produces the spike-and-wave seizure syndrome, it would be interesting to determine at what age the individual elements of the rhythmically oscillating thalamocortical network become inherently "capable" of sustaining a classical spike-wave discharge pattern, perhaps by regional application of a proepileptic agent. Unfortunately, no selective agonist for this cortical discharge pattern in an unaffected nervous system has been described, and the homology between drug-induced rhythmic spiking at various frequencies and the pathological patterns of spike-and-wave rhythm generation are unknown. Nevertheless, the ontogeny of "spike-and-wave–like" discharges has been examined, and 6 c/s rhythmic cortical spiking can be elicited in the rat at postnatal day 12 using a low dose of pentylenetetrazol (Mares et al., 1982) and at day 14 using γ-butyrolactone, a drug metabolized to γ-hydroxybutyrate, itself a GABA

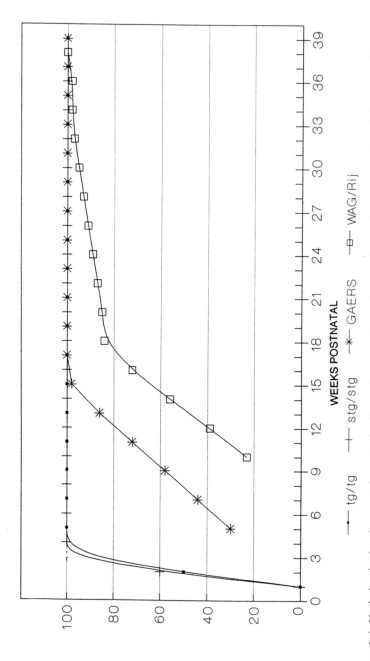

Figure 3-4. Variation in developmental onset of spike-and-wave seizures in experimental genetic models of absence epilepsy. Two recessive gene mutations in the mouse, *tottering* (*tg*) and *stargazer* (*stg*), both demonstrate an early onset of seizure discharges. Seizures (6 spikes per second) begin in all mice during the third postnatal week of life and rapidly attain their characteristic adult seizure frequencies (*tg*, mean 45–60 discharges per hour; *stg*, 60–120/h). Two inbred rat strains, GAERS (Strasbourg) and WAG/Rij (Nijmegen), show a later onset of seizures (7–11 spikes per second) at varying adult discharge frequencies (WAG/Rij, 15/h; GAERS, 80/h). In all models, the seizures persist throughout adulthood. (Data from Coenen and Van Luitjelaar, 1987; Noebels, 1984; Qiao and Noebels, 1991; and Vergnes et al 1986.)

metabolite (Snead, 1984). Depending on the dose, both these compounds produce a full spectrum of cortical activation in the adult, starting with a stage of continuous EEG spiking, progressing to a period of rapid spike-and-wave activity, and culminating in a depressed EEG pattern with slow spikes and burst suppression (Snead, 1988). Since the drugs were systemically administered, there are no localizing data to ascertain the maturity of individual elements of the oscillating circuit, and thus it remains unclear how these patterns relate to the ontogeny of specific absence syndromes. Most studies agree that the typical reproducible EEG patterns and brain metabolic responses of other seizure types, including limbic and generalized convulsive seizures, are present in rodent brain by the third postnatal week (Cherubini et al., 1983; Daval, 1992; Zouhar et al., 1989; also see Chapter 2).

Taken together, the genetic models reveal that spike-and-wave epilepsies can arise either during the final stages of brain immaturity or in the postmature brain. Interestingly, in both rodent model systems studied so far, the spike-and-wave discharges persist throughout adulthood, unlike the outcome in childhood absence epilepsy, where remission rates approach 75 percent (Aicardi, 1986). The neuronal mechanisms mediating this persistence of hyperexcitability provide an interesting area for future study.

Diversity of Intervening Neuronal Excitability Defects

The genetic and developmental heterogeneity in the models described previously raises the critical question of whether there exists a single definable neural network for cortical spike-wave seizure electrogenesis that comprises the final common target for epileptogenic lesions. At present there is no direct evidence for such a simplified pathway or mechanism. Rather, three converging lines of evidence suggest that independent neuronal excitability defects at different neuroanatomical sites might constitute a sufficient stimulus for pathological cortical spike-wave oscillations.

First, in vivo lesion studies have defined at least three model circuits that suffice for spike-wave generation: those that depend on altered synaptic modulation from ascending brainstem afferents (Mirsky and Oshima, 1973; Noebels, 1984; Steriade, 1992); those that depend on intact inputs from reticular nuclei of the thalamus (Avanzini et al., 1993; Avoli and Gloor, 1981; Jasper and Droogleever-Fortuyn, 1947); and those that result purely from the transcallosal interaction of two or more cortical foci, without pathologic participation of the thalamus (Marcus and Watson, 1966). In the intact brain, this anatomic distinction may be less relevant than defining exactly how the epileptogenic molecular defect interacts with normal brain mechanisms of rhythmic oscillation. The dynamic aspects of cortical circuit behavior leading to the expression of rhythmic EEG oscillations is well described, particularly as it is influenced by cycles of brain arousal (Steriade et al., 1993); this property is shared by epileptogenic discharges, as illustrated by the modulation of spindles and spike-wave discharges during the sleep cycle (Kellaway et al., 1990). There is striking evidence, however, that sleep spindles and 3 c/s spike-and-wave bursts are pharmacologically separable, since they are differentially affected by ethosuximide (Kellaway et al., 1991). This finding suggests a complex, if not entirely independent, relationship between normal and abnormal thalamocortical oscillations studied in humans.

Second, different absence seizure syndromes show selective differences in spike firing patterns and neuromodulation within the oscillating network. For example, spike-and-wave seizures in the mouse are critically dependent on excess noradrenergic innervation of the forebrain, since the seizures are prevented by neonatal noradrenergic depletion (Noebels, 1984), while those in the *stg* (Qiao and Noebels, 1991) and the Strasbourg rat (Marescaux et al., 1992a) are not. Extracellular recordings from pyramidal neurons in hippocampal slices of the two recessive mouse models reveal that the hypernoradrenergic *tg* cells show prolonged discharges that occur at a normal (similar to the wild type) frequency during potassium-induced network bursting; the pattern is reversed (i.e., normal burst duration but higher than normal burst frequency) in the nonhypernoradrenergic *stg* neurons (Fig. 3-5). Intracellular studies of the network burst defect in *tg* neurons show that the long burst duration is due to a prolongation of the paroxysmal depolarizing shift (Helekar and Noebels, 1991). One component of this prolongation was shown to coincide in appearance with the developmental onset of seizures, suggesting a possible role in epileptogenesis (Helekar and Noebels, 1992).

Electrophysiological evidence suggests that not all inherited excitability defects predispose the same regions of the brain to involvement in the spike-and-wave discharge pattern. For example, spike-and-wave discharges are seen in depth EEG recordings in the hippocampus of *tg* and *stg* mice, in the feline generalized penicillin model of spike-wave (Fisher and Prince, 1977), and in humans (Angeleri et al., 1964; Niedermayer et al., 1969); but they are not present in the Strasbourg rat model (Vergnes et al., 1990). The explanation for this difference remains unclear; however, the spike discharges in the Strasbourg rat typically occur at higher frequencies (7–11 c/s) and may differ in other respects. This variation in regional expression of the seizure may also be accompanied by a range of secondary alterations in neural circuitry in different absence syndromes, since the synchronous spike-and-wave discharge, like its focal convulsive counterparts, is associated with lasting alterations in the synaptic organization of the developing brain (see below).

Third, studies of the membrane actions of drugs effective in the treatment of generalized absence epilepsies are beginning to provide evidence for pharmacologic heterogeneity in different experimental models. Recently workers in several laboratories have proposed that the low-threshold calcium current in thalamic neurons could be potentiated by GABA acting on the GABA$_B$ receptor subtype, and that within certain ranges of depolarization this could alter the spike firing mode from repetitive to burst firing mode (Crunelli and Leresche, 1991). Ethosuximide produces a 30 percent block of the low-threshold calcium current, as does dimethsuximide. This reduction in a de-

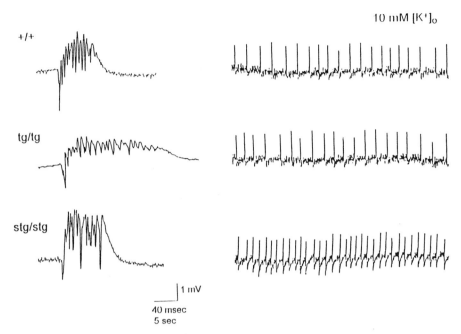

10 mM [K$^+$]$_0$

+/+

tg/tg

stg/stg

1 mV

40 msec
5 sec

Figure 3-5. Distinct network excitability defects in mutant mice with spike-and-wave epilepsy. In vitro hippocampal bursting induced by elevated potassium was used as an assay system to compare network excitability between the two mutant phenotypes. In *tg/tg* neurons, individual bursts were greatly prolonged compared to age-matched wild type (+/+) cells (left traces), while the rate of spontaneous bursting (right traces) was unaltered. In *stg/stg* neurons, the pattern was reversed (normal burst duration, accelerated spontaneous burst frequency), suggesting distinct defects in network repolarization mechanisms. (From Nangung and Noebels, 1991, and unpublished data.)

layed, depolarizing membrane current that is significantly involved in the generation of cyclical neuronal bursting has been proposed to explain its broad effectiveness in all experimental models of spike-and-wave discharge studied to date (Coulter et al., 1989). In particular, spike-and-wave discharges in the defined genetic mouse mutants *tottering, stargazer,* and *lethargic* and in the Strasbourg rat are all readily blocked by ethosuximide. In contrast, an experimental antagonist of the GABA$_B$ receptor, CGP 35348, blocks the discharges in the Strasbourg rat (Marescaux, Vergnes, and Bernasconi, 1992) and in *lethargic* (Hosford et al., 1992), but not in *stargazer* mutants, even at high doses (Qiao and Noebels, 1992). These data point strongly toward molecular heterogeneity of the underlying disorders, as well as toward the presence of multiple distinct sites available as potential targets for the pharmacologic inhibition of the spike-wave synchronization defect. For example, intrathalamic cadmium, a T-type calcium channel blocker, inhibits spike-and-wave discharges in the Strasbourg rat (Avanzini et al., 1993), despite the fact that no abnormalities were detected in the low-threshold calcium currents themselves in the thalamic neurons (Guyon et al., 1993).

Developmental Brain Plasticity and Primary
Generalized Absence Epilepsy

Substantial evidence now shows that intense focal seizures evoked by a variety of convulsant agents or electrical stimulation are linked to cell death, glial activation, and synaptic reorganization in the adult brain. While a major component of this seizure-induced damage is thought to be excitotoxic, a portion is associated with the transynaptic activation of new patterns of gene expression in neurons (Gall et al., 1991), and this cascade of secondary alterations in the bursting circuit, including the phenomenon of aberrant axonal sprouting and neosynaptogenesis in the dentate mossy fiber system, has been shown to possess age-dependent properties (Sankar, Wasterlain, and Sperber, Chapter 10).

In the *stargazer* mutant, it has been recently demonstrated that a long history of nonconvulsive 6 c/s spike-and-wave seizures is accompanied by a dramatic level of mossy fiber sprouting in the temporal hippocampus (Qiao and Noebels, 1993). The synaptic reorganization is similar in character and intensity to that described in human and experimental focal hippocampal seizures (Houser et al., 1990; Sutula et al., 1989); but with no evidence for the gliosis or prior cell loss that accompanies the axonal outgrowth in those models (Fig. 3-6). This finding strongly suggests that the repeated hypersynchronous spike bursts are sufficient to induce structural plasticity in axon terminals of associative brain areas, as they do in developing sensory pathways (see Schwartzkroin, Chapter 9; Swann, Chapter 8). It is interesting, however, that as seen in focal hippocampal seizures, the onset of this abnormal growth is delayed by several weeks following the onset of the seizure disorder (postnatal day 17–18). Although the mechanisms underlying this latency remain to be defined, the lack of fiber outgrowth in the first month of seizures corresponds with evidence that at least one activity-dependent hippocampal axonal growth factor, BDNF, is also refractory to seizure-induced expression during the same developmental time period (Dugich-Djordjevic et al., 1992).

Alterations in neurotransmitter phenotype provide a second general category of neuronal plasticity following experimental focal hippocampal (Marksteiner et al., 1990) and generalized electroshock (Wahlestedt et al., 1990) seizures that can also be found in the brain with spike-and-wave epilepsy. Immunohistochemical localization of neuropeptide Y (NPY) in the *stg* mutant reveals aberrant expression of NPY in the axons of dentate granule cells, whereas the mossy fibers in control +/+ mice normally devoid of this peptide neurotransmitter (Fig. 3-7). The intensity of aberrant mossy fiber NPY staining in young and adult *stg* mutants varied independently of their age. In normal rat brain, mRNA levels of the NPY gene can rise and fall within days following single hippocampal seizures, suggesting that the ab-

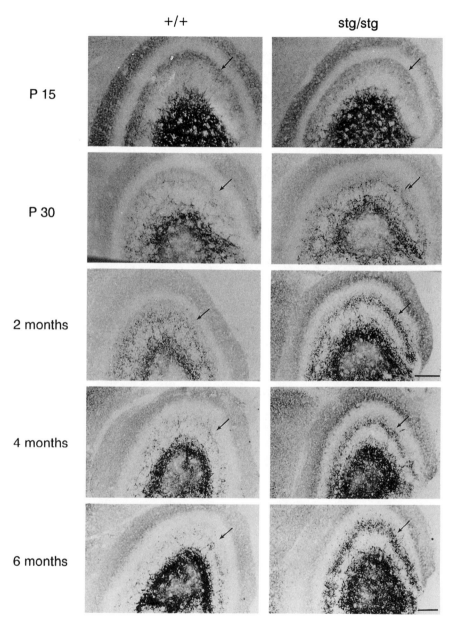

Figure 3-6. Axon sprouting and synaptic reorganization linked with spike-and-wave epilepsy in the *stargazer* mutant mouse. Serial selenium staining of zinc-rich mossy fiber pathway at different developmental stages in age-matched +/+ and *stg/stg* hippocampus reveals no sprouting in the dentate inner molecular layer (IML, arrows) at postnatal day 15 prior to seizure onset (P17–18). At P30, which is 12 days post–seizure onset, some sprouting in *stg* is barely visible, but not significantly different from control. At 2 months postnatal, IML zinc staining is clearly more intense in the *stg* and steadily increases with continuing seizure activity through 6 months of age. Scale bars, 100 μm. (From Qiao and Noebels, 1993.)

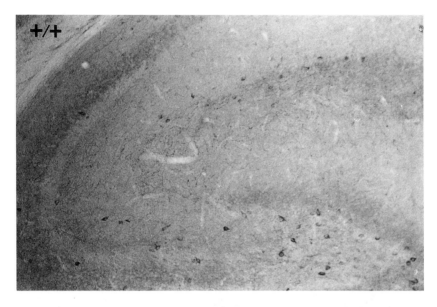

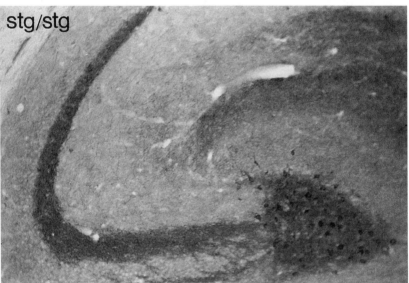

Figure 3-7. Plasticity of neurotransmitter phenotype linked with spike-and-wave epilepsy in the *stargazer* mutant mouse. Immunohistochemistry for neuropeptide Y shows dark immunostaining of scattered NPY+ local circuit neurons in the hilar region of the dentate gyrus and hippocampal formation in wild-type mice (+/+). There is no staining of the mossy fiber pathway. In *stargazer* hippocampus, there is dense aberrant staining in the hilus and throughout the stratum lucidum, matching the axon trajectories of the mossy fiber pathway. Ectopic NPY staining was found in all ages of stargazer mutants, but the intensity varied from mutant to mutant. (From Chafetz and Noebels, unpublished data.)

solute level of aberrant NPY expression in the *stg* mossy fiber system is graded, and it may reflect the integrated seizure history over a brief preceding interval. Since NPY exerts various pre- and postsynaptic effects on synaptic transmission (Brooks et al., 1987; Colmers et al., 1987), this specific example may exemplify a constellation of seizure-induced alterations in neural network excitability that could secondarily contribute to phenotypic complexity in a single-gene epilepsy syndrome.

No evidence has yet been obtained in *stg* mutants for the development of a second clinical seizure phenotype (e.g., focal hippocampal or generalized convulsive seizures) after the onset of spike-and-wave epilepsy; nevertheless, it seems likely that reactive axon reorganization, neosynaptogenesis, and plasticity in neurotransmitter phenotypes may contribute to other forms of abnormal interictal signaling in the epileptic brain. If a similar degree of neuronal plasticity occurs in children with spike-and-wave seizures, specific patterns of secondary brain changes may contribute to the clinical complexity of human absence epilepsy syndromes.

Conclusion

The pathological generation of cortical spike-and-wave discharges in the EEG is linked to a variety of clinical absence seizure phenotypes arising at distinct stages of brain development. Human disorders have been grouped by clinical and EEG criteria into four or more age-related hereditary syndromes; however, the genes and intervening mechanisms responsible have not yet been isolated, and it is not yet known whether the age at the time of the first seizure is a reliable marker for a specific disease gene. These issues are unlikely to be settled in human epilepsies until the age of seizure onset in a syndrome is reliably shown to be uniquely linked to a specific epileptic locus, and the identity of the mutant gene product is determined. Mutational analysis of inherited generalized spike-and-wave seizures in the mouse demonstrates that single genes can cause spike-wave epilepsy phenotypes, although their genetic homology to the human syndromes remains to be explored. In the mouse, the nonconvulsive spike-and-wave seizure pattern is under the independent control of at least five distinct genes, and they produce the abnormal synchronous discharges through different intervening neuromodulatory defects in the brain.

Three fundamental questions related to brain development and mechanisms of spike-wave epileptogenesis pose interesting challenges for future research. The first concerns the extent to which the developmental onset of seizures is dictated by the specific gene error inherited, or the remainder of the genetic background of the affected individual. The second centers on whether the seizure threshold is lowered, and subsequently raised, by the developmental expression of a single molecular defect in the oscillating thalamocortical neurons, by seizure-dependent patterns of neural gene expression, or by the normal maturation of other brain synaptic processes. The third asks whether there are critical developmental periods when the brain is vulnerable to epileptogenic synaptic reorganization in the brain, and seeks to explain why the natural history of several absence epilepsy phenotypes is typically self-limited. By allowing comparisons with the timetable of normal molecular and synaptic maturation in brain circuits, the developmental profiles of absence syndromes may help to pinpoint the identity of the underlying biological excitability defects and provide important clues into the mechanisms responsible for its disappearance.

Acknowledgments

The authors thank the Blue Bird Circle Foundation for Pediatric Neurology. This work was also supported by NIH NS 29709 and 11535 (J.L.N.).

References

Aicardi, J. (1986) *Epilepsy in Children*. New York: Raven Press, pp. 79–99.

Angeleri, F., Ferro-Milone, F., and Parigi, S. (1964) Electrical activity and reactivity of the rhinencephalic, pararhinencephalic and thalamic structures: Prolonged implantation of electrodes in man. *Electroencephalogr. Clin. Neurophysiol. 16:*100–129.

Avanzini, G., Vergnes, M., Spreafico, R., and Marescaux, C. (1993) Calcium-dependent regulation of genetically determined spike and waves by the reticular thalamic nucleus of rats. *Epilepsia 34:*1–7.

Avoli, M., and Gloor, P. (1981) The effects of transient functional depression of the thalamus on spindles and on bilateral synchronous epileptic discharges of feline generalized penicillin epilepsy. *Epilepsia 22:*443–452.

Bencze, K., Troupin, A., and Prockop, L. (1988) Reflex absence epilepsy. *Epilepsia 29:*48–51.

Berkovic, S. F., Andermann, F., Andermann, E., and Gloor, P. (1987) Concepts of absence epilepsies: Discrete syndromes or biological continuum? *Neurology 37:*993–1000.

Brooks, P. A., Kelly, J. C., Allen, J. M., Smith, D. A. S., and Stone, T. W. (1987) Direct excitatory effects of neuropeptide Y (NPY) on rat hippocampal neurones in vitro. *Brain Res. 408:*295–298.

Cavazzuti, G., Ferrari, F., Galli, V., and Benatti, A. (1989) Epilepsy with typical absence seizures with onset during the first year of life. *Epilepsia 30:*802–806.

Cherubini, E., De Feo, M. R., Mecarelli, O., and Ricci, G. F. (1983) Behavioral and electrographic patterns induced by systemic administration of kainic acid in developing rats. *Dev. Brain Res. 9:*69–77.

Coenen, A. M. L., and Van Luitjelaar, E. L. J. M. (1987) The WAG/Rij rat model for absence epilepsy: Age and sex factors. *Epilepsy Res. 1:*297–301.

Colmers, W. F., Lukowiak, K., and Pittman, Q. J. (1987) Presynaptic action of neuropeptide Y in area CA1 of the rat hippocampal slice. *J. Physiol. 383:*285–299.

Commission on Classification and Terminology of the International League against Epilepsy. (1989) Proposal for revised classification of epilepsies and epileptic syndromes. *Epilepsia 30:*389–399.

Connors B. W., and Gutnick M. J. (1990) Intrinsic firing patterns of diverse neocortical neurons. *TINS 13:*99–103.

Covanis, A., Skiadas, K., Loli, N., Lada, C., and Theodorou, V., et al. (1992) Absence epilepsy: Early prognostic signs. *Seizure 1:*281–289.

Coulter, D., Huguenard, J., and Prince, D. A. (1989) Characterization of ethosuximide reduction of low-threshold calcium current in thalamic neurons. *Ann. Neurol. 25:*582–593.

Crunelli, V., and Leresche, N. (1991) A role for GABA$_b$ receptors in excitation and inhibition of thalamocortical cells. *TINS 14:*16–21.

Crunelli, V., Lightowler, S., and Pollard, C. E. (1989) A T-type Ca^{++} current underlies low threshold CA^{++} potentials in cells of the cat and rat lateral geniculate nucleus. *J. Physiol. 413:*543–561.

Dalby, M. A. (1969) Epilepsy and 3 per second spike wave rhythms: A clinical, EEG, and prognostic analysis of 346 patients. *Acta Neurol. Scand. 40:*1–183.

Daval, J.-L., Pereira de Vasconcelos, A., El Hamdi, G., Werck, M.-C., and Nehlig, A. (1992) Quantitative autoradiographic measurements of functional changes induced by generalized seizures in the developing rat brain: Central adenosine and benzodiazepine receptors and local cerebral glucose utilization. *Epilepsy Res. S9:*83–93.

Degan, R., and Degan, H. (1990) Some genetic aspects of rolandic epilepsy: Waking and sleep EEGs in siblings. *Epilepsia 31:*795–801.

Delgado-Escueta, A., Greenberg, D., Weissbecker, K., et al. (1990) Gene mapping in the idiopathic generalized epilepsies: Juvenile myoclonic epilepsy, childhood absence epilepsy, epilepsy with grand mal seizures and early childhood myoclonic epilepsy. *Epilepsia 31* (Suppl.):S19–S29.

Doose, H. (1992) Myoclonic astatic epilepsy of early childhood. In J. Roger, M. Beireau, C. Dravet, F. Dreifuss, D. Perret, and P. Wolf (eds.), *Epileptic Syndromes in Infancy, Childhood and Adolescence.* London: John Libby, pp. 103–114.

Doose, H., and Baier, W. (1989) Generalized spikes and waves. In G. Beck-Mannagetta, V. Anderson, and D. Janz (eds.), *Genetics of the Epilepsies.* Berlin: Springer-Verlag, pp. 95–103.

Doose, H., and Gerken, H. (1973) On the genetics of EEG anomalies in childhood: IV. Photoconvulsive reaction. *Neuropaediatrie 3:*386–401.

Doose, H., Gerken, H. Horstmann, T., and Volzke, E. (1973) Genetic factors in spike-wave absences. *Epilepsia 14:*57–75.

Dreifuss, F. E. (1981) Proposal for revised clinical and electroencephalographic classification of epileptic seizures. *Epilepsia 22:*489–501.

Dugich-Djordjevic, M. M., Tocco, G., Willoughby, D. A., Najm I., Pasinetti, G., Thompson, R. F., Baudry, M., Lapchack, P. A., and Hefti, F. (1992) BDNF mRNA expression in the developing rat brain following kainic acid–induced seizure activity. *Neuron 8:*1127–1138.

Durner, M., Sander, T., Greenberg, D. A., Johnson, K., Beck-Mannegetta, G., and Janz, D. (1991) Localization of idiopathic generalized epilepsy on chromosome 6p in families of juvenile myoclonic epilepsy patients. *Neurology 41:*1651–1655.

Engel, J., Jr, Kuhl, D. E., and Phelps, M. E. (1985) Local cerebral metabolic rate for glucose during petit mal absences. *Ann. Neurol. 17:*121–128.

Fisher, R. S., and Prince, D. A. (1977) Spike-wave rhythms in cat cortex induced by parental penicillin: I. Electroencephalographic features. *Electroencephalogr. Clin. Neurophysiol. 42:*608–624.

Gall, C., Lauterborn, J., Bundman, M., Murray, K., and Isackson, P. (1991) Seizures and the regulation of neurotrophic factor and neuropeptide gene expression in brain. In V. E. Anderson, W. A. Hauser, I. E. Leppik, J. L. Noebels, and S. S. Roth (eds.), *Genetic Strategies in Epilepsy Research.* Amsterdam: Elsevier, pp. 225–245.

Gastaut, H. (1970) Clinical electroencephalographical classification of epileptic seizures. *Epilepsia 11:*102–113.

Gibbs, F. A., Davis, H., and Lennox, W. G. (1935) The electro-encephalogram in epilepsy and in conditions of impaired consciousness. *Arch. Neurol. Psychiatr. 34:*1133–1148.

Gloor, P. (1979) Generalized epilepsy with spike and wave discharge: A reinterpretation of its electro-encephalographic and clinical manifestations. *Epilepsia 20:*571–588.

Gloor, P., and Fariello, R. (1988) Generalized epilepsy: Some of its cellular mechanisms differ from those of focal epilepsy. *TINS 11:*63–68.

Gomez, M. R., and Westmoreland, B. F. (1987) Absence seizures. In H. Luders and R. P. Lesser (eds.), *Clinical Medicine and the Nervous System: Epilepsy: Electroclinical Syndromes.* New York: Springer-Verlag, pp. 105–129.

Gordon, N. (1979) Petit mal epilepsy and cortical epileptogenic foci. *Electroencephalogr. Clin. Neurophysiol. 11:*151–153.

Greenberg, D. A., and Delgado-Escueta, A. (1993) The chromosome 6p epilepsy locus: Exploring mode of inheritance and heterogeneity through linkage analysis. *Epilepsia 34:*S12–S18.

Greenberg, D. A., Delgado-Escueta, A. V., Widelitz, H., Sparkes, R. S., Treiman, L., Maldonado, H. M., Park, M. S., and Terasaki, P. I. (1988) Juvenile myoclonic epilepsy (JME) may be linked to the BF and HLA loci on human chromosome 6. *Am. J. Med. Genet. 31:*185–192.

Guerrini, R., Bureau, M., Mattei, M.-G., Battaglia, A., Galland, M.-C., and Roger, J. (1990) Trisomy 12p syndrome: A chromosomal disorder associated with generalized 3-Hz spike and wave discharges. *Epilepsia 31:*557–566.

Guyon, A., Vergnes, M., and Leresche, N. (1993) Thalamic low threshold calcium current in a genetic model of absence epilepsy. *Neuroreport 4:*1231–1234.

Helekar, S., and Noebels, J. L. (1991) Synchronous hippocampal bursting unmasks latent network excitability alterations in an epileptic gene mutation. *Proc. Natl. Acad. Sci. 88:*4736–4740.

Helekar, S. A., and Noebels, J. L. (1992) A burst-dependent excitability defect elicited by potassium at the developmental onset of spike-wave seizures in the *tottering* mutant. *Dev. Brain Res. 65:*205–210.

Holmes, G., McKeever, M., and Adamson, M. (1987) Absence seizures in children: Clinical and electroencephalographic features. *Ann. Neurol. 21:*268–273.

Hosford, D. A., Clark, S., Cao, Z., Wilson, W., Lin, F.-H., Morisett, R. A., and Huin, A. (1992) The role of GABA$_B$ receptor activation in absence seizures of *lethargic (lh/lh)* mice. *Science 257:*398–401.

Houser, C. R., Miyashiro, J. E., Swartz, B. E., Walsh, G. O., Rich, J. R., and Delgado-Escueta, A. V. (1990) Altered patterns of dynorphin immunoreactivity suggest mossy fiber reorganization in human hippocampal epilepsy. *J. Neurosci. 10:*267–282.

Huguenard, J. R., and Prince, D. A. (1992) A novel T-type current underlies prolonged Ca^{2+}-dependent burst firing in GABAergic neurons of the rat thalamic reticular nucleus. *J. Neurosci. 12:*3804–3817.

Italian League against Epilepsy Genetic Collaborative Group. (1993) Concordance of clinical forms of epilepsy in families with several affected members. *Epilepsia 34:*819–826.

Janz, D., Durner, M., Beck-Mannagetta, G., and Pantazis, G. (1989) Family studies on the genetics of juvenile myoclonic epilepsy (epilepsy with impulsive petit mal). In G. Beck-Mannagetta, V. Anderson, and D. Janz (eds.), *Genetics of the Epilepsies.* Berlin: Springer-Verlag, pp. 43–66.

Jasper, H. H., and Droogleever-Fortuyn, J. (1947) Experimental studies of the functional anatomy of petit mal epilepsy. *Assoc. Res. Nerv. Ment. Dis. Proc. 26:*272–298.

Kaufmann, W., and Galaburda, A. (1989) Cerebrocortical microdysgenesis in neurologically normal subjects: A histopathological study. *Neurology 39:*238–244.

Kellaway, P., Frost, J., and Crawley, J. (1990) The relationship between sleep spindles and spike-and-wave bursts in human epilepsy. In M. Avoli, P. Gloor, G. Kostopoulos, and R. Naquet (eds.), *Generalized Epilepsy: Neurobiological Approaches.* Boston: Birkhauser, pp. 36–48.

Kellaway, P., Frost, J. D., Jr., and Mizrahi, E. M. (1991) Ethosuximide effects on thalamic oscillating mechanisms, spindles, and generalized 3 Hz spike-and-wave bursts. *Ann. Neurol. 30:*293.

Lennox, W. J. (1960) *Epilepsy and Related Disorders,* Vol 1. Boston: Little Brown.

Livingston, S., Torres, H., Pavli, L., and Rider, R. V. (1965) Petit mal epilepsy. Results of a prolonged follow-up study of 117 patients. *JAMA 194:*227–232.

Lytton, W. W., and Sejnowski, T. J. (1992) Computer model of ethosuximide's effect on a thalamic neuron. *Ann. Neurol. 32:*131–139.

Marcus, E. M., and Watson, C. W. (1966) Bilateral synchronous spike-wave electroencephalographic patterns in the cat: Interaction of bilateral cortical foci in the intact, the bilateral cortical-callosal and adiencephalic preparation. *Arch. Neurol. 14:*601–605.

Mares, P., Maressova D., Trojan, S., and Fischer, J. (1982) Ontogenetic development of rhythmic thalamocortical phenomena in the rat. *Brain Res. Bull. 8:*765–769.

Marescaux, C., Vergnes, M., and Bernasconi, R. (1992) *Generalized Non-convulsive Epilepsy: Focus on GABA$_B$ Receptors.* Vienna: Springer-Verlag.

Marescaux, C., Vergnes, M., and Depaulis, A. (1992) Genetic absence epilepsy in rats from Strasbourg: A review. *J. Neurol. Trans. Suppl. 35:*37–69.

Marksteiner, J., Ortler, M., Bellman, R., and Sperk, G. (1990) Neuropeptide Y biosynthesis is markedly induced in mossy fibers during temporal lobe epilepsy of the rat. *Neurosci. Lett. 112:*143–148.

Martin, J. B. (1993) Molecular genetics in neurology. *Ann. Neurol. 34:*757–773.

Meencke, H.-J. (1985) Neuron density in the molecular layer of the frontal cortex in primary generalized epilepsy. *Epilepsia 26:*450–454.

Metrakos, K., and Metrakos, J. D. (1961) Genetics of convulsive disorders: II. Genetic and electrographic studies in centrencephalic epilepsy. *Neurology 11:*474–483.

Mirsky, A. F., and Oshima H. J. (1973) Effects of subcortical alumina cream lesions on attentive behavior and the electroencephalogram in monkeys. *Exp. Neurol. 39:*1–18.

Namgung, U., and Noebels, J. L. (1991) Hippocampal CA3 pyramidal cells of the epileptic mutant mouse *stargazer* display a distinctive gene-linked hyperexcitability. *Soc. Neurosci. Abstr. 17:*170.

Nehlig, A., Vergnes, M., Marescaux, C., Boyer, S., and Lannes, B. (1991) Local cerebral glucose utilization in rats with petit mal–like seizures. *Ann. Neurol. 29:* 72–77.

Niedermeyer, E., Laws, E. R., and Walker, A. E. (1969) Depth EEG findings in epileptics with generalized spike-wave complexes. *Arch. Neurol. 21:*51–58.

Noebels J. L. (1979) Analysis of inherited epilepsy using single locus mutations in mice. *Fed. Proc. 38:*2405–2410.

Noebels J. L. (1984) A single gene error in noradrenergic axon growth synchronizes central neurons. *Nature 10:*409–411.

Noebels J. L. (1992) Molecular genetics and epilepsy. In T. Pedley and B. Meldrum (eds.), *Recent Advances in Epilepsy.* London: Churchill Livingstone, pp. 1–15.

Noebels, J. L., and Sidman, R. L. (1979) Inherited epilepsy: Spike-wave and focal motor seizures in the mutant mouse *tottering. Science 204:*1334–1336.

Ochs, R. F., Gloor, P., Tyler, J. L., Wolfson, T., Worsley, K., Andermann, F., Diksic, M., Meyer, E., and Evans, A. (1987) Effect of generalized spike and wave discharge on glucose metabolism measured by positron emission tomography. *Ann. Neurol. 21:*458–464.

Panayiotopoulos, C., Obeid, T., and Waheed, G. (1989) Differentiation of typical absence seizures in epileptic syndromes. *Brain 112:*1039–1056.

Penry, J. K., Porter, R. J., and Dreifuss, F. E. (1975) Simultaneous recording of absence seizures with videotape and electroencephalography. *Brain 98:*427–440.

Qiao, X., and Noebels, J. L. (1991) Genetic heterogeneity of inherited spike-wave epilepsy: Two mutant gene loci with independent cerebral excitability defects. *Brain Res. 555:*43–50.

Qiao, X., and Noebels, J. L. (1992) GABA$_B$ receptor-independent spike-wave epilepsy in the mutant mouse *stargazer. Pharmacol. Abstr. 18:*553.

Qiao, X., and Noebels, J. L. (1993) Developmental analysis of hippocampal mossy fiber outgrowth in a mutant mouse with inherited spike-wave seizures. *J. Neurosci. 13:*4622–4635.

Quesney, L., Andermann, F., Lal, S., and Prelevic, S. (1980) Transient abolition of generalized photosensitive epileptic discharge in man by apomorphine, a dopamine-receptor agonist. *Neurology 30:*1169–1174.

Roger, J. (1974) Prognostic features of petit mal absence. *Epilepsia 15:*433.

Sato, S., Dreifuss, F., and Penry, J. K. (1983) Long-term follow-up of absence seizures. *Neurology 33:*1590–1595.

Snead, O. C. (1984) Ontogeny of γ-hydroxybutyric acid: II. Electroencephalographic effects. *Dev. Brain Res. 15:*89–96.

Snead, O. C. (1988) γ-Hydroxybutyrate model of generalized absence seizures: Further characterization and comparison with other absence models. *Epilepsia 29:*361–368.

Steriade, M. (1992) Spindling, incremental thalamocortical responses, and spike-wave epilepsy. In M. Avoli, P. Gloor, G. Kostopoulos, and R. Naquet (eds.), *Generalized Epilepsy: Neurobiological Approaches.* Boston: Birkhauser, pp. 161–180.

Steriade, M., Jones, E. G., and Llinas, R. R. (1990) *Thalamic Oscillations and Signaling.* New York: John Wiley and Sons.

Steriade, M., McCormick, D. A., and Sejnowski, T. J. (1993) Thalamocortical oscillations in the sleeping and aroused brain. *Science 262:*679–685.

Sundaram, M., Hill, A., and Lowry, N. (1985) Thyroxine-induced petit mal status. *Neurology 35:*1792–1793.

Sutula, T., Cascino, G., Cavazos, J., Parada, I., and Ramirez, L. (1989) Mossy fiber synaptic reorganization in the epileptic human temporal lobe. *Ann. Neurol. 26:*321–330.

Thomas, P., Beaumanoir, A., Genton, P., Dolisi, C., and Chatel, M. (1992) "De novo" absence status of late onset. *Neurology 42:*104–110.

Vergnes, M., Marescaux, C., and Depaulis, A. (1990) Mapping of spontaneous spike and wave discharges in Wistar rats with genetic generalized non-convulsive epilepsy. *Brain Res. 523:*87–91.

Vergnes, M., Marescaux, C., Depaulis, A., Micheletti, G., and Warter, J. M. (1986) Ontogeny of spontaneous petit mal-like seizures in Wistar rats. *Dev. Brain Res. 30:*85–87.

Von Krosigk, M., Bal, T., and McCormick, D. A. (1993) Cellular mechanisms of a synchronized oscillation in the thalamus. *Science 261:*361.

Wahlestedt, C., Blendy, J. A., Kellar, K. J., Heilig, M., Widerlov, E., and Ekman, R. (1990) Electroconvulsive shocks increase the concentration of neocortical and hippocampal neuropeptide Y (NPY)-like immunoreactivity in the rat. *Brain Res. 507:*65–68.

Williams, D. (1953) A study of thalamic and cortical rhythms in "petit mal." *Brain 76:*50–69.

Wolf, P., and Inoue, Y. (1984) Therapeutic response of absence seizures in patients of an epilepsy clinic for adolescents and adults. *J. Neurol. 231:*225–229.

Yohai, D., and Barnett, S. (1989) Absence and atonic seizures induced by piperazine. *Pediatr. Neurol. 5:*393–394.

Zhang, X., Ju, G., and Le Gal La Salle, G. (1991) Fos expression in GHB-induced generalized absence epilepsy in the thalamus of the rat. *Neuroreport 2:*469–472.

Zouhar, A., Mares, P., Liskova-Bernaskova, K., and Mudrochova, M. (1989) Motor and electrocorticographic epileptic activity induced by bicuculline in developing rats. *Epilepsia 30:*501–510.

4

Developmental Neuropathology and Childhood Epilepsies

VERNE S. CAVINESS, JR.
MARY E. HATTEN
SUSAN K. McCONNELL
TAKAO TAKAHASHI

The threshold for virtually all seizure manifestations is at its lowest in early childhood (Aicardi, 1986; Lennox, 1969; Roger et al., 1984). Further, the primary generalized epilepsies such as grand mal, absence, and certain of the myoclonic disorders invariably arise before adulthood. Should these seizure disorders be regarded generically as a variant electrophysiologic state that is associated with normal brain ontogeny? Neuropathological analysis argues otherwise. The histologic studies of Meencke (1985, 1989) identified pathologic correlates for the major classes of the childhood epilepsies, including both the primary and secondary generalized seizure disorders. Evidence from these studies suggests that there is a general correlation between the gravity of the seizure disorder and the extent of the associated anatomic anomalies. In this chapter we first survey the primary neuropathologic data from human postmortem studies in order to establish a set of guiding inferences; we then review the experimental studies of brain development, which provide a framework for understanding the complex disturbances of neural organization that may arise in childhood epilepsies.

Neuropathologic Correlates of Childhood Epilepsy

The neuropathologic survey of Meencke included 591 brains obtained postmortem from epileptic subjects, as well as 7,374 brains from subjects not known to have had seizures (Meencke, 1985, 1989). Of particular interest are his findings relating to four epilepsy syndromes of infancy and childhood: two secondary generalized epilepsies, West syndrome or infantile spasms ($n = 40$, age at onset with average = 2–12 months, 3.5 months) and Lennox-Gastaut syndrome ($n = 12$, age at onset with average = 1.5–5.0 years, 3.1 years); and two primary generalized epilepsies, childhood absence ($n = 12$, average age at onset, 7.5 years) and juvenile myoclonic epilepsy ($n = 3$, average age at onset 15.5 years). These syndromes are presented in the approximate order of their age of onset, severity, intractability, and clinical outcome independent of the seizure course. By each of these criteria, West syndrome is the most sinister, with the primary generalized epilepsies the least sinister. Meencke demonstrated explicit anatomic abnormalities in a substantial portion of brains representative of each disorder. It must be emphasized, however, that no abnormalities were found in at least a few of the brains from children who had West syndrome, the gravest of the secondary generalized seizure disorders.

West Syndrome

Among these epileptic syndromes, West syndrome is associated with the broadest spectrum of pathoanatomic abnormalities (Meencke, 1985, 1989). Some of the anomalies are most consistent with disruptions of early (intra-uterine) histogenetic events; where this is the case, the onset of seizures is within the first half of the first year of life. Other classes of pathoanatomic abnormality appear to be more consistent with the consequences of inter-current destructive processes to which the brain had been exposed late in gestation, in the perinatal period, or subsequent to birth. Where the pathological process seems to have struck around the time of birth or later in postnatal life, the onset of seizures is more typically delayed to the second half of the first year of life.

Approximately 70 percent of brains representing West syndrome were associated with the gravest pathoanatomic anomalies encountered in the series, 20 percent with explicit though less grave pathoanatomic abnormalities, and 10 percent with no evident pathoanatomic abnormality. The full set of classes of pathoanatomic abnormalities with their specific representations associated with West syndrome is as follows:

1. Dysraphic states, anomalies considered to be a reflection of abnormalities of primary segmentation or of neural tube closure, and represented in this series of brains specifically by encephalocele.
2. Major disruptions of neuronal migration, expressed in terms of heterotopic accumulations of cells along the customary migratory route, and represented in this series of brains specifically by pachygyria.
3. Severe reduction in brain weight, which in this series of brains averaged approximately 30 percent less than normal brain weight. In a few specimens microcephaly was already evident at birth, but otherwise reflected nongrowth or retarded growth of the brain in the earliest months of postnatal life. Typically, reduced brain weight was not associated with

increased neuron density, implying a substantial reduction in neuron number.

4. Focal or multifocal regions of neuronal necrosis, in some brains expressed in frank tissue dissolution and in others suggested by the presence of calcification. The traces of neuronal necrosis were most prevalent in the cerebral cortices and cerebellum but were also encountered in basal ganglia, thalamus, and brainstem. The patterns of necrotic distribution predicted neither age of onset nor severity of the associated pattern of infantile spasms. In most instances these findings were attributable to perinatal or postnatal hypoxia-ischemia, but in a few they were probably the direct or indirect consequences of infections.

5. Microdysgenesis, a heterogeneous taxonomic grouping. As applied by Meencke to the pathologic anatomy of West syndrome, microdysgenesis included increase in density of neurons in the neocortical molecular layer where the most marked expression included focal neuronal accumulations and the mildest was characterized by a more diffuse (i.e., nonclustered) increase of neurons in this layer; increase in density of subcortical neurons; disruptions in the patterns of alignment and differentiation of the neocortical laminae, encountered as protrusions of layer 2 into layer 1, as malregistration of the neurons of the infragranular layers, and as diminished differentiation of the boundary of layer 6 with the subcortical white matter.

Lennox-Gastaut Syndrome

The brains representative of the Lennox-Gastaut syndrome presented a high proportion of explicit pathoanatomic anomalies which, though substantial and heterogeneous, tended to be less severe than those of the West syndrome. Small foci of neuronal necrosis within widespread forebrain cortical and subcortical structures and cerebellum and microdysgenesis involving principally layer 1 were characteristic of approximately 90 percent of these specimens. The wider range of histogenetic lesions and salient zones of tissue necrosis associated with this syndrome in other studies (Viani et al., 1977) were not encountered by Meencke. The larger group of intracortical and subcortical dysgenesis typical of West syndrome was also absent in brains from the Lennox-Gastaut syndrome.

Primary Generalized Epilepsies: Childhood and Juvenile Myoclonic Absence

Mild, diffuse increases in density of neurons in neocortical layer 1 were observed in 13 of 15 brains in the Meencke series. Given this high proportion of abnormalities established by observation, taken together with the fact that the observations were based upon examination of a relatively small sample of the neocortex, it is probable that none of the brains were normal by the pathoanatomic criteria applied by Meencke. However, the brain weights were normal, and no other pathoanatomic correlates of these syndromes have been described.

Pathoanatomic Correlates of Epilepsies of Childhood: Selected Inferences

We propose here a brief set of inferences drawn from the pathoanatomic study of brains by Meencke. These inferences are designed to bridge the clinical world of epilepsy and basic themes central to the developmental neurobiology of the mammalian central nervous system. These are working inferences, based on the available set of observations; they are not proposed here to be comprehensive or confidently establish principles of pathophysiology. This disclaimer is a necessary recognition of the great complexity of the clinical and anatomic phenomena providing the observational base, as well as the limitations dictated by the biased population sample selection (including only the deceased) and the relatively small size of this population sample.

Inference 1. All classes of pathoanatomic abnormality affecting the developing cerebrum may increase the likelihood of epilepsy; all epilepsies are associated with some class of pathoanatomic abnormality.

Inference 2. The gravity of the pathoanatomic disruption, and not its specific anatomic or etiologic nature, determines the relative age of onset of the epileptic disorder. The graver the disruption, the earlier the age of onset.

Inference 3. The age of onset of an epileptic disorder is the principal determinant of both the clinical characteristics of the seizure syndrome and the ultimate level of resulting behavioral disability. The earlier the onset, the more aggressive the seizure disorder and the graver the associated behavioral disability.

Major Steps in Brain Development: Intersection with Epilepsy Syndromes

The pathology of epilepsy invites a consideration of principles of normal and abnormal development of the central nervous system far too comprehensive for the present limited review. We will instead focus on a schematic framework of normal histogenetic sequence, and where this sequence may be inferred (from the pathologic evidence) to have gone awry in brains representative of childhood epilepsies.

Histogenetic Sequence

Schematically considered, development of the mammalian central nervous system advances through four overlapping histogenetic epochs (Fig. 4-1; Sidman and Rakic, 1982):

1. *Regional determination and segmentation* is followed by
2. *Cytogenesis* and then by

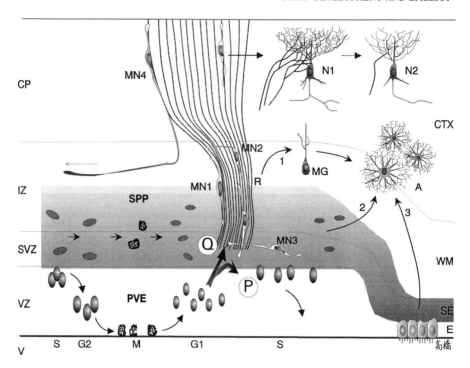

Figure 4-1. Cell ontogeny in cerebral wall. Two proliferative populations located within the ventricular (VZ), subventricular (SVZ), and intermediate (IZ) zones of the cerebral wall, the pseudostratified ventricular epithelium (PVE) and the secondary proliferative population (SPP, shaded area), give rise to the general neuronal and astroglial cell lineages. The phases of a complete cell cycle read linearly from left to right at the ventricular (V) surface: S–G2–M–G1–S. Cycling cells are represented only as nuclei. Interkinetic nuclear movement occurs in the PVE but not the SPP. In the PVE there is progressive dispersion of closely adjacent cells with successive cycles. After mitosis, a portion of the daughter cells will leave the cycle (Q fraction, Q) while the remainder will enter the next cycle (P fraction, P). The proliferative activity is continued through multiple cycles. Eventually mitoses within the PVE give rise to only Q fraction cells and the epithelium is transformed into the nonproliferative ependyma (E).

Cells of the astroglial lineage (A) probably arise within PVE and SPP. Before and during cortical histogenesis large numbers of these have the form of radial glial cells (R; ascending processes represented) whose processes, spanning ventricular and pial surfaces, support migrations of postmitotic neurons (MN1). As neurons ascend through the radial glial fiber system, they may pass from fiber to fiber (MN2) or even bolt tangentially across the fiber system for substantial distances (MN3). Axons may issue from the cell before migrations are completed (MN4, arrow).

Postmigratory neurons (N1) within the cortical plate (CP) grow and differentiate an "exuberance" of dendritic and axonal processes which are eventually "pruned" (broken arrow indicating N2) to form operation neural networks. Astrocytes (A) arise by monopolar transformation (MG, arrow 1) of radial glial cells or by proliferation of other astrocyte progenitors of the SPP (arrow 2) or, later, of the subependymal region (SE, arrow 3). These will spread through subcortical white matter (WM) and cortex (CTX).

3. *Cell migration,* which then yields to the events of
4. *Growth and differentiation.*

As far as the human forebrain is concerned, the first three of these sequences are accomplished by the end of the second trimester, at which time the brain weighs some 100 g, that is, about 25 percent of its weight at term and less than 10 percent of its adult weight (Gilles et al., 1983; Lemire et al., 1975; Sidman and Rakic, 1982). The developmental events of growth and differentiation are only beginning to surge ahead at the end of the second trimester. They accelerate in pace through the final trimester and continue strongly well beyond term through the early years of life. The cellular events of this final epoch contribute overwhelmingly to the final mass of the brain and also to the details of its form.

The Earliest Developmental Events

Pathologic processes may intersect and deflect the course of this histogenetic sequence at virtually any stage, including disruptions of karyotype or of single genes which predate conjunction of paternal and maternal genotypes. Whereas such deflections of pre–third trimester development are of substantial theoretical interest, they probably cast only a pale shadow over the postnatal preoccupations of clinical epilepsy. This is because their consequences are inordinately grave, generally leading to involution of conceptus or miscarriage, depending upon the developmental stage when the abnormal process declares itself (Friede, 1989). Thus some 40 percent of concepti probably involute before implantation because of the catastrophic consequences of aneuploidy.

Disorders of segmentation and regional specification, similarly set in motion in the prehistory of implantation or within a week or two of this event, also involute at an early stage. Infants with the most severe defects, for example, holoprosencephaly or anencephaly (Friede, 1989), only infrequently survive to term. The disorders of segmentation and regional specification more commonly encountered among surviving infants, such as the Chiari malformations and other malformations associated with encephalocele, probably reflect primarily disruptions of mesenchymal ontogeny and only secondarily disruptions of central nervous system ontogeny (Marin-Padilla, 1978).

Among this group, the Chiari malformations, which may include seizures, figure prominently among the causes of severe disability in postnatal life. For complex reasons (Caviness, 1976), the principal effect of the dysraphic process upon cerebral development is probably felt primarily beyond midgestation. Although such malformations may be associated with epilepsy, the aberrations of forebrain development set in motion in the final development epoch (the epoch of growth and differentiation) are probably most relevant to the ontogeny of seizure disorders.

Cytogenesis and Cell Migration

Judging from Meencke's observations, these processes figure more prominently in the pathoanatomic substrate of childhood epilepsies than do the earlier events of segmentation and regional determination. Here the disorders that lead to major disruptions of migration, represented by subcortical heterotopia, must be distinguished from minor disruptions leading to the spectrum of microdysgeneses. Heterotopia most likely reflect the consequences of disruption of the cellular mechanisms of neuronal migration rather than the prior events of cytogenesis or those which determine the architectonic character of cortex during the principal migratory trajectory. Lissencephaly, encountered by Meencke in a single specimen representative of West syndrome (and associated in about half the population with a deletion on chromosome 17p; Dobyns, 1987; Dobynes et al., 1983), is prototypical of malformations of this caste. Other rare cytogenetic and migrational defects recognized for their association with epileptic disorders of childhood include pachygyria ("band heterotopia"), the Walker-Warburg malformation, and the Zellweger syndrome (Caviness et al., 1989).

Paradoxically, the microdysgeneses, though the consequence of disorders less catastrophic for the overall shape of the brain and the patterns of cell distribution within the cerebral hemispheres, may in a certain sense be developmentally more complex. This spectrum of histopathologic abnormalities may result from the disruption of events to be described later: during cytogenesis, migration, and positional "fine-tuning" in the final phase of migration.

Basic Neurobiological Insights into Brain Development

Precursor Populations

The majority of young neurons destined to populate cerebral cortical structures arise in pseudostratified proliferative epithelium (PVE), which lines the cerebral ventricular cavities and more or less corresponds to the cytoarchitectonically defined ventricular zone (VZ) (Fig. 4-1; His, 1889; Sauer, 1936; Sidman and Rakic, 1973). Precursors of the glial populations also arise from this epithelium; however, precursors of the astroglial, and possibly the oligodendroglial, lineages appear to proliferate secondarily in a subventricular location (secondary proliferative population [SPP]; Misson, Takahashi, and Caviness, 1991; Sidman and Rakic, 1982; Takahashi et al., 1993). The pace of proliferation in both these populations is intense. The proportion of cycling cells—that is, the growth fraction—approximates 100 percent for much of the cytogenetic epoch (Takahashi et al., 1993; Waechter and Jaensch, 1972). The length of the cell cycle, initially approximately 10 hours in mice, increases to a value nearly double that at the outset as cell formation continues (Caviness et al., 1991). This increase in length primarily reflects a progressive prolongation of the G1 phase of the cycle. At the same time that G1 is lengthening, the proportion of cells that will leave the cycle following division (Q fraction) is also increasing (Takahashi et al., 1991, 1994). Early in the cytogenetic epoch, the Q fraction is less than 50 percent, with the result that cell proliferation contributes more to augmentation of the neuronal precursor population (Takahashi et al., 1991, 1993b); later it exceeds 50 percent, resulting in the involution of the proliferative zone as the delivery of neurons to the cortex accelerates.

Whereas these general attributes of cell cycle control are reflected in the cytogenetic behavior of both the PVE and the SPP, the former largely runs through its cycle to completion before there is significant output from the latter (Takahashi et al., 1992). That is, the neurons of the cerebral cortex are largely born before the glial cells which come to populate the cerebral wall. This dissociation in the proliferative behavior of neuronal and glial elements reflects fundamental cell lineage determinations achieved during the earliest phases of cytogenesis.

Fate Determination

Critical aspects of fate determination within the neuronal population may also be achieved in the course of its cell cycle within the proliferative epithelium (McConnell 1988a, 1989a, 1991; McConnell and Kaznowski, 1991). ^{3}H-thymidine "birthdating" studies have been performed to assess the order in which neurons of the cerebral cortex are normally generated (Angevine and Sidman, 1961; Jackson et al., 1989; Luskin and Shatz, 1985a; Rakic, 1974). These studies have revealed that the first neurons to become postmitotic and leave the PVE migrate toward the pial surface, forming a single layer, termed the "preplate" (Luskin and Shatz, 1985b; Marin-Padilla, 1971). The subsequent generation of neurons destined for the cortical plate, beginning with layer 6, splits the preplate into two regions: the marginal zone (future layer 1, just underneath the pia), and the subplate, located subjacent to the cortical plate (Kostovic and Rakic, 1980; Luskin and Shatz, 1985b). The subplate is a transient structure; the majority of its constituent neurons are eliminated by a wave of programmed cell death in the first weeks to months of postnatal life (Chun and Shatz, 1989b; Kostovic and Rakic, 1980; Woo et al., 1990). Within the cortical plate proper, the remaining neurons of the permanent cortical layers are generated in an inside-first, outside-last sequence in all mammals that have been studied. Following their migration into the cortical plate, these neurons undergo dendritic differentiation, form axonal projections, and acquire their characteristic sets of axonal inputs (reviewed in McConnell, 1988a).

The correlation between a neuron's birthday (time of final mitosis) and its ultimate laminar destination has enabled McConnell and coworkers to test the relative contributions of cell lineage and cell environment to the establishment of layer-specific phenotypes (McConnell, 1988b; McConnell and Kaznowski, 1991). They transplanted neurons or their progenitors from animals in which deep-layer neurons were being generated into host animals in which deep-layer neurogenesis was complete and upper-layer neurons were in the process of mitosis and migration. The transplanted neurons were thereby presented with a choice as they migrated out into the host environment (Fig. 4-2). If these cells were multipotent and had yet to receive instructions as to their ultimate laminar fate, they should migrate to the upper layers along with host neurons and develop axonal connections to other regions of cortex, as are typical of neurons in layers 2 and 3. If, however, the transplanted neurons were committed at the time of transplantation to the deep-layer fates characteristic of their birthday, they should migrate specifically to layer 6 of the host and form subcortical axonal projections.

Cell Cycle Determines Fate

These transplantation experiments have revealed that whether a presumptive deep-layer neuron has undergone a commitment to its normal fate or

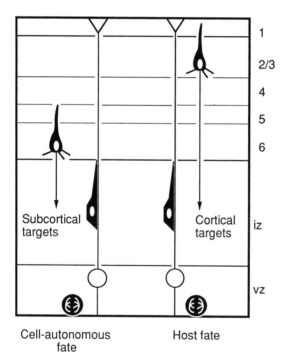

Figure 4-2. Two possible outcomes of the transplantation of young, presumptive layer 6 neurons into an older host brain, in which upper-layer neurons are being generated. If transplanted cells are committed to their normal laminar fates (left), they should develop autonomously within the novel environment, migrate to layer 6 (the destination appropriate for their birthday), and form subcortical projections. If, however, environmental factors determine laminar fate, transplanted neurons should adopt the host fate (right) by migrating to the upper layers 2 and 3, and sending axons to cortical targets. iz, intermediate zone; vz, ventricular zone.

not depends on its position in the cell cycle at the time of transplantation (McConnell and Kaznowski, 1991). If cells are transplanted while still in the S phase of the cell cycle, prior to their terminal mitotic division, the neurons generated from that division will apparently switch fates and migrate to the upper layers, along with the cohort of surrounding host neurons. If, however, the transplanted neuron is grafted later in the cell cycle, at any time at or after G2, it displays a commitment to its normal laminar phenotype; these neurons migrate to cortical layer 6 and can form the thalamic axonal projections typical of their birthday (McConnell, 1988b; McConnell and Kaznowski, 1991). Thus there appears to be a cell cycle–dependent plasticity within the cortical ventricular zone: progenitor cells in S phase of the cell cycle are multipotent and can give rise to daughters of many laminar phenotypes. Under the influence of environmental signals, however, the progenitor makes a commitment as to the fate of its daughter, roughly at the time that it transmits into G2 of the cell cycle. Daughter neurons transplanted at or after this point have been endowed with the information they need to "home" to the cortical layer appropriate for their birthday and form axonal projections characteristic of that layer.

Origin of Environmental Fate-Determining Signals

The molecular nature of the environmental cues that signal the acquisition of particular cell fates is not yet known. One source of environmental input to multipotent progenitor cells during S phase may be the previously generated differentiating neurons. According to this model, based on studies of retinal neurogenesis by Reh and Tully (1986), there may be control over neurogenesis by daughter cells, such that the act of producing neurons of a given layer might feed back onto parent progenitor cells, in effect saying "enough of this layer, get on with the next." Evidence consistent with this general scheme has recently been obtained by Price and coworkers (Gillies and Price, 1993). They interfered with the production of deep-layer neurogenesis in the mouse by treating young embryos with the cytotoxic agent methylazoxymethanol acetate, which kills dividing precursor cells. The ventricular zone recovered from drug treatment within a few days, but instead of resuming its normal laminar production schedule the system reset and replaced the missing deep-layer neurons. The resulting cortex was thinner and contained fewer cells overall, but all layers and their axonal projections were present.

What might be the cellular source of feedback from differentiating neurons in the cortical plate to the PVE? One possibility has been raised by studies in which developing axons were traced using the lipophilic fluorescent tracer DiI (Kim et al., 1991; McConnell et al., 1993). When DiI is placed into the preplate or cortical plate of fixed embryonic brains, it labels the axons and growth cones of cortical neurons. These studies show that along the initial part of their trajectory, cortical growth cones travel directly along the surface of the ventricular zone—notably, just above the region where the cell bodies of multipotent cortical progenitor cells are found. This juxtaposition of growing axons and precursor cell bodies raises the possibility that axons deliver a feedback signal from differentiating neurons in the cortical plate to the progenitor cells below. This hypothesis, however, remains to be tested directly.

Cell–Cell Contacts Regulate Neuronal Proliferation and Differentiation

The developing cerebellar cortex, with a clear zone of neurogenesis in the external granule layer (EGL), provides a simplified model system to study further the mechanisms of extrinsic signaling and the specification of cell identity. One approach to identifying the signals that regulate cell differentiation is to identify markers that are specifically expressed in discrete zones of the EGL. Recent studies have identified genes with a pattern of expression that is restricted to the outer layer, the proliferative zone of the EGL (Kuhar et al., 1993). Other analyses indicate that expression of late neuronal markers commences in the deeper layers of the EGL, where cells are exiting the cell cycle and initiating neurite extension. These markers include the axonal glycoprotein TAG-1 (Furley et al., 1990), the neuron–glia adhesion system astrotactin (Edmondson et al., 1988; Stitt and Hatten, 1990), and the neuronal intermediate filament protein, α-internexin (Kaplan et al., 1990).

To examine how the interactions among neuronal precursor cells contribute to the specification of identity in cerebellar granule cells, Hatten and colleagues have developed a purified EGL precursor cell differentiation system, cultured as a dispersed cell monolayer; a three-dimensional collagen gel where the cells would be present at high cell density yet prevented from forming contacts; or in cellular reaggregates, where the cells would form cell–cell physical contacts. Three general hypotheses could be tested with these in vitro systems. According to one hypothesis, neurogenesis would occur by an intrinsic program of gene expression; in this model, neuronal differentiation might proceed "on schedule" when the cells were dispersed in cell culture. In two alternative hypotheses, local signals among cells in the EGL might modify neurogenesis either by diffusible or by membrane-bound signals.

When immature granule cells, purified from P5 mouse cerebellum (Hatten, 1985, 1987), were plated as a dispersed monolayer, low levels of DNA synthesis were detected by ^{3}H-thymidine uptake assays. When the cells were plated as freshly purified granule cells at high cell density (1×10^7 cells/mL) in a collagen matrix, DNA synthesis levels remained low, comparable to those observed for dispersed cells, suggesting that even high concentrations of a soluble factor were ineffective in triggering gene expression. In contrast, cells cultured in large cellular reaggregates (500–2,000 cells) showed high levels of DNA synthesis. These data suggest that local interactions among EGL cells provide a signal that promotes precursor cell proliferation.

To determine whether the signal for granule cell neuronal differentiation was cell-autonomous, granule cells with a specific defect in neuronal differentiation from the neurological mutant mouse *weaver* were analyzed. *Weaver* granule cell precursors proliferate normally in the superficial layer of the EGL (Rezai and Yoon, 1972) and move into the deepest layers of the EGL (Rakic and Sidman, 1973), but they fail to extend neurites or to migrate away from the EGL (Hatten et al., 1983; Rakic and Sidman, 1973; Sotelo and Changeux, 1974). Using a reaggregate culture system (Gao, Heintz, and Hatten, 1991), purified EGL precursor cells from the midline of the cerebellar cortex of *weaver* mice (wv/wv) failed to extend neurites, as seen in vivo (Hatten, 1985, 1987; Hatten et al., 1986). However, when wild-type EGL precursor cells were mixed with *weaver* granule cell precursors, *weaver* cells extended neurites to the same extent as wild-type neurites (Gao et al., 1992). This observation suggested that cell–cell interactions with wild-type EGL cells rescued the phenotypic defect in *weaver* neurite extension by providing a signal that induces neurite extension. To examine whether mixing *weaver* neuronal precursor cells with wild-type neuronal precursor cells would rescue the cell migration defect, labeled *weaver* EGL cells were mixed with wild-type EGL cells; wild-type astroglial cells were added to provide a substrate for migration (Hatten and Sidman, 1978). After transplantation into cellular reaggregates of wild-type cells, the labeled mutant cells migrated onto the glial fascicles interconnecting the reaggregates. Fluorescence microscopy of dye-labeled *weaver* cells showed that labeled mutant cells expressed the normal cytological features of migrating granule cells, including the formation of a close apposition with the glial fiber and the extension of a leading process. The finding that cell–cell interactions with neuronal precursors rescue the migration of *weaver* cells along astroglial fibers (Gao et al., 1992) suggests that cell–cell interactions among EGL neuronal precursors induce the expression of genes required for cell migration (Fig. 4-3).

Migration Guidance

The majority of neuronal lineages destined for the neocortex undergo their full allotment of cell division within the proliferative zone, and each division may be viewed as the point of initiation of a "clone" of cells. The relationship of clonal mechanics to the ultimate disposition of neurons within the cortex is apparently complex. The simplest entry in the equation appears to be the proliferative zone-to-cortex leg of the excursion. This leg, the migratory trajectory proper, appears to be guided by adherence to the surfaces of specialized radial glial cells whose ascending and descending processes, collectively, span the full width of the cerebral wall (Fig. 4-1; Misson, Austin, et al., 1991; Rakic 1972, 1990; Rakic et al., 1974).

Evidence that radial glial fibers form a substratum for the guidance of neuronal migration was obtained originally from electron microscopic observations of the primate intermediate zone, in which close and intimate cellular appositions were observed between radial glial fibers and cells that had the morphological characteristics of migrating neurons (Rakic, 1971a, 1972). In support of this view, Hatten and coworkers found that purified

GRANULE NEURON DIFFERENTIATION

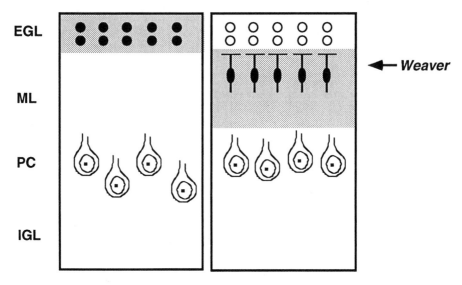

Figure 4-3. The *weaver* gene disrupts the differentiation of granule cells in the developing mouse cerebellar cortex. Whereas wild-type cells undergo each of the major steps in development, neurogenesis, axon outgrowth, migration and synaptogenesis in discrete layers of the cerebellar cortex, weaver EGL (external granule layer) development is arrested prior to axon extension (arrow). (*Left*) EGL precursor cells undergoing mitosis (filled cells) are located at the pial surface. (*Right*) Postmitotic cells undergoing axon extension and glia-guided migration through the molecular layer (ML) are located below the proliferating precursor cell population. IGL, internal granule layer.

granule neurons from the cerebellum migrate actively along Bergmann glial fibers in vitro (Edmondson and Hatten, 1987).

Radial Fibers Guide Migration

The cerebellar cortex has provided a clear model for studies on CNS migration because of its relatively small number of principal neurons and well-established pattern of histogenesis. As described by Ramón y Cajal (1911), there is a unique, displaced proliferative zone, the external granule layer (EGL), which generates the granule cell, the most numerous neuron of the cerebellar cortex. Neuroanatomic studies (Altman, 1972; Fugita, 1967; Fugita et al., 1966; Miale and Sidman, 1961) indicate that cells within the EGL are organized into two discrete zones, a superficial zone, one to two cells thick, containing mitotic figures; and an underlying zone of postmitotic cells. It is in the deeper zone where the first evidence of neuronal differentiation can be seen: the extension of granule cell axons, formation of parallel fibers, and the inward migration of the soma of immature granule cells along the radially aligned processes of the Bergmann glial cells (Fig. 4-4; Edmondson and Hatten, 1987; Gregory et al., 1988; Hatten, 1990; Rakic, 1971b).

Features of Migrating Neurons

In microcultures, astroglial cells differentiate into highly elongated, radial forms resembling the glial forms that support neuronal migration in brain (Rakic, 1971b). By video-enhanced differential interference contrast microscopy, the migration of living neurons along single glial fibers can be observed in real time (Edmondson and Hatten, 1987; Hatten et al., 1983). The migrating neurons express a bipolar extension along the glial fiber and extend a leading process in the direction of migration (Edmondson and Hatten, 1987; Gasser and Hatten, 1990; Gregory et al., 1988; Hatten, 1990).

Although the leading process resembles the growth cone of a neurite in its motility, it differs in several aspects. First, whereas the growth cone is an expansive ending of a thin neurite, the leading process is contoured to the dimensions of the glial fiber. Second, whereas the growth cone is the site of growth and extension, the leading process is simply a tapered rostral portion

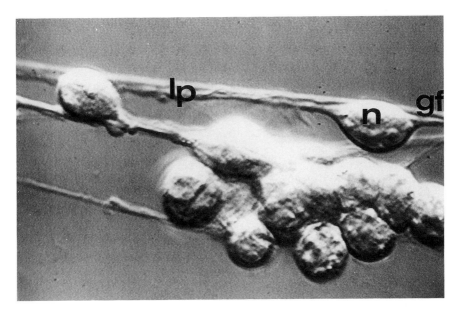

Figure 4-4. Cytology and neuron–glia relationship of a cerebellar granule cell migrating along an astroglial fiber. Cerebellar cells were dissociated from early postnatal mouse cerebellar tissue and cultured in microwells for 24 hours prior to observation with video-enhanced differential interference contrast microscopy. The granule neuron (n) closely apposes the glial fiber (gf) along the length of the neuronal cell soma and extends a leading process (lp) in the direction of migration along the glial guide (modified from Edmondson and Hatten, 1987.)

of the cell. Third, whereas the growth cone is the site of adhesion of the growing neurite, the cell body is the site of adhesion of the migrating neuron. A common feature of the growth cone and the leading process is that both guide the directionality of the neuron.

To define neuron–glia adhesion mechanisms in glial-guided neuronal migration, an antibody, antiastrotactin, was identified that blocks neuronal migration in vitro (Edmondson et al., 1988; Fishell and Hatten, 1991). Western blot and immunoprecipitation analysis indicate that the blocking antibodies recognize a neuronal glycoprotein with an apparent molecular mass of approximately 100,000 (Edmondson et al., 1988). Antiastrotactin antibodies block the binding of neuronal membranes to glial cells (Stitt and Hatten, 1990) and the establishment of neuron–glia contacts in vitro (Edmondson et al., 1988); they also show rapid effects on migrating cells. Within 15 minutes of antibody application, streaming of cytoplasmic organelles into the leading process is arrested, the nucleus is shifted from a caudal to a central position, and the extension of filopodia and lamellopodia along the leading process ceases. Correlated video and electron microscopy suggests that the mechanism of arrest by antiastrotactin antibodies involves the failure to form new adhesion sites along the leading process and the disorganization of cytoskeletal components. These results suggest that astrotactin acts as a neuronal receptor for granule neuron migration along astroglial fibers (Fishell and Hatten, 1991).

Neuronal Derailment from Radial Guides

Radial glia may not, however, provide the exclusive route for neuronal migration, as demonstrated by analysis of the dynamic behaviors of neurons migrating in a histotypically normal, three-dimensional environment in living brain slices. Using time-lapse confocal microscopy, O'Rourke and colleagues tracked the migration of individual DiI-labeled cells in the intermediate zone of neocortex. The majority of labeled cells (around 80 percent) moved along a radial trajectory; the leading processes dynamically extended and retracted filopodia, and the cell somas moved in a saltatory manner, as do migrating granule neurons in vitro. Subsequent immunostaining of the slices revealed that radially oriented migrating cells were closely aligned with vimentin-positive radial glia (O'Rourke et al., 1992).

A fraction of migrating cells, however, diplayed a surprising behavior: roughly 13 percent of the cells imaged were found traveling in directions orthogonal to the radial glia. These cells had the characteristic morphologies of migrating neurons. Some were viewed as they changed orientation from radial to orthogonal or from orthogonal to radial. Nonradially migrating cells generally moved at rates three times faster than radially oriented cells. The cellular or extracellular substrate that supports nonradial migration is not yet known. Glial fibers are unlikely suspects, since preliminary electron microscopic observations reveal no consistent apposition between orthogonally oriented migrating cells and glial processes (C. E. Kaznowski, N. A.

O'Rourke, and S. K. McConnell, unpublished observations). Candidate substrates include axons that populate the intermediate zone and extracellular matrix molecules such as fibronectin (Chun and Shatz, 1988a; Sheppard et al., 1991; Stewart and Pearlman, 1987). Thus there appears to be no specific commitment of migrating cell to a single glial fiber. On the contrary, cells appear to slip across the surfaces of multiple fibers in their ascent, and cells arising from a common point at the ventricular origin appear to become substantially separated from each other by journey's end (Misson, Austin, et al., 1991a).

In summary, disruption of the VZ-to-cortex leg of this journey may result from processes that destroy the guiding glial fiber system (Caviness et al., 1989). It may also be disrupted by more subtle molecular mechanisms that disturb the adhesive affinity between migrating cell and glial fibers (Caviness et al., 1989; Gao, Liu, and Hatten, 1991; Pinto-Lord et al., 1982; Rakic, 1978, 1988a). Both these classes of mechanisms probably contribute to the complex array of specific disorders associated with gross subcortical heterotopia in epileptic disorders of infancy and childhood.

Clonal Behavior

Less well understood is the operation of clonal mechanics within the PVE, prior to the initiation of migration proper, and the events which determine the final architectonic details at the final or intracortical phases of migration (Luskin et al., 1988; Price and Thurlow, 1988; Rakic, 1988b; Walsh and Cepko, 1988, 1990, 1992). There appear to be two classes of clonal behavior within the PVE, an interpretation suggested by two different but complementary types of experiments. When separate lineages are marked in the course of proliferation in such a way that the issue of each clone may be unambiguously distinguished after they complete their migrations, two quite different patterns of distribution are revealed. As expected, some cells of shared lineage cluster close, but never immediately adjacent to each other after the cortex is constructed. The degree of separation is not surprising given the propensity to tangential "slippage" through the glial fiber system in the course of ascent (Austin and Cepko, 1990; Misson, Austin, et al., 1991; Rakic et al., 1974).

Other cells arising from the same lineage, remarkably, are widely separated to a degree that cannot be explained by either the degree of tangential slippage (Misson, Austin, et al., 1991) or frank tangential migration (O'Rourke et al., 1992) that occurs during ascent (Walsh and Cepko, 1990, 1992). An additional mechanism of dispersion which must be considered is tangential movement of proliferating progenitor cells occurring within the PVE (Fig. 4-1; Fishell et al., 1992; O'Leary and Bomgasser, 1992). This phenomenon may occur increasingly at later stages of cytogenesis within the PVE (Fishell et al., 1992; O'Leary and Bomgasser, 1992; Walsh and Cepko, 1992). In fact one might imagine that progenitor cells still in the exponential growth mode could move widely, perhaps freely, through the PVE. These wandering progenitors would in time give rise to a widely scattered secondary population of daughter cells. These secondary offspring would then be the proximate progenitors of cells that would initiate migrations following a terminal division. Patterns of dispersion of proliferating cells within the PVE, directly observed by enhanced time-lapse video in vitro preparations, are consistent with this complex histogenetic sequence (Fishell et al., 1992; O'Leary and Bomgasser, 1992; Walsh and Cepko, 1992).

In theory, any of the cytogenetic and histogenetic events occurring within the PVE and overlying cerebral wall—cell production, lineage assignment, and postmitotic cell distribution—might be disrupted as a consequence of genetic accident or intercurrent pathologic processes. The consequences, if not lethal, might be antecedents to the range of microdysgeneses associated with childhood epilepsies. Thus too few cells might be formed or survive, as in the case of early microcephaly. The cell class profile may be anomalous—that is, with not enough inhibitory interneurons or not enough of the pyramidal cell classes, the principal set of cerebral cortical neurons of projection. Anomalies in migration, or in the stabilization of cell position after migration within the cortical plane itself, might be antecedent to an anomalous cortical lamination pattern. For example, experimental evidence in animals now supports the hypothesis that the neuroglial ectopias associated with collections of neurons in the molecular layer and/or malregistration of the cells of subjacent layers may be provoked by superficial cortical injury in and around the time that the cortical layers are being assembled by migration (Caviness et al., 1978; Caviness and Williams, 1984; Caviness et al., 1989; Galaburda and Kemper, 1979; Sherman et al., 1989). This histological pattern of abnormality, abundant in the anatomic specimens surveyed by Meencke, has also been associated with dyslexia and other cognitive disabilities independently of seizure disorders (Galaburda and Kemper, 1979; Sherman et al., 1989).

Growth and Differentiation

Growth and *differentiation* are terms applied to the full range of cell transformations and interactions underlying the assembly of the normal mature brain. These are considered to be initiated *following,* rather than before the termination of cytogenesis and cell migration, although it is clear that certain cells come to their postmigratory positions well after they have elaborated their primary axonal arbors (Schwartz et al., 1991) while others may arrive armed with functional receptor and transmitter signaling systems (Chun et al., 1987; Chun and Shatz 1989a; Schwartz and Meencke, 1992). Several fundamental points should be emphasized.

"Mapping" of Cortical Structure

First, the migrating cells, particularly those completing migrations late in this epoch of histogenesis, are recruited to a neuronal community that is already "mapped" (Caviness, 1988; Crandall and Caviness, 1984; Ghosh et al., 1990; O'Leary, 1992). The architectonic subdivisions and their positions relative to each other are realized in skeletal sets of connections that are topologically equivalent to those of the adult brain. The earliest postmitotic and postmigratory cells participate in this primordial organization. The determinants of this map and their antecedents in development are unknown. To some extent single neurons or even microcircuits appear to be interchangeable between mapped domains (Frost, 1988; O'Leary, 1992; O'Leary et al., 1992). No experimental manipulations have been discovered that can rearrange the topology of the intact map. However, selective ablations of the subplate during early phases of cortical histogenesis appear also to ablate secondarily corresponding portions of the overlying map (Ghosh et al., 1990).

The subplate appears to act as a way station for ingrowing thalamic afferents. Axons from the thalamus of cats and primates arrive in the cortex long before their final target neurons in cortical layer 4 have been delivered to the cortical plate. During the intervening period, which lasts for weeks in the cat and months in the primate, the axons appear to "wait" within the subplate, where they establish functional synaptic contacts with subplate neurons (Chun and Shatz, 1988b; Chun and Shatz, 1989a; Friauf et al., 1990; Friauf and Shatz, 1991; Herrmann et al., 1991; Kostovic and Rakic, 1980; Wahle and Meyer, 1987). The arrival of layer 4 neurons within the cortical plate is closely followed by the ingrowth of the thalamic axons into this layer; subsequently, the vast majority of subplate neurons are eliminated by cell death (Chun et al., 1987; Chun and Shatz, 1989b; Kostovic and Rakic, 1980; Valverde and Facal-Valverde, 1987; Wahle and Meyer, 1987; Woo et al., 1990). The subplate appears to play an essential role in establishing the normal topography of thalamocortical projections.

Portions of the map can, of course, be destroyed outright. Injection of the neurotoxin kainic acid has been used to ablate selectively subplate neurons during the waiting period in which thalamic axons are arriving in the subplate. Following the loss of subplate neurons, thalamic axons fail to invade their normal cortical target, instead growing past the appropriate area into regions of white matter that they would normally have failed to encounter (Ghosh et al., 1990; Ghosh and Shatz, 1992). These observations are consistent with the hypothesis that there is topographic information present within the subplate; how the subplate may have acquired this information, however, is not yet understood. The architectonic character of cortex may be further modified, or local circuit properties may be altered, by disruption of normal patterns of afferent activity (Hubel et al., 1977; Purves, 1988; Rakic, 1977).

The experimental perspective relating to normal and pathologic development thus informs us that the critical choices available to the postmigratory cell are substantially imposed by the cell environment. The cell increases massively in size, and its shape evolves dramatically as the axonal arbor establishes synaptic contact with targets and as its dendritic and somatic surfaces synaptically engage converging axons. Powerful constraints, probably in the form of both diffusible and cell surface–fixed molecular tropic cues, act to determine the pattern of deployment of these effector and receptor surfaces of the cell (Fischbach, 1992; Koester and O'Leary, 1992; O'Leary, 1992; Shatz, 1992). These factors may differ in kind and distribution as they act upon initial, or "pioneer," process deployment and as they ensure the subsequent deployment of follower processes (Ghosh and Shatz, 1992; McConnell, 1989b).

It appears to be a general property of assembling neural systems that an initial exuberant surge of process elaboration and synaptogenesis is succeeded by a regression in this deployment (Huttenlocher et al., 1982; Innocenti, 1991; O'Leary, 1992; Oppenheim, 1991; Purves, 1988). The regression is expressed not only in the classes of interconnected structures (i.e., the central nodes of the wiring diagram), but also in the patterns of cell survival and synapses. As such, this process exercises decisive control over the final density and topology of synaptic placement on the surfaces of surviving cells. The overall "stepdown" in cellular and synaptic elements in the fulfillment of these regressive processes typically attains 50 percent of the starting number (Finlay et al., 1986; Huttenlocher et al., 1982; Oppenheim, 1991).

Changing Patterns of Gene Expression Define Distinct Stages of Neuron Differentiation

Neuronal migration is one step in a program of neuronal differentiation, a step that takes the young neuron through a matrix of epigenetic cues that signal specific stages of development. Using the cerebellar system as a model to identify markers for cells in different stages of neuronal development, Hatten and colleagues constructed cDNA expression libraries from immature granule cells, purified from mouse cerebellum on postnatal days 3–5 (Hatten, 1985), and used novel antibody screening methods to identify cDNA clones that mark specific stages of granule neuron differentiation (Kuhar et al., 1993). Northern blot analysis of poly(A+) RNA purified from various brain regions and developmental stages revealed that of 34 clones analyzed, all were expressed at high levels in cerebellum. Four of the clones were expressed at higher levels in the cerebellum and forebrain; three clones were detectable only in cerebellum. In situ analysis of the expression of developmentally regulated clones in cerebellar tissue at postnatal day 8 offered the opportunity to visualize individual cells in each of the stages of granule neuron development. As shown in Figure 4-5, a restricted pattern of expression was observed for 8 clones, suggesting that different cDNAs were expressed at different stages of granule neuron differentiation (Kuhar et al., 1993). The program of gene expression in cerebellar granule cells revealed in this analysis demonstrates that there are at least four distinct stages of granule cell differentiation. Further analysis of the regulation of these novel cDNAs should allow the identification of the epigenetic signals for granule neuron differentiation. In particular, they should allow the identification of

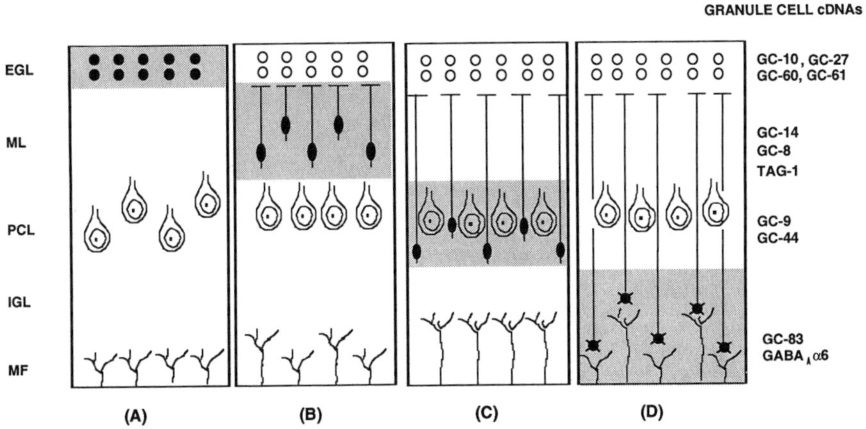

GRANULE CELL cDNAs

EGL

ML

PCL

IGL

MF

GC-10, GC-27
GC-60, GC-61

GC-14
GC-8
TAG-1

GC-9
GC-44

GC-83
GABA$_A$ α6

(A)   (B)   (C)   (D)

Figure 4-5. Changing patterns of gene expression define four stages of granule neuron development. In situ hybridization analysis of the pattern of expression of cDNAs expressed in granule cells during development indicates a discrete pattern of localization for four classes of cDNAs. (A) At postnatal day 7, GC-10, GC-27, GC-60, and GC-61 mRNA are localized to proliferating granule cells in the superficial layer of the EGL (solid circles in shaded zone). (B) GC-1, GC-8, and TAG-1 mRNA are localized to postmitotic and migrating granule cells at the internal surface of the EGL and in the molecular layer, respectively (solid circles in shaded zone). (C) GC-9 and GC-44 mRNA are both localized to a previously undescribed transient layer of granule cells (solid circles in shaded zone) terminating migration just below the Purkinje cell bodies. (D) mRNAs, for GC83 and for the α6 subunit of the GABA$_A$ receptor are localized in the IGL. In situ hybridizations were performed as described for the Genius system (Boehringer-Mannheim) and processed for colorimetric detection using NBT and X-phosphate (Kuhar et al., 1993). Ingrowing afferent axons, the mossy fibers, are shown at the bottom of each panel. (For details, see Kuhar et al., 1993.)

membrane-associated signals that regulate precursor cell proliferation and induce neuronal differentiation (Gao, Heintz, Hatten, 1991; Gao et al., 1992) and of transcription factors that regulate the expression genes at specific stages of granule neuron differentiation.

Synaptic Activity Regulates Differentiation

The potentials for growth and differentiation inherent in each neuron are modulated by the full set of converging influences that constitute the cells' environment. These modulating forces play a role in determining which elements will persist, and they regulate the functional state of the emerging network. The seemingly infinite flexibility offered by such modulation may be essential to optimize the cellular composition and the dynamic information-processing properties of neural systems. Thus even at the ultimate level of resolution of the individual synapse, the issue of the appropriateness of its persistence appears to be determined by the presence or absence of corollary discharge. Specific transmitter–receptor interactions, for example, those driven by the NMDA receptor, appear to play a central role in this "strategic" secondary reorganization of the developing nervous system in the course of histogenesis (Constantine-Patton et al., 1990). Similar mechanisms mediated by trophic factors that act via cell surface receptors coupled to G protein systems complement the voltage-dependent systems related directly to neural activity. Both classes of modulatory systems appear continually to refine the synaptic composition of neural systems (see Swann, Chapter 8).

The Visible and Invisible Worlds of Biology in the Developing Epileptic Brain

The distinctive seizure phenomena by which epileptic disorders are characterized are readily observable by the clinician. The pathoanatomic correlates so far revealed in postmortem specimens of representative cases also represent abnormalities that have actually been observed, albeit within the relatively insensitive limits of routine pathologic analysis that are even further constrained by the exigencies of tissue sampling. This "visible world" of the clinician and pathologist describes the workings of neural systems, on the one hand, and the histologic outcome of a complex and extended developmental history on the other.

Neither this biology nor history is fully visible in the living human brain with epilepsy. Though seizures proceed in "real time," their most informative details are invisible within the realm of sensitivity of the available tools of clinical neurophysiology and imaging, and the initiating pathologic events of development that began in the fetus are no longer accessible. Since any abnormality seen by conventional histopathologic techniques is a marker for the molecular derangements that underlie the origin and propagation of the epileptic discharge, the current data leave ambiguous the specific relation of any given recognized histopathologic abnormality and the known basic mechanisms of seizure generation.

These visible and invisible worlds must therefore be spanned by conceptual bridges—that is, by extrapolation to experimental study in animals. Developmental models will need to be constructed that test the reference principles of developmental neurobiology derived from the types of experiments in cortical organization outlined in this chapter, and they must be compared with human disorders for a plausible fit to the available pathologic record. The general correlation between the gradient in severity of cerebral pathology and that of the age of onset of a seizure disorder—the severity of attack pattern and the gravity of its consequences for a normal behavioral repertoire—is readily predicted from the principles of developmental neurobiology. The transitional, exuberant developmental state of neural organization is exquisitely vulnerable to any structural or functional perturbation in the course of development. It is presumed that any pathologic process which intersects forebrain development with such force as to leave visible, macroscopic traces will wreak havoc with histogenetic phenomena. It is to be expected that the more cataclysmic the intrusion, the more salient the effect. Onslaughts suffered early should be expected to be more drastic in their effects than those suffered later. Thus the earlier the disruption occurs, the greater will be the expected consequences in terms of the roster of surviving neural elements and the epileptogenic potential of the nervous system.

Acknowledgments

The authors gratefully acknowledge the contributions of W.-Q. Gao, G. Fishell, S. Kuhar, L. Feng, and N. Heintz and the support of NIH grants NS 15429 and NS12005, and a grant from the PEW Neuroscience Program (M.E.H.).

References

Aicardi, J. (1986) *Epilepsy in Children.* New York: Raven Press.

Altman, J. (1972) Postnatal development of the cerebellar cortex in the rat: I. The external germinal layer and the transitional molecular layer. *J. Comp. Neurol. 145:*353–514.

Angevine, J. B., Jr., and Sidman, R. L. (1961) Autoradiographic study of cell migration during histogenesis of cerebral cortex in the mouse. *Nature 192:*766–768.

Austin, C. P., and Cepko, C. L. (1990) Cellular migration patterns in the developing mouse cerebral cortex. *Development 110:*713–732.

Caviness, V. S., Evrard, P., and Lyon, G. (1978) Radial neuronal assemblies, ectopia and necrosis of developing cortex: A case analysis. *Acta Neuropathol. 41:*67–72.

Caviness, V. S., and Williams, R. S. (1984) Cellular patterns in developmental malformations of neocortex: Neuron–glial interactions. In M. Arima, Y. Suzuki, and H. Yabuuchi (eds.), *The Developing Brain and Its Disorders.* Tokyo: University of Tokyo Press, pp. 43–67.

Caviness, V. S., Jr. (1976) The Chiari malformations of the posterior fossa and their relation to hydrocephalus. *Dev. Med. Child. Neurol. 18:*103–116.

Caviness, V. S., Jr. (1988) Architecture and development of the thalamocortical projection in the mouse. In M. Bentivoglio and R. Spreafico (eds.), *Cellular Thalamic Mechanisms.* Amsterdam: Elsevier Science Publishers, pp. 489–499.

Caviness, V. S., Jr., Misson, J.-P., and Gadisseux, J.-F. (1989) Abnormal neuronal patterns and disorders of neocortical development. In A. M. Galaburda (ed.), *From Reading to Neurons.* Cambridge, Mass.: MIT Press, pp. 405–439.

Caviness, V. S., Jr., Takahashi, T., and Nowakowski, R. S. (1991) Cytokinetic parameters of the ventricular zone in developing mouse neocortex. *Soc. Neurosci. Abstr. 17:*29.

Chun, J. J., Nakamura, M. J., and Shatz, C. J. (1987) Transient cells of the developing mammalian telencephalon are peptide-immunoreactive neurons. *Nature 325:*617–620.

Chun J. J. M., and Shatz, C. J. (1988a) A fibronectin-like molecule is present in the developing cat cerebral cortex and is correlated with subplate neurons. *J. Cell Biol. 106:*857–872.

Chun, J. J. M., and Shatz, C. J. (1988b) Redistribution of synaptic vesicle antigens is correlated with the disappearance of a transient synaptic zone in the developing cerebral cortex. *Neuron 1:*297–310.

Chun, J. J. M., and Shatz, C. J. (1989a) The earliest-generated neurons of the cat cerebral cortex: Characterization by MAP2 and neurotransmitter immunohistochemistry during fetal life. *J. Neurosci. 9:*1648–1667.

Chun, J. J. M., and Shatz, C. J. (1989b) Interstitial cells of the adult neocortical white matter are the remnant of the early generated subplate neuron population. *J. Comp. Neurol. 282:*555–556.

Constantine-Patton, M., Cline, H. T., and Debski, E. (1990) Patterned activity, synaptic convergence, and the NMDA receptor in developing visual pathways. In W. M. Cowan, E. M. Shooter, C. F. Stevens, and R. F. Thompson (eds.), *Annual Review of Neuroscience.* Palo Alto, Calif.: Annual Reviews, pp. 129–154.

Crandall, J. E., and Caviness, V. S., Jr. (1984) Thalamocortical connections in newborn mice. *J. Comp. Neurol. 228:*542–556.

Dobyns, W. B. (1987) Developmental aspects of lissencephaly and the lissencephaly syndromes. *Birth Defects 23:*225–241.

Dobyns, W. B., Stratton, R. F., Parke, J. T., Greenberg, F., Nussbaum, R. L., and Ledbetter, D. H. (1983) Miller-Dieker syndrome: Lissencephaly and monosomy 17p. *J. Pediatr. 102:*552–558.

Edmondson, J. C., and Hatten, M. E. (1987) Glial-guided granule neuron migration in vitro: A high-resolution time-lapse video microscopic study. *J. Neurosci. 7:*1928–1934.

Edmondson, J. C., Liem, R. K. H., Kuster, J. E., and Hatten, M. E. (1988) Astrotactin, a novel cell surface antigen that mediates neuron–glia interactions in cerebellar microcultures. *J. Cell Biol. 106:*505–517.

Finlay, B. L., Sengelaub, D. R., and Berian, C. A. (1986) Control of cell number in the developing visual system: I. Effects of monocular enucleation. *Dev. Brain Res. 28:*1–10.

Fischbach, G. D. (1992) Mind and brain. *Sci. Am. 267:*48–57.

Fishell, G., and Hatten, M. E. (1991) Astrotactin provides a receptor system for CNS neuronal migration. *Development 113:*755–765.

Fishell, G., Mason, C. A., and Hatten, M. E. (1992) Lateral dispersion of premigratory, neural progenitors within the ventricular zone of cerebral cortex. *Soc. Neurosci. Abstr. 18:*926.

Friauf, E., McConnell, S. K., and Shatz, C. J. (1990) Functional circuits in the subplate during fetal and early postnatal development of cat visual cortex. *J. Neurosci. 10:*2601–2613.

Friauf, E., and Shatz, C. J. (1991) Changing patterns of synaptic input to subplate and cortical plate during development of visual cortex. *J. Neurophysiol. 6:*2059–2071.

Friede, R. L. (1989) *Developmental Neuropathology,* 2nd ed. New York: Springer-Verlag.

Frost, D. O. (1988) Mechanisms of structural and functional development in the thalamus: Retinal projections to the auditory and somatosensory systems in normal and experimentally manipulated hamsters. In M. Bentivoglio and R. Spreafico (eds.), *Cellular Thalamic Mechanisms.* Amsterdam: Elsevier Scientific Publishers, pp. 447–464.

Fugita, S. (1967) Quantitative analysis of cell proliferation and differentiation in the cortex of the postnatal mouse cerebellum. *J. Cell Biol. 32:*277–287.

Fugita, S., Shimada, M., and Nakanuna, T. (1966) ³H-thymidine autoradiographic studies on the cell proliferation and differentiation in the external and internal granular layers of the mouse cerebellum. *J. Comp. Neurol. 128:*191–209.

Furley, A. J., Morton, S. B., Manalo, D., Karagogeos, D., Dodd, J., and Jessell, T. M. (1990) The axonal glycoprotein TAG-1 is an immunoglobulin superfamily member with neurite outgrowth-promoting activity. *Cell 61:*157–170.

Galaburda, A. M., and Kemper, T. L. (1979) Cytoarchitectonic abnormalities in developmental dyslexia: A case study. *Ann. Neurol. 6:*94–100.

Gao, W.-Q., Heintz, N., and Hatten, M. E. (1991). Cerebellar granule cell neurogenesis is regulated by cell–cell interactions in vitro. *Neuron 6:*705–715.

Gao, W.-Q., Liu, X.-L., and Hatten, M. E. (1991) The weaver gene acts non-autonomously in granule neuron differentiation in vitro. *Soc. Neurosci. Abstr. 17:*533.

Gao, W.-Q., Liu, X.-L., and Hatten, M. E. (1992) The weaver gene encodes a nonautonomous signal for CNS neuronal differentiation. *Cell 68:*841–854.

Gasser, U. E., and Hatten, M. E. (1990) CNS neurons migrate on astroglial fibers from heterotypic brain regions in vitro. *Proc. Natl. Acad. Sci. 87:*4543–4547.

Ghosh, A., Antonini, A., McConnell, S. K., and Shatz, C. J. (1990) Requirement for subplate neurons in the formation of thalamocortical connections. *Nature 347:*179–181.

Ghosh, A., and Shatz, C. J. (1992) Pathfinding and target selection by developing geniculocortical axons. *J. Neurosci. 12:*39–55.

Gilles, F. H., Leviton, A., and Dooling, E. C. (1983) *The Developing Human Brain.* Boston: John Wright, PSG.

Gillies, K., and Price, D. J. (1993) The fates of cells in the developing cerebral cortex of normal and methylazoxymethanol acetate-lesioned mice. *Eur. J. Neurosci. 5:*73–84.

Gregory, W. A., Edmondson, J. C., Hatten, M. E., and Mason, C. A. (1988) Cytology and neuron-glial apposition of migrating cerebellar granule cells in vitro. *J. Neurosci. 8:*1728–1738.

Hatten, M. E. (1985) Neuronal regulation of astroglial morphology and proliferation in vitro. *J. Cell Biol. 100:*384–396.

Hatten, M. E. (1987) Neuronal regulation of astroglial proliferation is membrane-mediated. *J. Cell Biol. 104:*1353–1360.

Hatten, M. E. (1990) Riding the glial monorail: A common mechanism for glial-guided migration in different regions of the developing brain. *Trends Neurosci. 13:*179–187.

Hatten, M. E., Liem, R. K. H., and Mason, C. A. (1983) Defects in specific associations between astroglia and neurons occur in microcultures of weaver mouse cerebellar cells. *J. Neurosci. 4:*1163–1172.

Hatten, M. E., Liem, R. K. H., and Mason, C. A. (1986) Weaver mouse cerebellar granule neurons fail to migrate on wild-type astroglial processes in vitro. *J. Neurosci. 9:*2676–2683.

Hatten, M. E., and Sidman, R. L. (1978) Cell reassociation behavior and lectin-induced agglutination of embryonic mouse cells in different brain regions. *Exp. Cell Res. 113:*111–125.

Herrmann, K., Antonini, A., and Shatz, C. J. (1991) Thalamic axons make synaptic contacts with subplate neurons. *Soc. Neurosci. Abstr. 17:*899.

His, W. (1889) Die Neuroblasten und deren Entstehung im embryonalen Mark. *Abh. Math. Phys. CC. Kql. Sächs. Ges. Wiss. 15:*313–372.

Hubel, D. H., Wiesel, T. N., and LeVay, S. (1977) Plasticity of ocular dominance columns in monkey striate cortex. *Phil. Trans. R. Soc. London B 278:*377–409.

Huttenlocher, P. R., de Courten C., Garey, L. J., and Van der Loos, H. (1982) Synaptogenesis in the human visual cortex: Evidence for synapse elimination during normal development. *Neurosci. Lett. 33:*247–252.

Innocenti, G. M. (1991) The development of projections from cerebral cortex. *Prog. Sens. Physiol. 12:*65–114.

Jackson C. A., Peduzzi, J. D., and Hickey, T. L. (1989) Visual cortex development in the ferret: I. Genesis and migration of visual cortical neurons. *J. Neurosci. 9:*1242–1253.

Kaplan, M. P., Chin, S. S. M., Fliegner, K. H., and Liem, R. K. H. (1990) Alpha internexin, a novel neuronal intermediate filament protein, precedes the low molecular weight neurofilament protein (NF-L) in the developing rat brain. *J. Neurosci. 10:*2735–2748.

Kim, G. J., Shatz, C. J., and McConnell, S. K. (1991) Morphology of pioneer and follower growth cones in the developing cerebral cortex. *J. Neurobiol. 22:*629–642.

Koester, S. E., and O'Leary, D. D. (1992) Functional classes of cortical projection neurons develop dendritic distinctions by class-specific sculpting of an early common pattern. *J. Neurosci. 12:*1382–1392.

Kostovic, I., and Rakic, P. (1980) Cytology and time of origin of interstitial neurons in the white matter in infant and adult human and monkey telencephalon. *J. Neurocytol. 9:*219–242.

Kuhar, S., Feng, L., Vidan, S., Ross, E. R., Hatten, M. E., and Heintz, N. (1993) Developmentally regulated cDNAs define four stages of cerebellar granule neuron differentiation. *Development 112:*97–104.

Lemire, R. J., Loeser J. D., Leech, R. W., and Alvord, E. C., Jr. (1975) *Normal and Abnormal Development of the Human Nervous System.* Hagerstown, Md.: Harper and Row.

Lennox, W. G. (1969) *Epilepsy and Related Disorders.* Boston: Little, Brown.

Luskin, M. B., Pearlman, A. L., and Sanes, J. R. (1988) Cell lineage in the cerebral cortex of the mouse studied in vivo and in vitro with a recombinant retrovirus. *Neuron 1:*635–647.

Luskin M. B., and Shatz, C. J. (1985a) Neurogenesis of the cat's primary visual cortex. *J. Comp. Neurol. 242:*611–631.

Luskin, M. B., and Shatz, C. J. (1985b) Studies of the earliest generated cells of the cat's visual cortex: Cogeneration of subplate and marginal zones. *J. Neurosci. 5:*1062–1075.

Marin-Padilla, M. (1971) Early prenatal ontogenesis of the cerebral cortex (neocortex) of the cat *(Felis domestica).* A Golgi study: I. The primordial neocortical organization. *Z. Anat. Entwicklungsgesch. 134:*117–145.

Marin-Padilla, M. (1978) Clinical and experimental rachischisis. In P. J. Vinken and G. W. Bruyn (eds.), *Congenital Malformations of the Spine and Spinal Cord.* Amsterdam: North-Holland, pp. 159–191.

McConnell, S. K. (1988a) Development and decision-making in the mammalian cerebral cortex. *Brain Res. Rev. 13:*1–23.

McConnell, S. K. (1988b) Fates of visual cortical neurons in the ferret after isochronic and heterochronic transplantation. *J. Neurosci. 8:*945–974.

McConnell, S. K. (1989a) The determination of neuronal fate in the cerebral cortex. *Trends Neurosci. 12:*342–349.

McConnell, S. K. (1989b) Subplate neurons pioneer the first axon pathway from the cortex. *Science 245:*978–982.

McConnell, S. K. (1991) The generation of neuronal diversity in the central nervous system. In W. M. Cowan, E. M. Shooter, C. F. Stevens, and R. F. Thompson (eds.), *Annual Review of Neuroscience*. Palo Alto, Calif.: Annual Reviews, pp. 269–300.

McConnell, S. K., Ghosh, A., and Shatz, C. J. (1993) Subplate pioneers and the formation of descending connections from cerebral cortex. *J. Neurosci. 14:*1892–1907.

McConnell, S. K., and Kaznowski, C. E. (1991) Cell cycle dependence of laminar determination in developing neocortex. *Science 254:*282–285.

Meencke, H.-J. (1985) Neuron density in the molecular layer of the frontal cortex in primary generalized epilepsy. *Epilepsia 26:*450–454.

Meencke, H.-J. (1989) Pathology of childhood epilepsies. *Cleveland Clin. J. Med. 56* (Suppl., Part 1):111–120.

Miale, I., and Sidman, R. L. (1961) An autoradiographic analysis of histogenesis in the mouse cerebellum. *Expl. Neurology 4:*277–296.

Misson, J.-P., Austin, C. P., Takahashi, T., Cepko, C. L., and Caviness, V. S., Jr. (1991) The alignment of migrating neuronal cells in relation to the murine neopallial radial glial fiber system. *Cereb. Cortex 1:*221–229.

Misson, J.-P., Takahashi, T., and Caviness, V. S., Jr. (1991) Ontogeny of radial and other astroglial cells in murine cerebral cortex. *Glia 4:*138–148.

O'Leary, D. D. (1992) Development of connectional diversity and specificity in the mammalian brain by the pruning of collateral projections. *Curr. Opin. Neurobiol. 2:*70–77.

O'Leary, D. D., Schlaggar, B. L., and Stanfield, B. B. (1992) The specification of sensory cortex: Lessons from cortical transplantation. *Exp. Neurol. 115:*121–126.

O'Leary, D. D. M., and Bomgasser, N. N. L. (1992) Minimal dispersion of neuroepithelial cells and their progeny during generation of the cortical preplate. *Soc. Neurosci. Abstr. 18:*925.

Oppenheim, R. W. (1991) Cell death during development of the nervous system. In W. M. Cowan, E. M. Shooter, C. F. Stevens, and R. F. Thompson (eds.), *Annual Review of Neuroscience*. Palo Alto, Calif.: Annual Reviews, pp. 453–501.

O'Rourke, N. A., Dailey, M. E., Smith, S. J., and McConnell, S. K. (1992) Diverse migratory pathways in the developing cerebral cortex. *Science 258:*299–302.

Pinto-Lord, M. C., Evrard, P., and Caviness, V. S. (1982) Obstructed neuronal migration along radial glial fibers in the neocortex of the reeler mouse: A Golgi-EM analysis. *Dev. Brain Res. 4:*379–393.

Price, J., and Thurlow, L. (1988) Cell lineage in the rat cerebral cortex: A study using retrovirus-mediated gene transfer. *Development 104:*473–482.

Purves, D. (1988) *Body and Brain*. Cambridge, Mass: Harvard University Press.

Rakic, P. (1971a) Guidance of neurons migrating to the fetal monkey neocortex. *Brain Res. 33:*471–476.

Rakic, P. (1971b) Neuron–glia relationship during granule cell migration in developing cerebellar cortex: A golgi and electronmicroscopic study in Macacus Rhesus. *J. Comp. Neurol. 141:*283–312.

Rakic, P. (1972) Mode of cell migration to the superficial layers of fetal monkey neocortex. *J. Comp. Neurol. 145:*61–84.

Rakic, P. (1974) Neurons in the rhesus monkey visual cortex: Systematic relationship between time of origin and eventual disposition. *Science 183*:425–427.

Rakic, P. (1977) Prenatal development of the visual system in rhesus monkey. *Phil. Trans. R. Soc. London B 278*:245–260.

Rakic, P. (1978) Neuronal migration and contact guidance in the primate telencephalon. *Postgrad. Med. J. 54*:25–40.

Rakic, P. (1988a) Defects of neuronal migration and the pathogenesis of cortical malformations. *Prog. Brain Res. 73*:15–37.

Rakic, P. (1988b) Specification of cerebral cortical areas. *Science 241*:170–176.

Rakic, P. (1990) Principles of neural cell migration. *Experientia 46*:882–891.

Rakic, P., and Sidman, R. L. (1973) Sequence of developmental abnormalities leading to granule cell deficit in cerebellar cortex of weaver mutant mice. *J. Comp. Neurol. 152*:103–132.

Rakic, P., Stensaas, L. J., Sayer, E. P., and Sidman, R. L. (1974) Computer aided three-dimensional reconstruction and quantitative analysis of cells from serial electron microscopic montage of foetal monkey brain. *Nature 250*: 31–34.

Ramón y Cajal, S. (1911) *Histologie du Système Nerveux de l'Homme et des Vertebres.* Paris: Maloine; reprint, Madrid: Consejo Superior de Investigaciones Cientificas, 1955.

Reh, T. A., and Tully, T. (1986) Regulation of tyrosine-hydroxylase-containing amacrine cell number in the larval frog retina. *Dev. Biol. 114*:463–469.

Rezai, Z., and Yoon, C. H. (1972) Abnormal rate of granule cell migration in cerebellum of "weaver" mutant mice. *Dev. Biol. 29*:17–26.

Roger, J., Dravet, C., Bureau, M., Dreifuss, F. F., and Wolf, P. (1984) *Les Syndromes Épileptiques de l'Enfant et de l'Adolescent.* Paris: John Libbey.

Sauer, F. C. (1936) The interkinetic migration of embryonic epithelial nuclei. *J. Morphol. 60*:1–11.

Schwartz, M. L., and Meencke, D. L. (1992) Early expression of GABA-containing neurons in the prefrontal and visual cortices of rhesus monkeys. *Cereb. Cortex 2*:16–37.

Schwartz, M. L., Rakic, P., and Goldman-Rakic, P. S. (1991) Early phenotype expression of cortical neurons: Evidence that a subclass of migrating neurons have callosal axons. *Proc. Natl. Acad. Sci. 88*:1354–1358.

Shatz, C. J. (1992) The developing brain. *Sci. Am. 267*:60–67.

Sheppard, A. M., Hamilton, S. K., and Pearlman, A. L. (1991) Changes in the distribution of extracellular matrix components accompany early morphogenetic events of mammalian cortical development. *J. Neurosci. 11*:3928–3942.

Sherman, G. F., Rosen, G. D., and Galaburda, A. M. (1989) Animal models of developmental dyslexia: Brain lateralization and cortical pathology. In A. M. Galaburda (ed.), *From Reading to Neurons.* Cambridge, Mass.: MIT Press.

Sidman, R. L., and Rakic, P. (1973) Neuronal migration with special reference to developing human brain: A review. *Brain Res. 62*:1–35.

Sidman, R. L., and Rakic, P. (1982) Development of the human central nervous system. In W. Haymaker and R. D. Adams (eds.), *Histology and Histopathology of the Nervous System.* Springfield, Ill.: Charles C Thomas, pp. 3–145.

Sotelo, C., and Changeux, P. (1974) Bergmann fibers and granule cell migration in the cerebellum of homozygous weaver mutant mouse. *Brain Res. 77*:484–491.

Stewart, G. R., and Pearlman, A. L. (1987) Fibronectin-like immunoreactivity in the developing cerebral cortex. *J. Neurosci. 7*:3325–3333.

Stitt, T. N., and Hatten, M. E. (1990) Antibodies that recognize astrotactin block granule neuron binding to astroglia. *Neuron 5:*639–649.

Takahashi, T., Nowakowski, R. S., and Caviness, V. S., Jr. (1991) Cell output of the ventricular zone of the E14 mouse neocortex. *Soc. Neurosci. Abstr. 17:*29.

Takahashi, T., Nowakowski, R. S., and Caviness, V. S., Jr. (1992) Cytogenesis in the secondary proliferative population of the murine cerebral wall. *Soc. Neurosci. Abstr. 18:*30.

Takahashi, T., Nowakowski, R. S., and Caviness, V. S., Jr. (1993) Cell cycle parameters and patterns of nuclear movement in the neocortical proliferative zone of the fetal mouse. *J. Neurosci. 13:*820–833.

Takahashi, T., Nowakowski, R. S., and Caviness, V. S., Jr. (1994) Mode of cell proliferation in the developing mouse neocortex. *Proc. Natl. Acad. Sci. 91:*375–379.

Valverde, F., and Facal-Valverde, M. V. (1987) Transitory population of cells in the temporal cortex of kittens. *Dev. Brain Res. 32:*283–288.

Viani, F., Strada, G. P., Riboldi, A., Manghi, E., Rossotti V., and Allegranza, A. (1977) Aspetti neuropathologici della sindrome di Lennox-Gastaut: Considerazioni su tre casi. *Rev. Neurol. 47:*1–35.

Waechter, R. V., and Jaensch, B. (1972) Generation times of the matrix cells during embryonic brain development: An autoradiographic study in rats. *Brain Res. 46:*235–250.

Wahle, P., and Meyer, G. (1987) Morphology and quantitative changes of transient NPY-ir neuronal populations during early postnatal development of the cat visual cortex. *J. Comp. Neurol. 161:*165–192.

Walsh, C., and Cepko, C. L. (1988) Clonally related cortical cells show several migration patterns. *Science 242:*1342–1345.

Walsh, C., and Cepko, C. L. (1990) Cell lineage and cell migration in the developing cerebral cortex. *Experientia 46:*940–947.

Walsh, C., and Cepko, C. (1992) Generation of widespread cerebral cortical clones. *Soc. Neurosci. Abstr. 18:*925.

Walsh, C., and Cepko, C. L. (1992) Widespread dispersion of neuronal clones across functional regions of the cerebral cortex. *Science 255:*434–440.

Woo, T. U., Beale, J. M., and Finlay, B. L. (1990) Dual fate of subplate neurons in the rodent. *Soc. Neurosci. Abstr. 16:*836.

5

Neuronal Identity, Neuronal Migration, and Epileptic Disorders of the Cerebral Cortex

CHRISTOPHER A. WALSH

For most of the twentieth century there has been an appreciation that brains of some epileptics show developmental abnormalities (Alzheimer, 1907). However, the relationship between abnormalities of cortical development and epilepsy has remained controversial, in part because normal brains occasionally show developmental abnormalities and in part because epileptic tissue is not characterized by consistent pathology. Whereas there are severe forms of cortical malformation that are very frequently associated with epilepsy, the relationship between more subtle disorders of the cortex and epilepsy has been less certain. Recently an experimental framework based on investigation from human neuropathology, molecular genetics, and developmental biology has begun to provide a broad context for interrelating human cortical development with epilepsy. In addition, the application of improved clinical imaging and electrophysiologic techniques is generating new evidence to relate specific cellular disturbances to defined pediatric epilepsy syndromes. This chapter summarizes these recent developments, many of which are also discussed in Chapter 4.

Developmental Disturbances in Epileptic Brains

Disturbances of cerebral cortical development are frequent findings in epileptic brains, especially in the most severe pediatric epilepsy syndromes that start at early ages. Postmortem studies of epileptic brains have allowed the broadest study of cortical structure but have the potential drawback that detailed knowledge of the seizure type and the brain region affected is often limited. In infantile spasms, perhaps the most severe type of childhood epilepsy (see Chapters 1 and 4), about half of epileptic brains show structural abnormalities suggestive of developmental disturbances of cortical development (Meencke and Gerhard, 1985). Brains of children with milder forms of epilepsy also display developmental abnormalities, but at a lower frequency and generally lesser severity. Thus childhood absence epilepsy, Lennox-Gastaut syndrome (Meencke, 1989), and primary generalized epilepsy (Meencke, 1985) are characterized by developmental abnormalities in 15–20 percent of autopsy cases. The interpretation of apparent developmental disturbances in epileptic brains is complicated by the relatively frequent finding of similar mild disturbances in nonepileptic brains (Lyon and Gastaut, 1985; Meencke and Veith, 1992). Therefore, careful quantitative evaluation is important. According to Mennecke and Veith (1992), the incidence of pathological findings is five- to tenfold higher in epileptic brains than in normals, consistent with a specific association between developmental disturbances and pediatric epilepsy syndromes.

The relation of developmental disturbances to seizures is strengthened by the frequent finding of developmental abnormalities in brain tissue that is surgically removed for treatment of epilepsy. In the last several decades, localized removal of regions of cerebral cortex has become routine in the treatment of severe intractable epilepsy at specialized epilepsy surgery centers. Epileptic foci are carefully mapped using EEG (Andermann et al., 1987) or CT or MRI scanning; more recently, PET (Chugani et al., 1990) and SPECT analyses (Harvey et al., 1993) have been used. In several large surgical studies, removal of the brain tissue has been correlated with reduction in electrophysiologic abnormalities and in seizure frequency (Robitaille et al., 1992), suggesting that the removed surgical tissue was epileptogenic. Surgical studies of epilepsy pathology thus have the advantage that resected cortical tissue is more easily correlated with known epileptic activity; however, histological analysis is generally more limited in surgical studies than in postmortem analysis. The incidence of developmental abnormalities in resected epileptic cortex parallels results from postmortem studies; developmental abnormalities are seen most commonly in tissue removed in severe pediatric epilepsy syndromes. In one study of brain tissue removed for treatment of symptomatic infantile spasms (see Chapters 1 and 3) 9 of 13 cases showed cortical malformation or dysplasia (Vinters et al., 1992). In another study, about half the cases of intractable childhood epilepsy of diverse types (Farrell et al., 1992) were associated with cortical dysplasia, heterotopic neurons, or gyral abnormalities. In seizure disorders originating from the temporal lobe, 42 percent of specimens showed developmental abnormalities; no comparable abnormalities were seen in control specimens (Hardiman et al., 1988). The specific histological changes reported in epileptic brains are surprisingly variable, however, and are discussed later.

Therefore, several lines of evidence suggest that developmental disturbances of the cortex are associated with epileptic foci. But of course, not all humans with inferred developmental disturbances of the cortex have epilepsy. Furthermore, dramatic disturbances in neocortical development in the mutant mouse *reeler* (Caviness, 1982) and experimentally induced cortical migrational disturbances (Rosen et al., 1992) are not associated with epilepsy. Thus, while disordered cortical development and epilepsy are connected, the association is not invariant, and the mechanistic relationships between the two are not well understood. What are the possible cause–effect relationships between the two? A review of recent data about cortical development may provide a perspective to approach this question.

Formation and Radial Migration of Cortical Neurons

Neurons of the cortex are formed in specific proliferative zones located deep in the brain—far from where they reside in the adult brain. Cortical neurons are produced by sequential division of progenitor cells, in regions known as the ventricular zone and the subventricular zone (Boulder-Committee, 1970). As the first cortical neurons are formed, they migrate only a short distance from the proliferative zones and then differentiate to form an initial cortical organization termed the "primitive plexiform layer" (Marin-Padilla, 1978), or "preplate" (Allendorfer and Shatz, 1994). Neurons in the preplate show precocious morphological (Marin-Padilla, 1971) and neurochemical development (Chun et al., 1987), and they may form a scaffolding for development of later born neurons (Allendorfer and Shatz, 1994).

After formation of the preplate, later born cortical neurons show a different pattern of migration. Neurons destined for layers II–VI of the mature cortex migrate radially from the proliferative zones and settle into the middle of the preplate. The progressive accumulation of immature neurons, forming the cortical plate, divides the preplate into two layers. The outer layer differentiates into layer I of the mature cortex, while the deeper layer forms the subplate (Allendoerfer and Shatz, 1994). Subplate cells become highly differentiated during embryonic development and form widespread connections (Allendoerfer and Shatz, 1994). At later stages subplate cells (as well as some layer I cells) regress, and they may die as cells from the cortical plate mature.

An important feature of cortical plate development is that neurons in the cortical plate (that give rise to layers II–VI of the adult structure) are generated in a stereotyped sequence. Cells destined for layers VI, V, IV, III, and II are generated in rough sequence, and each new cohort of neurons migrates past older neurons, producing an "inside-out" pattern of cortical generation (Berry and Rogers, 1965). Cortical plate development also differs from development of the preplate in that preplate cells differentiate relatively close to the proliferative zones. Cortical plate cells must migrate from where they become postmitotic to where they differentiate.

Morphological studies originally suggested that migration from the proliferative zones to the cortical plate is guided by long, radially oriented glial fibers (Rakic, 1972). These unique cells have somata in the proliferative layers and long processes that stretch to the pial surface. Elongated cells, presumably migrating cortical neurons, were observed to be closely apposed to these radial glial cells. Not all immature migrating cortical cells, however, are in contact with radial glial cells (Shoukimas and Hinds, 1978). Furthermore, complete three-dimensional reconstructions of immature cortical cells have shown that some presumably migrating cells contact multiple radial glial fibers, suggesting that migrating cells might not follow one single radial glial fiber faithfully (Rakic et al., 1974). Radial glial–guided migration has since been studied directly using time-lapse video in dissociated single cells (Edmondson and Hatten, 1987) and in tissue slices (O'Rourke et al., 1992), confirming the importance of radial glia in guiding cortical neurons.

Radial glial–guided migration provides a potential mechanism that could sort cortical cells in clonal fashion, with the daughters of different progenitor cells being kept separate on their route to the cortex (Rakic, 1978, 1988b). In principle, such a model, referred to as the *radial unit hypothesis* (Rakic, 1988b), could produce a cortical structure in which clonally related sibling cells formed tight, functionally related clusters in the adult cerebral cortex. However, for such clonal sorting to occur, several conditions must be met in addition to radial glia acting as guides for migrating cortical cells. Clonal sorting would require that progenitor cells that generate a clone of cortical cells remain fixed with respect to a single glial fascicle, generating serial progeny that migrate to the same region of cortex. Moreover, clonal sorting would require not only that cortical neurons follow radial glia, but that serial daughter cells of a common progenitor follow the same radial glial fascicle, all with a high degree of fidelity. Recent studies suggest that although radial glia are essential guides for cortical neuronal migration, not all of these conditions are met, producing substantial clonal intermingling in the developing cerebral cortex.

Radial and Nonradial Cell Migration Shown in the Cortex of Chimeric Mice

In addition to the radial migration of postmitotic cortical neurons, recent studies have revealed several nonradial modes of cell migration in the cortex. Initial evidence for nonradial migration came from studies of chimeric mice containing cells of two distinguishable species or strains. If cortical cells migrated strictly radially from the ventricular zone to the cortex, then such chimeras should contain columnar bands of cells of one type or the other. Studies from three labs all failed to find such a simple, columnar organization of cells of similar genotype (Crandall and Herrup, 1990; Fishell et al., 1990; Goldowitz, 1987). On the contrary, neurons in upper and deeper cortical layers in any given cortical zone tended to have distinct origins, suggesting that spatially restricted cortical domains are not clonally uniform.

A more recent study obtained slightly different results using a variant on the chimera approach (Tan and Breen, 1993), produced by a fortuitous insertion of a β-galactosidase transgene into the X chromosome. During development, one X chromosome is inactivated in cells of the female brain. The choice of which X chromosome is inactivated appears to be random but is subsequently inherited as cells divide. Therefore, the female brain constitutes a chimera of cells expressing one or the other X chromosome, and the β-galactosidase transgene allows cells expressing one X chromosome or the other to be distinguished. The β-galactosidase staining revealed some cortical regions that contained as much as 70 percent of one genotype and 30 percent of the other. Sharply bordering regions had opposite composition. This study provided support for the hypothesis that there are imperfect radial constraints on the migration of some cell types. However, since other cortical regions did not show such sharply divided clonal domains, this study also suggests the absence of constraints on other migrating cells. The identity and precise proportions of cortical cells that do and do not show radial constraints are not known; furthermore, it is not clear why these results differ from the earlier chimera studies.

Retrovirus Studies of Cell Lineage and Clonal Dispersion

Direct study of patterns of cell lineage in the cortex has been possible with the use of retroviral vectors (Sanes et al., 1986; Turner and Cepko, 1987). Retroviruses infect dividing cells, such that a DNA copy of the retroviral genome becomes integrated stably into the DNA of the infected cell; thus the retroviral tag is passed on to all the progeny of the originally infected cell in a simple, Mendelian fashion. Retroviral vectors that encode histochemical markers such as β-galactosidase allow clonal progeny to be visualized histochemically (Cepko et al,. 1993). The virus is injected into the developing brain of early embryos, where it infects dividing progenitor cells, and the development of the embryo is then allowed to proceed normally for various survival times. The animal is then sacrificed, and the brain is sectioned and stained to reveal the histochemical marker. Clonal patterns must be inferred from the patterns of distribution of histochemically labeled cells.

Early retroviral studies suggested that histochemically labeled cortical glial cells form tight clusters, whereas labeled cortical neurons frequently form loose clusters, suggesting that cortical sibling cells could be grouped spatially. However, there were conflicting interpretations about the degree of dispersion of clustered sibling neurons (Austin and Cepko, 1990; Luskin et al., 1988; Price and Thurlow, 1988; Walsh and Cepko, 1988), and it was not possible to demonstrate convincingly that all cortical clones formed clusters or whether some cortical clones might not be clustered (Walsh and Cepko, 1988). Differences of interpretation arose because retroviral vectors are unable to distinguish between histochemically labeled cells arising from different progenitors, and because the number of labeled clones in a given experiment cannot be strictly controlled or independently determined (Walsh and Cepko, 1990). Therefore, histochemically labeled cells from different clones might disperse widely or intermingle in patterns that would be undetectable.

Libraries of Retroviruses Reveal Clustered and Widespread Clonal Patterns

One attempt to define retrovirally labeled clones directly has used libraries of retroviral vectors (Fig. 5-1). Each member of a retroviral library is designed to carry a histochemical marker gene (to allow retrovirally labeled cells to be identified) as well as a distinct DNA "tag." The DNA tags can be amplified by using the polymerase chain reaction (PCR) to provide a DNA fingerprint that distinguishes labeled cells in one clone from labeled cells in another clone (Walsh and Cepko, 1992). Cortical progenitors are labeled by injecting the retroviral library into the brain of fetal rats. Depending on how many distinct members there are in the retroviral library used, distinct progenitor cells are most likely to be infected by retroviruses carrying different DNA fingerprints. Again rats are allowed to develop for variable periods of time (3 days or more) before the brains are removed and processed histochemically to identify the retrovirally labeled cells. Then, after the labeled cells are studied anatomically, the cells are physically removed from the tissue sections by a simple dissection procedure, dissolved in a protease solution, and processed for the PCR amplification, and the DNA tags are analyzed on agarose gels. Cells in each clone are uniquely marked regardless of patterns of migration or dispersion (Walsh and Cepko, 1992, 1993). Results from such experiments need to be carefully interpreted to avoid misinterpretation, which would arise from the coincidental infection of two different clones by retroviruses carrying the same DNA fingerprint (Walsh et al,. 1992). Moreover, major findings need to be confirmed by independent methods. However, this retroviral library approach has provided important insight into several different aspects of cortical development.

Retrovirally labeled clones can also be distinguished by virtue of the fact that the site of integration of a retrovirus varies from clone to clone. Whereas retroviral integration sites probably occur randomly throughout the genome, some research suggests a few hundred to a thousand preferred sites of integration (Goff, 1992; Sandmeyer et al., 1990). The retroviral integration site can be amplified and analyzed by using a variant of PCR called inverse PCR (Snyder et al., 1992; Walsh, 1994). However, inverse PCR does not appear to have sufficient sensitivity to reliably amplify single DNA molecules from histochemical preparations. Moreover, newer retroviral libraries can be designed which have essentially unlimited complexity (Walsh, 1994), containing thousands of distinct tags, so that retroviral libraries can (if

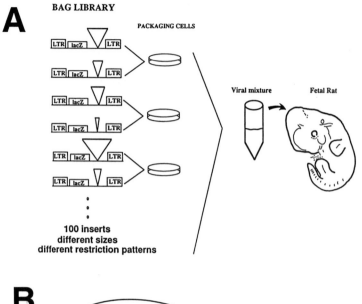

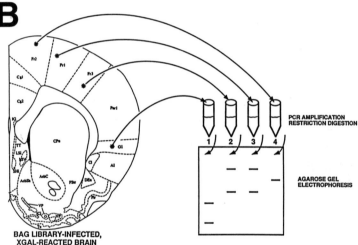

Figure 5-1. Construction and use of a retroviral library. Retroviral vectors encoding histochemical marker genes (in this case, the lacZ gene encoding β-galactosidase) are useful as lineage markers, since the histochemical marker is inherited in clonal fashion by the progeny of infected cells. Distinct clones can be differentiated by using a library of retroviral vectors.

(A) Construction of a retroviral library. In addition to the lacZ gene, each vector contains a short piece of DNA that is distinctive in either its size or DNA sequence. The DNA fragments serve as genetic "fingerprints." They can be distinguished by amplification of the DNA fingerprint even from single β-galactosidase-positive cells. The fingerprints are amplified by performing the polymerase chain reaction (PCR) using oligonucleotide primers that are complementary to DNA sequences in the viral "backbone" (arrowheads), so that one pair of primers amplifies all the fingerprints. The original retroviral library (BAG), shown here, contained 100 members, and pairs of retroviral constructs were transfected into viral "producer cells" pairwise, to produce 50 viral solutions that were then combined to generate the library. In more needed) exceed the number of preferred integration sites in the genome, providing the optimum ability to distinguish clonal relationships.

Recent studies of cell lineage in the rodent cortex using retroviral libraries have shown surprisingly complex patterns of cellular migration. For 3 days after retroviral labeling, most cells in cortical clones remain in the proliferative layers (VZ, SVZ). At these stages, clones contain up to four to five cells, and sibling cells are tightly clustered (Walsh and Cepko, 1993), confirming earlier reports with single retroviral markers (Austin and Cepko, 1990; Luskin et al., 1988; Walsh and Cepko, 1988). Even after an additional 3 days, approximately half the retrovirally labeled cortical clones still show tight clustering of sibling cells. However, the other half of the marked clones display very wide dispersion of clonally related cells across broad cortical regions. Some of this dispersion undoubtedly occurs within the proliferative zones, since sibling cells can be dispersed for several millimeters within these layers (Walsh and Cepko, 1993). Similar patterns of clonal clustering and clonal dispersion are found to persist during the early postnatal period and beyond. Among clones labeled at embryonic day 15 and analyzed perinatally (E21, or 3 days after birth), about half of cortical clones represented single cells or clusters of sibling cells within 1 mm of each other, while widespread dispersion occurred in the other half of the clones. In the adult, widespread clones were found to be dispersed across cytoarchitectonic zones of the cortex (Walsh and Cepko, 1992). In addition, some cortical clones showed dispersion of sibling cells from neocortical regions into the olfactory bulb (Luskin 1993; Walsh and Cepko, 1993). The finding of both clustered and widely dispersed clones forms an intriguing parallel to the chimera evidence of Tan and Breen (1993), since there appear to be radial constraints upon the migration of some cell types but not others.

Time-Lapse Video Analysis of Radial and Nonradial Migration

Studies using time-lapse video analysis of cultured neurons provide data complementary to the retroviral studies of cell dispersion and also allow direct analysis of the mechanisms of cortical migration and clonal disper-

---

recent studies retroviral libraries contain more distinct members and different histochemical markers, and they have been prepared by slightly different protocols (Walsh 1994). (Reproduced with permission from Walsh and Cepko, 1992.)

(B) The retroviral library is injected into the fetal rat brain, where distinct progenitor cells are infected with viruses carrying different fingerprints. Analysis of clonal relationships is done after sectioning and histochemically staining the brain to reveal the retrovirally infected cells. Histochemically labeled cells (asterisks) are identified, dissected directly out of the tissue sections, and transferred into tubes where PCR amplification of the viral fingerprints is carried out. Digestion of the PCR products with restriction enzymes creates a characteristic fingerprint of bands that are visible when the DNA fragments are separated by gel electrophoresis.

sion. Fishell et al. (1993) have developed a novel explant preparation to study the proliferative zone of the cortex directly. They removed the presumptive cortex from mice during the age of cortical plate formation (E17), and they cultured the cortex with the proliferative zones up. Cells of the proliferative zone were labeled directly using the lipophilic dye diI; then time-lapse photography was used to track movements of labeled cells during an 8-hour observation period. In striking contrast to previous assumptions that proliferative zone cells were stationary, Fishell et al. showed that the proliferative zone was a dynamic environment populated by cells undergoing migration in many directions (see Fig. 5-2). Many ventricular zone cells were found to undergo migration perpendicular to the radial glial fibers, some at rates up to 100 μm/h. No obvious substrate guidance for this migration was observed. After division of cortical progenitor cells, clonal progeny appeared to behave independently from each other in their subsequent migration. Progenitor cells appeared to migrate in random directions over the short period of observation with one exception; there was an apparent barrier to cell migration that separated the cortical and subcortical proliferative zones of the telencephalon from other each.

At earlier stages of development, the cortical proliferative zone shows very different patterns of migration. Studies essentially identical to those of Fishell et al. have been performed by O'Leary and Borngasser (1992) in the same mouse explant system, but these researchers used tissue from less mature cortex at embryonic day 12, during development of preplate and subplate cells. Labeled ventricular zone cells remained remarkably stationary throughout long periods of observation, with no cells observed to migrate nonradially by more than 50 μm. The more precise radial restriction of cells of the preplate may simply reflect the shorter distance that these cells migrate. Moreover, the persistent clustering of labeled preplate cells is consistent with the suggestion that preplate cells may form a "protomap" of the cortex (O'Leary 1989; Rakic 1988b), with neighbor relationships between progenitor and preplate cells apparently maintained at this early stage, despite the fact that this highly rigid pattern does not seem to be maintained during formation of the cortical plate. Thus preplate cells may form a scaffold not only for later development of regionally specific cortical connections, but perhaps also for migrating cortical plate cells (Allendorfer and Shatz, 1994). Comparably early periods of cortical development have thus far not been studied using retroviral labeling, since the embryo is not surgically accessible to retroviral labeling at the ages of generation of preplate cells.

O'Rourke et al. (1992) studied coronal slices of the developing cerebral cortex and analyzed labeled cortical cells destined for the cortical plate at a slightly later developmental stage, during the migration from the proliferative zone up to the incipient cortical plate. Their data confirmed the importance of radial glia in guiding the migration of most (88 percent) cells. However, a significant minority of cells destined for the cortical plate were observed to leave the radial glia and migrate at rapid speeds perpendicular to radial glia. Thus migration perpendicular to radial glia occurs in at least

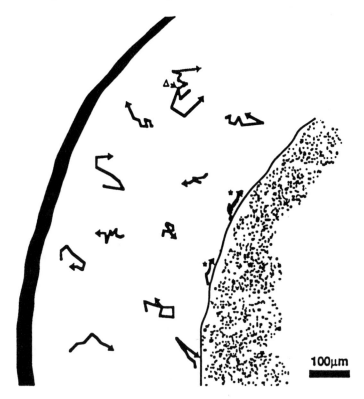

Figure 5-2. Nonradial patterns of migration in the ventricular zone of the cerebral cortex. This schematic summary drawing shows patterns of migration of single ventricular zone cells that were labeled with DiI and observed with time-lapse video imaging for up to 8 hours. Labeled cells migrated at rates of up to 100 μm/h in widely varying directions, in a pattern that closely resembled a random walk. Cells that divided (Δ) produced progeny that appeared to migrate independently from one another. One exception to the random walk of ventricular cells might be the pattern of cell movement when migrating cells encounter the boundary between cortical and subcortical ventricular zones (solid line; asterisks). In this case, migrating cells did not cross the boundary; they directed their movement longitudinally (either rostrally or caudally) along the boundary. (Reproduced with permission from Fishell et al., 1993.)

two different regions—within the proliferative zone and above the proliferative zone in the intermediate zone that separates the proliferative zone from the cortex. While our knowledge of the detail of patterns of cortical migration is incomplete, the picture is clearly much more complicated than originally assumed (see Fig. 5-3).

How can the elegant confirmation of the importance of radial glial fibers be reconciled with equally persuasive evidence of multiple forms of migration that do not appear to depend upon radial glial fibers? Preliminary data suggest that migratory movements in the developing cerebral cortex may consist of several types. During generation of the cortical plate, dividing

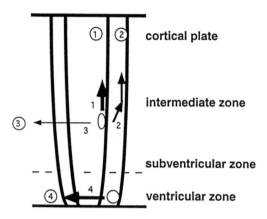

Figure 5-3. Schematic summary of patterns of migration during cortical development. A schematic coronal section of immature cerebral cortex is illustrated, with directions of migration indicated by arrows. The width of the arrow provides a very rough indication of relative frequency of distinct modes of cell migration based on current data. The major mode of migration in the intermediate zone (1) involves postmitotic cortical neurons that migrate radially in relation to radial glial fascicles (vertical lines). During radial glial–guided migration, fewer migrating cells leave one radial glial fascicle and join another, nearby fascicle (2). Approximately 12 percent of radially migrating cells leave their radial guides altogether and appear to migrate perpendicular to radial fibers at rapid rates; the substrate for this nonradial migration in the intermediate zone is not known (3) (O'Rourke et al., 1992). In contrast to the behavior of postmitotic cells in the intermediate zone, the predominant mode of cell migration in the ventricular zone during cortical plate formation appears to be parallel to the ventricular surface (4) and perpendicular to radial glial fibers (Fishell et al., 1993).

progenitor cells in the ventricular zone and/or subventricular zone seem to migrate perpendicular to radial glia at rapid rates, producing widespread dispersion of the eventual offspring of these primitive progenitors. In sharp contrast, the postmitotic progeny of most progenitor cells migrate largely in contact with radial glia. This radial migration is not always perfect, with the strict radial path further degraded as some migrating neurons shift from one radial fiber to another, or temporarily leave the radial path altogether (O'Rourke et al., 1992). However, the net outcome of migration of postmitotic neurons is generally radial, in that they are translated from the proliferative zone to the cerebral cortex. Current research is now focused on how various types of cellular migration are controlled in the developing forebrain, and how these relate to the formation of cortical cells.

Cell Migration and Cell Fate: A Second Layer of Complexity

Another layer of complexity is introduced by the fact that the ventricular and subventricular zones also contain cells that are making decisions about their ultimate fate. In the *reeler* mouse brain (Caviness, 1982), postmitotic neurons migrate to inappropriate laminar locations, so that cortical laminae are inverted and less precisely defined than in normal mice. In *reeler* mice the preplate is not split normally by cortical plate cells. Instead, cortical plate cells accumulate beneath the preplate, not within it (Ogawa et al., 1992). Nonetheless, cells formed at a given developmental age in *reeler* choose the same cell fate as normal cells, suggesting that the disordered migration of cortical neurons does not affect their choice of cell fate (Caviness, 1982). These data have been interpreted as suggesting that cell fate is fixed before cortical neurons begin their radial migration. Interpretation of human pathological conditions (Caviness, 1987) has supported a similar interpretation.

Elegant studies by McConnell (1988), which clearly suggest that neuronal precursors become committed to particular fates before they migrate radially, have allowed some definition of when and how this choice of fate occurs. Cortical precursor cells are initially multipotential: if a precursor is transplanted from a younger brain into the proliferative region of an older brain, the precursor will produce cells characteristic of the older brain—but only if transplantation takes place early in the cell cycle (G1-S phase) (McConnell and Kaznowski, 1991). In contrast, transplantation of neuronal precursors later in the cell cycle has shown that precursors at this stage have already decided what cell type to produce and cannot be respecified by external cues. Thus specification of cortical neurons to cell type seems to occur late in their final cell division but is complete before cortical cells begin their migration from the proliferative zone to the cortex.

Retroviral studies also support such a model of changing potentials of cortical progenitors during development. Some cortical progenitors appear to produce clusters of uniform neuronal types over several cell divisions (Parnevelas et al., 1991), or produce only neurons or only glial cells (Luskin et al., 1993). In contrast, other cortical progenitors can produce multiple neuronal types, including both neurons and glial cells (Price and Thurlow, 1988; Walsh and Cepko, 1992). However, it remains to be demonstrated just how the movement of cells from proliferative layers to the cortical plate relates to the changing fate of cortical cells or how the widespread patterns of clonal dispersion relate to the formation of the many cells types of the cerebral cortex. This knowledge is key to relating patterns of cortical pathology to the normal development of the cortex.

Defects in Cortical Development Related to Epilepsy-Associated Pathology

Whereas developmental disorders of the cortex that are associated with epilepsy have often been referred to as neuronal migration disorders, it seems clear that several different types of developmental abnormalities can cause these lesions. The wide variety of such developmental disorders that are associated with epilepsy includes examples of apparent abnormalities of radial migration, neural cell fate determination, neuronal differentiation, and normal regressive processes such as morphogenetic neural cell death. Pathological analyses of epileptic brains may also shed light on the role of non-radial migration in human brain.

Abnormalities of Radial Glial Fibers

Rakic (1988a) and others (Caviness, et al., 1989; see Chapter 4) have suggested that several migrational disorders can be produced by damage to radial glial fibers. Polymicrogyria in humans has been proposed to reflect damage to the radial glia from infarction or viral illness. Alternatively, polymicrogyria may arise from postmigrational damage to cortical cells (Barkovich et al., 1992). In rats, direct freeze lesions of the cerebral cortex produce microgyria, apparently by direct damage to radial glial fibers and cortical neurons (Rosen et al., 1992). In the *reeler* mouse, a faulty interaction between migrating neurons and radial glial fibers has been suggested to cause abnormalities of neuronal migration that affect the entire cerebral cortex as well as other brain structures that show radial glial–guided neuronal migration (Caviness, 1982).

Abnormalities of Cell Birth and Cell Death

Whereas gross abnormalities of neuronal migration occur in 10–20 percent of epileptic brains (Meencke and Gerhard, 1985), some epileptic brains show very subtle abnormalities, often termed "microdysgenesis" (Meencke, 1985). Microdysgenesis includes increased numbers of neurons persisting in the subcortical white matter or in layer I, abnormal clustering of neurons in otherwise normal cortical layers (Meencke, 1985), or subpial gliosis (Hardiman et al., 1988). For the most part, microdysgenetic lesions do not appear to be disorders of neuronal migration, since cells are in approximately the correct location. Instead, microdysgenetic lesions may reflect abnormal proliferation of cells or persistence of neurons of the preplate or subplate that normally are removed by morphogenetic cell death (Chun et al., 1987).

Abnormal Neural Differentiation

A third type of epilepsy-associated lesion, the focal cortical dysplasias, may involve faulty neuronal differentiation among cells that are distributed in roughly radial fashion. Focal cortical dysplasias characteristically show localized accumulations of dysplastic neurons over cortical zones that are sometimes limited to one lobe of a hemisphere. The sometimes bizarre cells contained in these dysplasias suggest abnormalities of fate determination as well as differentiation. For example, focal cortical dysplasias contain large neurons that are abnormally rich in neurofilaments but which migrate to roughly a "normal" location in the cortex (Farrell et al., 1992). In addition, some focal cortical dysplasias show large, abnormal cells, termed "balloon cells" (De Rosa, Farrell, et al., 1992). Balloon cells resemble astrocytes, but sometimes are immunoreactive for both neuronal and glial markers (De Rosa, Secor, et al., 1992; Stefansson and Wollmann, 1981). Further, dysplastic neurons show abnormal patterns of cortical lamination. In focal cortical dysplasias dysplastic neurons can overlap with normal neurons in regions that are millimeters in length (Farrell et al., 1992). Whereas focal dysplasias have not been reported to be limited to one cytoarchitectonic region, abnormal neuronal and glial elements often radiate from a localized point near the subcortical ventricular zone in striking patterns (Barkovich and Kjos, 1992a). This pattern is consistent with generally radial migration that arises from a source in or near the proliferative zone (Sarnat, 1992). Dystrophic cells suggest that fundamental developmental processes such as the commitment of cells to neuronal or glial cell phenotypes may be abnormal in some epileptic brains, and that further characterization of epilepsy-associated lesions may provide important insight into normal and abnormal cortical development.

Abnormal Progenitor Cells

Since both radial and nonradial migrations seem to be important in normal cortical development, both types of migration might be affected in pathologic conditions of the human cortex. The major type of nonradial migration may occur in the proliferative zone, whereas radial migration predominates in the intermediate zone and white matter, so that the locus of lesions affecting the two processes may differ, as does their geometry. Are there other epilepsy-associated lesions that might involve abnormalities in nonradially migrating cells? In some epileptic brains, histologic abnormalities are found that involve broad areas of the cortex with no obvious radial orientation. One example is periventricular heterotopias. Heterotopias are defined as collections of cerebral cortical cells found in abnormal locations—usually beneath the cortex. Periventricular heterotopias are collections of neuronal and/or glial cells that are found near the lateral ventricles, in regions corresponding to the proliferative zones. Periventricular heterotopias (PHs) come in several morphologically and genetically distinct varieties. For example, tuberous sclerosis shows periventricular heterotopias that are characteristically large and focal, containing cells that can stain for both neuronal and glial markers (Stefansson and Wollmann, 1981). In contrast, a recently described type of periventricular heterotopia can involve the entire ventricular and subventricular zone of the human cortex with continuous nodules of abnormal cells (Barkovich and Kjos, 1992a). Perhaps periventricular heterotopias reflect a disorder of progenitor cells that are undergoing nonradial movements, so that abnormal cells are dispersed over broader areas. The continuous periventricular heterotopias have recently been reported to the familial (Dimario et al., 1993; Huttenlocher et al., 1994; Oda et al., 1993); thus they might reflect abnormalities in genes that regulate proliferation of cortical progenitors or give rise to signals that direct cortical neuroblasts to begin their radial ascent. An alternative explanation is that PH involves failure of radial migration of certain types of cells.

Neuronal Signal Transduction Defects and the Developmental Expression of Epilepsy

Fundamental information about the relationship between abnormalities of cortical development and epileptic disorders may be gained from analysis of inherited disorders which are characterized by both abnormalities of cortical development and seizures. For example, the lissencephalic brain (type I) shows extensive failure of normal cortical migration from the ventricular zone to the cortex, with large numbers of heterotopic neurons remaining in the subcortical white matter (Dobyns et al., 1984). Patients with lissencephaly usually show severe mental retardation and intractable seizures. In the four-layered lissencephalic cortex (Dobyns et al., 1984), there is (1) an outer, cell-poor layer similar to layer I of normal cortex; (2) a layer of relatively normal-appearing pyramidal neurons that may represent cells normally destined for the deep layers of the cortex; (3) a cell-poor layer with some myelinated fibers; and (4) the deepest layer, consisting of large numbers of heterotopic cortical neurons with abnormal morphology and orientation. The heterotopic neurons may represent neurons destined for the middle and upper layers of the normal cortex (Sarnat, 1992). In lissencephaly, the normal inside-out relationship between cellular age and cortical layer may be inverted, in a way that superficially resembles the *reeler* abnormality in mice (Caviness and Rakic, 1978).

Recently the gene for lissencephaly of the Miller-Dieker type was cloned (Reiner et al., 1993). The gene, *LIS-1*, encodes a protein identical to a regulatory subunit of Platelet Activating Factor (PAF) acetylhydrolase (Hattori et al., 1994). *LIS-1* contains structural domains that suggest it may direct the formation of protein-protein interactions (Neer et al., 1993). PAF is a potent bioactive phospholipid first identified as an initiator of the acute inflammatory response. PAF alters the migratory behavior and shape of inflammatory cells (Hanahan, 1986). However, PAF is also synthesized and released in the brain, interacting with a specific receptor in neurons and glia that stimulates Ca^{2+} influx (Bito et al., 1993). Since PAF acetylhydrolase controls the level of PAF by degrading it (Elstad et al., 1989), *LIS-1* may regulate intercellular signaling by PAF. Mutations in *LIS-1* account for only 30–40 percent of cases of lissencephaly, and at least two other genes probably cause a similar phenotype (Doybns et al., 1992). Therefore, isolation of other genes involved in epileptic abnormalities of cortical development may provide rich insights into the genetic regulation of normal cortical development.

The gene mutated in neurofibromatosis type 1 (NF-1) may also be involved in intercellular signal transduction, since it encodes a protein, neurofibromin, homologous to *ras*GAP (Xu et al., 1990). Neurofibromin has been shown to modify signal transduction pathways that involve *ras,* a member of a family of small G proteins (Martin et al., 1990). G proteins are extremely important signaling proteins that can be cyclically activated by the binding of the guanine nucleotide, GTP, and subsequently inactivated by the hydrolysis of the bound GTP to GDP. NF-1 patients also frequently suffer from seizures (Kotagal and Rothner, 1993), and some NF-1 patients show developmental abnormalities of the cerebral cortex (Rosman and Pearce, 1967).

Another genetic disorder of the human cortex that is frequently associated with cortical malformations and seizures, tuberous sclerosis (TS), also may involve alterations in a protein that controls the small G proteins. Tuberous sclerosis is a common (1 case in about 10,000 births) disorder with multifaceted manifestations in many different tissues. Neurologic manifestations are most common, including seizures and mental retardation (Gomez, 1988). The cerebral cortex in TS shows three types of pathology that all seem to reflect abnormalities of neural cell differentiation: cortical tubers, focal cortical dysplasia (discussed previously), and periventricular heterotopias (Stefansson and Wollmann, 1981). Tuberous sclerosis can occur sporadically or can be inherited as an autosomal dominant trait. At least two distinct genetic loci have been identified, on chromosomes 9 and 16. The gene for the chromosome 16 locus was recently cloned (European Chromosome 16 Tuberous Sclerosis Consortium, 1993) and encodes a protein with a short sequence of amino acid homology to the GAP43 protein. GAP3 seems to modify a small GTP binding protein distinct from *ras,* called p21^{rap1}, for which neurofibromin binding has also been proposed but not yet tested (Martin et al., 1990). Together these various examples of developmental abnormalities suggest that dysfunction in critical G protein-related signal transduction pathways may give rise to structural abnormalities associated with seizure activity.

Recent in vitro experimental data also suggest that neuronal signal transduction may be very important to cortical proliferation and migration. For example, GABA, the major inhibitory transmitter in the adult central nervous system, is expressed at high levels in all regions of the developing neocortex (Meinecke and Rakic, 1992; Schwartz and Meinecke, 1992). Recent in situ hybridization studies indicate that several subunits of the GABA$_A$ receptor are expressed at high levels in the developing cortex (Laurie et al., 1992). Patch-clamp studies indicate that cells within the ventricular zone have functional GABA$_A$ channels (Lo Turco and Kriegstein, 1991). Researchers have speculated that the precocious functional expression of components of the GABA signaling system is involved in regulating cell division among cortical progenitors. Other signaling systems have also been implicated in cortical migration; for example, antagonists of NMDA receptors (Komuro and Rakic, 1993) and of *N*-type calcium channels interfere with radial migration in the cerebellum (Komuro and Rakic, 1992). Interestingly, *N*-type calcium channels also appear to be associated with a G protein-mediated pathway (Clapham and Neer, 1993), providing a possible connection between membrane-mediated and intracellular signaling.

The presence of the same signal transduction mechanisms in the developing and postnatal brain suggests a testable hypothesis for the relationship of heterotopias and epilepsy: perhaps the two phenomena are sometimes caused by common abnormalities in signal transduction processes that have different roles in the prenatal and postnatal brain. Thus heterotopias may be caused in some individuals by abnormalities in signal transduction that participate in early decisions about cell identity or control of neural cell migration. The same signal transduction mechanisms may serve different purposes in the more mature nervous system, where abnormalities of the same cellular mechanism may lead to mental retardation and/or epilepsy. Alternatively, other genetic causes of abnormal cortical development may involve mechanisms without a role in the adult, and such malformations may be inherently less epileptogenic. The *reeler* mouse is one example of an inherited, nonepileptogenic mutation of neuronal migration. A third possibility, however, is that inherited abnormalities (e.g., heterotopias), once expressed, may alter the normal course of brain development. Misplaced neurons by their presence in a region may lead to abnormal circuitry and epilepsy. Thus heterotopias might serve as important markers for epileptic brains, in addition to their direct pathogenic significance (Barkovich and Kjos, 1992b).

Deepening knowledge of cortical development has so far only revealed the complexity of even the most fundamental steps in neural cytogenesis. However, the tools are now available for a clearer cellular description of the process of cortical cytogenesis, allowing us to investigate both gene action and epigenetic processes. In the process, our knowledge of cortical development disorders will eventually lead to a classification based on molecular mechanisms. While some cortical abnormalities are well described by the term "neuronal migration disorders," other syndromes are not. Thus a broader framework for nomenclature might be the more neutral term "neuronal identity disorders." Neuronal identity is a term defined by Jessel (Kandel et al., 1991) to encompass a broad array of features, including a neuron's proper formation, migration, differentiation, and interconnection into larger functional ensembles. Studies to provide a clearer understanding of the mechanisms that generate cell identity in the cortex may thus also generate a clearer view of the relationship between cortical development and epilepsy.

Acknowledgments

The author gratefully acknowledges research support from the Klingenstein Foundation, the Rita Allen Foundation, and the NINDS. Thanks also to C. L. Cepko for permission to reproduce Figure 5-1B, and G. Fishell for permission to reproduce Figure 5-2. J. A. Golden and J. Lo Turco provided constructive comments on an earlier version of the manuscript.

References

Allendoerfer, K. L., and Shatz, C. J. (1994) The subplate, a transient neocortical structure: Its role in development of connections between thalamus and cortex. *Ann. Rev. Neurosci. 17:*185–218.

Alzheimer, A. (1907) Die Gruppierung der Epilepsie. *Allg. Z. Psychiatri. 64:*418–421.

Andermann, F., Olivier, A., Melanson, D., and Robitaille, Y. (1987) Epilepsy due to focal cortical dysplasia with macrogyria and the forme fruste of tuberous sclerosis: A study of fifteen patients. *Adv. Epileptology 16:*35–38.

Austin, C. P., and Cepko, C. L. (1990) Cellular migration patterns in the developing mouse cerebral cortex. *Development 110:*713–732.

Barkovich, A. J., Gressens, P., and Evrard, P. (1992) Formation, maturation, and disorders of brain neocortex. *Am. J. Neuroradiol. 13:*423–446.

Barkovich, A. J., and Kjos, B. (1992a) Gray matter heterotopias: MR characteristics and correlation with developmental and neurological manifestations. *Radiology 182:*483–499.

Barkovich, A. J., and Kjos, B. O. (1992b) Nonlissencephalic cortical dysplasias: Correlation of imaging findings with clinical deficits. *Am. J. Neuroradiol. 13:*95–103.

Berry, M., and Rogers, A. W. (1965) The migration of neuroblasts in the developing cerebral cortex. *J. Anat. 99:*691–709.

Bito, H., Nakamura, M., Honda, Z., Izumi, T., Iwatsubo, T., Seyama, Y., Ogura, A., Kudo, Y., and Shimizu, T. (1993) Platelet-activating factor (PAF) receptor in rat brain: PAF mobilizes intracellular Ca^{2+} in hippocampal neurons. *Neuron 9:*285–294.

Boulder-Committee, T. (1970) Embryonic vertebrate central nervous system: Revised terminology. *Anat. Rec. 166:*257–262.

Caviness, V. S., Jr. (1982) Neocortical histogenesis and *reeler* mice: A developmental study based upon [³H]thymidine autoradiography. *Dev. Brain Res. 4:*293–302.

Caviness, V. S., Jr. (1987) Neuronal migration and disorders of cerebral organization. *Neuroscience 22S:*1189W.

Caviness, V. S., Jr., Misson, J.-P., and Gadisseux, J.-F. (1989) Abnormal neuronal patterns and disorders of neocortical development. In A. M. Galaburda (ed.), *From Reading to Neurons.* Cambridge, Mass.: M.I.T. Press/Bradford Books, pp. 405–442.

Caviness, V. S., Jr., and Rakic, P. (1978) Mechanisms of cortical development: A view from mutations in mice. *Ann. Rev. Neurosci. 1:*297–326.

Cepko, C. L., Ryder, E. F., Austin, C. P., Walsh, C., and Fekete, D. M. (1993) Lineage analysis using retrovirus vectors. In P. S. Wassarman and M. L. DePamphilis (eds.), *Methods in Enzymology Guide to Mouse Techniques.* New York: Academic Press, pp. 933–960.

Chugani, H. T., Shields, W. D., Shewmon, D. A., Olson, D. M., Phelps, M. E., and Peacock, W. J. (1990) Infantile spasms: I. PET identifies focal cortical dysgenesis in cryptogenic cases for surgical treatment. *Ann. Neurol. 27:*406–413.

Chun, J. J., Nakamura, M. J., and Shatz, C. J. (1987) Transient cells of the developing mammalian telencephalon are peptide-immunoreactive neurons. *Nature 325:*617–620.

Clapham, D. E., and Neer, E. J. (1993) New roles for G-protein βγ-dimers in transmembrane signalling. *Nature 365:*403–406.

Crandall, J., and Herrup, K. (1990) Patterns of cell lineage in the cerebral cortex reveal evidence for developmental boundaries. *Exp. Neurol. 109:*131–139.

De Rosa, M. J., Farrell, M. A., Burke, M. M., Secor, D. L., and Vinters, H. V. (1992) An assessment of the proliferative potential of "balloon cells" in focal cortical resections performed for childhood epilepsy. *Neuropathol. Appl. Neurobiol. 18:*566–574.

De Rosa, M. J., Secor, D. L., Barsom, M., Fisher, R. S., and Vinters, H. V. (1992) Neuropathologic findings in surgically treated hemimegalencephaly: Immunohistochemical, morphometric, and ultrastructural study. *Acta Neuropathol. 84:*250–260.

Dimario, F. J., Cobb, R. J., Ramsby, G. R., and Leicher, C. (1993) Familial band heterotopias simulating tuberous sclerosis. *Neurology 43:*1424–1426.

Dobyns, W. B., Elias, E. R., Newlin, A. C., Pagon, R. A., and Ledbetter, D. H. (1992) Causal heterogeneity in isolated lissencephaly. *Neurology 42:*1375–1388.

Dobyns, W. B., Stratton, R. F., and Greenburg, F. (1984) Syndromes with lissencephaly: I. Miller-Dieker and Norman-Roberts syndromes and isolated lissencephaly. *Am. J. Med. Genet. 18:*509–526.

Edmondson, J. C., and Hatten, M. E. (1987) Glial-guided granule neuron migration in vitro: A high-resolution time-lapse video microscopic study. *J. Neurosci. 7:*1928–1934.

Elstad, M. R., Stafforini, D. M., McIntyre, T. M., Prescott, S. M., and Zimmerman, G. A. (1989) Platelet-activating factor acetylhydrolase increases during macrophage differentiation. A novel mechanism that regulates accumulation of platelet-activating factor. *J. Biol. Chem. 264:*8467–8470.

European Chromosome 16 Tuberous Sclerosis Consortium (1993) Identification and characterization of the tuberous sclerosis gene on chromosome 16. *Cell 75:*1305–1315.

Farrell, M. A., DeRosa, M. J., Curran, J. G., Lenard Secor, D., Cornford, M. E., Comair, Y. G., Peacock, W. J., Shields, W. D., and Vinters, H. V. (1992) Neuropathologic findings in cortical resections (including hemispherectomies) performed for the treatment of intractable childhood epilepsy. *Acta Neuropathol. 83:*246–259.

Fishell, G., Mason, C. A., and Hatten, M. E. (1993) Dispersion of neural progenitors within the germinal zones of the forebrain. *Nature 362:*636–638.

Fishell, G., Rossant, J., and Vanderkooy, D. (1990) Neuronal lineages in chimeric mouse forebrain are segregated between compartments and in the rostrocaudal and radial planes. *Dev. Biol. 141:*70–83.

Goff, S. P. (1992) Genetics of retroviral integration. *Ann. Rev. Genet. 26:*527–544.

Goldowitz, D. (1987) Cell partitioning and mixing in the formation of the CNS: Analysis of the cortical somatosensory barrels in chimeric mice. *Dev. Brain Res. 35:*1–9.

Gomez, M. (1988) *Tuberous Sclerosis.* New York: Raven Press.

Hanahan, D. J. (1986) Platelet-activating factor: A biologically active phosphoglyceride. *Ann. Rev. Biochem. 55:*483–509.

Hardiman, O., Burke, T., Phillips, J., Murphy, S., O'Moore, B., Staunton, H., and Farrell, M. A. (1988) Microdysgenesis in resected temporal neocortex: Incidence and clinical significance in focal epilepsy. *Neurology 38:*1041–1047.

Harvey, A. S., Hopkins, I. J., Bowe, J. M., Cook, D. J., Shield, L. K., and Berkovic, S. F. (1993) Frontal lobe epilepsy: Clinical seizure characteristics and localization with ictal 99mTc-HMPAO SPECT. *Neurology 43:*1966–1980.

Hattori, M., Adachi, H., Tsujimoto, M., Arai, H., and Inoue, K. (1994) Miller-Dieker lissencephaly gene encodes a subunit of brain platelet-activating factor acetylhydrolase. *Nature 370*:216–218.

Huttenlocher, P. R., Taravath, S., and Mojtahedi, S. (1994) Periventricular heterotopia and epilepsy. *Neurology 44*:51–55.

Kandel, E. R., Schwartz, J. H., and Jessel, T. M. (1991) *Principles of Neural Science*. Norwalk, Conn.: Appleton and Lange, pp. 887–907.

Komuro, H., and Rakic, P. (1992) Selective role of *N*-type calcium channels in neuronal migration. *Science 257*:806–809.

Komuro, H., and Rakic, P. (1993) Modulation of neuronal migration by NMDA receptors. *Science 260*:95–97.

Kotagal, P., and Rothner, A. D. (1993) Epilepsy in the setting of neurocutaneous syndromes. *Epilepsia 34*:S71–S78.

Laurie, D. J., Wisden, W., and Seeburg, P. H. (1992) The distribution of thirteen $GABA_A$ receptor subunit mRNAs in the rat brain: III. Embryonic and postnatal development. *J. Neurosci. 12*:4151–4172.

Lo Turco, J. J., and Kriegstein, A. R. (1991) Clusters of coupled neuroblasts in embryonic neocortex. *Science 252*:563–566.

Luskin, M. B. (1993) Restricted proliferation and migration of postnatally generated neurons derived from the forebrain subventricular zone. *Neuron 11*:173–189.

Luskin, M. B., Parnavelas, J. G., and Barfield, J. A. (1993) Neurons, astrocytes, and oligodendrocytes of the rat cerebral cortex originate from separate progenitor cells: An ultrastructural analysis of clonally related cells. *J. Neurosci. 13*:1730–1750.

Luskin, M. B., Pearlman, A. L., and Sanes, J. R. (1988) Cell lineage in the cerebral cortex of the mouse studies in vivo and in vitro with a recombinant retrovirus. *Neuron 1*:635–647.

Lyon, G., and Gastaut, H. (1985) Considerations on the significance attributed to unusual cerebral histological findings described in eight patients with primary generalized epilepsy. *Epilepsia 26*:365–367.

Marin-Padilla, M. (1971) Early prenatal ontogenesis of the cerebral cortex (neocortex) of the cat *(Felis domestica)*. A Golgi study: I. The primordial neocortical organization. *Z. Anat. Entwicklungsgesch. 134*:117–145.

Marin-Padilla, M. (1978) Dual origin of the mammalian neocortex and evolution of the cortical plate. *Anat. Embryol. 152*:109–126.

Martin, G. A., Visckochil, D., Bollag, G., McCabe, P. C., Crosier, W. J., Haubruck, H., Conroy, L., Clark, R., O'Connell, P., Cawthon, R. M., Innis, M. A., and McCormick, F. (1990) The GAP-related domain of the neurofibromatosis type 1 gene product interacts with ras p21. *Cell 63*:843–849.

McConnell, S. K. (1988) Fates of visual cortical neurons in the ferret after isochronic and heterochronic transplantation. *J. Neurosci. 8*:945–974.

McConnell, S. K., and Kaznowski, C. E. (1991) Cell cycle dependence of laminar determination in developing neocortex. *Science 254*:282–285.

Meencke, H.-J. (1985) Neuron density in the molecular layer of the frontal cortex in primary generalized epilepsy. *Epilepsia 26*:450–454.

Meencke, H.-J. (1989) Pathology of childhood epilepsies. *Cleveland Clin. Med. 56*:111–120.

Meencke, H.-J., and Gerhard, C. (1985) Morphological aspects of aetiology and the course of infantile spasms (West syndrome). *Neuropediatrics 16*:59–66.

Meencke, H.-J., and Veith, G. (1992) Migration disturbances in epilepsy. In J. J. Engel, C. G. Wasterain, E. A. Cavalheiro, and U. Heinemann (eds.), *Molec-*

ular Neurobiology of Epilepsy. Amsterdam: Elsevier Science Publishers, pp. 31–40.

Meinecke, D. L., and Rakic, P. (1992) Expression of GABA and $GABA_A$ receptors by neurons of the subplate zone in developing primate occipital cortex: Evidence for transient local circuits. *J. Comp. Neurol. 317:*91–101.

Neer, E. J., Schmidt, C. J., and Smith, T. (1993) LIS is more. *Nat. Genet. 5:*3–4.

Oda, T., Nagai, Y., Fuijimoto, S., Sobajima, H., Kobayashi, M., Togari, H., and Wada, Y. (1993) Hereditary nodular heterotopia accompanied by mega cisterna magna. *Am. J. Med. Genet. 47:*268–271.

Ogawa, M., Miyata, T., Yagyu, K., Nakajima, K., Ikenaka, K., et al. (1992) *Early morphogenesis in the neocortex: The Cajal-Retzius neuron plays a role in the lamina formation of cortical plate*. Fourth International Forum on the Frontier of Telecommunication Technology, Japan. Cited in Allendoerfer and Shatz (1994).

O'Leary, D. D. M. (1989) Do cortical areas emerge from a protocortex? *Trends Neurosci. 12:*400–406.

O'Leary, D. D. M., and Borngasser, D. J. (1992) Minimal dispersion of neuroepithelial cells during generation of the cortical preplate. *Soc. Neurosci. Abstr. 18:*925.

O'Rourke, N. A., Dailey, M. E., Smith, S. J., and McConnell, S. K. (1992) Diverse migratory pathways in the developing cerebral cortex. *Science 258:*299–302.

Parnevelas, J. G., Barfield, J. A., Franke, E., and Luskin, M. B. (1991) Separate progenitor cells give rise to pyramidal and nonpyramidal neurons in the rat telencephalon. *Cereb. Cortex 1:*1047–3211.

Price, J., and Thurlow, L. (1988) Cell lineage in the rat cerebral cortex: A study using retroviral-mediated gene transfer. *Development 104:*473–482.

Rakic, P. (1972) Mode of cell migration to the superficial layers of fetal monkey neocortex. *J. Comp. Neurol. 145:*61–84.

Rakic, P. (1978) Neuronal migration and contact guidance in primate telencephalon. *Postgrad. Med. J. 54:*25–40.

Rakic, P. (1988a) Defects of neuronal migration and the pathogenesis of cortical malformations. *Prog. Brain Res. 73:*15–37.

Rakic, P. (1988b) Specification of cerebral cortical areas. *Science 241:*170–176.

Rakic, P., Stensaas, L. J., Sayre, E. P., and Sidman, R. L. (1974) Computer-aided three-dimensional reconstruction and quantitative analysis of cells from serial electron microscopic montages of foetal monkey brain. *Nature 250:*31–34.

Reiner, O., Carrozzo, R., Shen, Y., Wehnert, M., Faustinella, F., Dobyns, W. B., Caskey, C. T., and Ledbetter, D. H. (1993) Isolation of a Miller-Dieker lissencephaly gene containing G protein β-subunit-like repeats. *Nature 364:*717–721.

Robitaille, Y., Rasmussen, T., Dubeau, F., Tampieri, D., and Kemball, K. (1992) Histopathology of nonneoplastic lesions in frontal lobe epilepsy: Review of 180 cases with recent MRI and PET correlations. In P. Chauvel, A. V. Delgado-Escueta, E. Halgren, J. Bancaud (eds.), *Frontal Lobe Seizures and Epilepsy*. New York: Raven Press, pp. 499–513.

Rosen, G. D., Press, D. M., Sherman, G. F., and Galaburda, A. M. (1992) The development of induced cerebrocortical microgyria in the rat. *J. Neuropathol. Exp. Neurol. 51:*601–611.

Rosman, N. P., and Pearce, J. (1967) The brain in multiple neurofibromatosis (von Recklinghausen's disease): A suggested neuropathological basis for the associated mental defect. *Brain 90:*829–838.

Sandmeyer, S. B., Hansen, L. J., and Chalker, D. L. (1990) Integration specificity of retrotransposons and retroviruses. *Ann. Rev. Genet. 24:*491–518.

Sanes, J. R., Rubenstein, J. L. R., and Nicolas, J.-F. (1986) Use of a recombinant retrovirus to study post-implantation cell lineage in mouse embryos. *EMBO J. 5:*3133–3142.

Sarnat, H. B. (1992) *Cerebral Dysgenesis: Embryology and Clinical Expression.* New York: Oxford University Press.

Schwartz, M. L., and Meinecke, D. L. (1992) Early expression of GABA-containing neurons in the prefrontal and visual cortices of rhesus monkeys. *Cereb. Cortex 2:*16–37.

Shoukimas, G. M., and Hinds, J. W. (1978) The development of the cerebral cortex in the embryonic mouse: An electron microscopic serial section section analysis. *J. Comp. Neurol. 179:*795–830.

Snyder, E. L., Deitcher, D. L., Walsh, C., Arnold-Aldea, S., Hartweig, E. A., and Cepko, C. L. (1992) Multipotent neural cell lines can engraft and participate in development of mouse cerebellum. *Cell 68:*33–51.

Stefansson, K., and Wollmann, R. (1981) Distribution of the neuronal specific protein, 14-3-2, in central nervous system lesions of tuberous sclerosis. *Acta Neuropathol. 53:*113–117.

Tan, S. S., and Breen, S. (1993) Radial mosaicism and tangential cell dispersion both contribute to mouse cortical development. *Nature 362:*638–640.

Turner, D., and Cepko, C. L. (1987) Cell lineage in the rat retina: A common progenitor for neurons and glia persists late in development. *Nature 328:*131–136.

Vinters, H. V., Fisher, R. S., Cornford, M. E., Mah, V., Lenard Secor, D., DeRosa, M. J., Comair, Y. G., Peacock, W. J., and Shields, W. D. (1992) Morphological substrates of infantile spasms: Studies based on surgically resected cerebral tissue. *Child's Nerv. Syst. 8:*8–17.

Walsh, C. (1994) PCR-based techniques for cell lineage analysis using retroviruses. In K. Adolph (ed.), *Methods in Molecular Genetics, Vol. 4: Molecular Virology.* Orlando, Fla.: Academic Press.

Walsh, C., and Cepko, C. L. (1988) Clonally related neurons show several patterns of migration in cerebral cortex. *Science 255:*1342–1345.

Walsh, C., and Cepko, C. L. (1990) Cell lineage and cell migration in the developing cerebral cortex. *Experientia 46:*940–947.

Walsh, C., and Cepko, C. L. (1992) Widespread dispersion of neuronal clones across functional regions of the cerebral cortex. *Science 255:*434–440.

Walsh, C., and Cepko, C. L. (1993) Widespread clonal dispersion in proliferative layers of cerebral cortex. *Nature 362:*632–635.

Walsh, C., Cepko, C. L., Ryder, E. F., Church, G. M., and Tabin, C. (1992) The dispersion of neuronal clones across the cerebral cortex: Response. *Science 258:*317–320.

Xu, G., O'Connell, P., Viskochil, D., Cawthon, R., Robertson, M., Culver, M., Dunn, D., Stevens, J., Gesteland, R., White, R., and Weiss, R. (1990). The neurofibromatosis type 1 gene product encodes a protein related to GAP. *Cell 62:*599–608.

6

Regulation of Excitability in Developing Neurons

NICHOLAS C. SPITZER

The immature nervous system is particularly vulnerable to epilepsy; more than two-thirds of all seizure problems commence in childhood. Moreover, seizures display the broadest range of forms during this age period. Accordingly, it has been of interest to ask if there are particular features of early neuronal development, features of the normal maturation of the nervous system, that could contribute to this early susceptibility. Since voltage-gated channels appear at very early stages in embryogenesis and the initial expression of these properties is often distinct from that observed in the adult nervous system, these early transient features of differentiation have been studied to evaluate their contribution to the pathophysiology of epilepsy.

A natural expectation from such studies is that we will be able to identify the general rules according to which different voltage-gated ion channels appear during differentiation of the central nervous system. Of specific value would be the time course of maturation of sodium, calcium, potassium, chloride, and hydrogen ion channels—in terms of their permeation and gating properties and changes in these parameters—which could be examined to assess correlations with abnormal electrical activity of the brain. Unfortunately, even after a substantial period of investigation, a clear and simple set of rules characterizing the maturation of the CNS is not only unavailable but currently seems unlikely to exist. Ion channels often appear in a stereotyped sequence within a class of neurons in a particular species but may vary from one cell type to the next and within the same cell type from species to species. A consequent expectation is the gradual compilation of an atlas documenting the maturation of excitability in particular classes of neurons within specific regions of the brain for a given species. At present, however, such an atlas would be a slender object with only a small number of entries.

An important conclusion nonetheless is that immature forms of excitability are often specialized to promote calcium influx that is utilized in directing programs of neuronal differentiation. This calcium influx is mediated by a constellation of voltage-gated ion channels, which will be reviewed in this chapter. A similar promotion of calcium influx is achieved through a variety of ligand-gated channels, including NMDA and GABA receptors, as discussed elsewhere in this volume (see Chapters 8 and 9). In immature neurons, the presence of voltage-gated calcium currents that have a low threshold for activation, coupled with the small size of potassium currents, allows repetitive firing and stimulation of greater calcium influx than is observed in mature neurons. Calcium may stimulate calcium release from intracellular stores to promote even greater calcium elevation; this mechanism may be particularly effective in immature cells since buffering of intracellular calcium is slower and less extensive than in mature neurons. Similar facilitation of calcium in immature neurons is produced by magnesium-resistant NMDA receptors and by GABA receptors with relatively positive reversal potentials. The sequelae of these calcium elevations may include abnormal bursts of action potentials, prolonged neurotransmitter release, and excitotoxicity.

Development of Ion Channels

We begin with consideration of the developmental changes in action potentials in the CNS. Impulses represent the integrated output of all the voltage-gated ion channels expressed in a cell. Furthermore, these events have been experimentally addressed over many years (Dietzel, 1994; Spitzer, 1979, 1985, 1991); substantially more information is available about the impulses generated by particular neurons during their development than the changes in voltage-gated currents they express. This picture should change rapidly now that the technology for whole-cell voltage clamp recordings from neurons in situ and in slice preparations has rendered this objective feasible (Blanton et al., 1989; Desarmenien et al., 1993; Sakmann et al., 1989).

The primary sensory neurons of amphibian embryos illustrate the early expression of calcium-dependent action potentials that are converted to brief sodium-dependent spikes during early maturation. In these cells, the Rohon-Beard neurons of the spinal cord, intracellular recordings demonstrate that the action potential may be hundreds of milliseconds in duration at the neural tube stage, allowing prominent calcium influx. By one further day of differentiation the action potential is brief and sodium-dependent, only a few milliseconds in duration (Baccaglini and Spitzer, 1977). A similar pattern is seen in amphibian motor neurons and in interneurons (Spitzer and Lamborghini, 1976; Willard, 1980) and in motor neurons from chick embryos (McCobb, Best, and Beam, 1990), amphibian and murine dorsal root ganglion cells (Baccaglini, 1978; Matsuda et al., 1978), and in rat sympathetic ganglion cells (Nerbonne and Gurney, 1989). Interestingly, this sequence of changes in excitability is also described for both cortical and brain nuclear neurons of the rat and chick (Ahmed et al., 1983; Mori-Okamoto et al., 1983; Pettigrew et al., 1988), as well as in neuroblastoma and pheochromocytoma (PC12) cell lines (Dichter et al., 1977; Miyake, 1978; O'Lague and Huttner, 1980; Ritchie, 1979). The stimulus-evoked decrease in extracellular calcium concentrations in postnatal kitten visual cortex is reduced during development, consistent with a larger calcium influx at early stages that may be related to experience-dependent modifications of neuronal response properties (Bode-Greuel and Singer, 1991).

In other instances, however, the ionic basis of the action potential is constant during development. In cells of the mesencephalic neural crest of quail embryos (Bader et al., 1985), for example, action potentials are relatively brief and sodium-dependent; long-duration, calcium-dependent impulses are not a feature of their early differentiation. This paradigm is observed for neural crest from chick embryos and for chick ciliary ganglion neurons (Bader, Bertrand, Dupin, and Kato, 1983; Bader, Bertrand, and Kato, 1983), for rat motor neurons (Walton and Fulton, 1986; Ziskind-Conhaim, 1988), and for murine spinal neurons (Krieger and Sears, 1988). Thus this fundamental form of excitability varies in its developmental pattern from one region of the CNS to another within the same animal and from animal to animal for the same neuronal type. A role for calcium influx in the early maturation of these neurons is not excluded by this form of differentiation, however. The relatively modest calcium influx that occurs through these briefer action potentials may still be sufficient to stimulate substantial calcium release from intracellular stores; alternatively, calcium influx may be stimulated in these cells by other means, such as the activity of ligand-gated channels.

Ca^{2+} Currents

During development, control of action potential duration and calcium influx appears in general not to be achieved by the direct regulation of expression of the calcium currents themselves. Instead, their expression is regulated by opposing outward potassium currents. In chick motor neurons the increase in high voltage–activated (HVA) calcium current density occurs prior to the time of naturally occurring cell death (McCobb et al., 1989). In contrast, HVA calcium currents in mouse motor neurons increase in density at a later stage of differentiation during the time of synapse elimination (Mynlieff and Beam, 1992), again illustrating a species-specific difference in the developmental program for the same class of neuron. Once calcium currents have appeared, the aggregate current is stable in its density or may even increase somewhat. The largest of these currents, carrying the greater fraction of the current, are typically the HVA N and L currents, which appear not to change with further development (Barish, 1986; Gottmann et al., 1988; Lovinger and White, 1989; McCobb et al., 1989; O'Dowd et al., 1988; Yaari et al., 1987). Low voltage–activated (LVA) calcium T currents are often expressed at early stages of differentiation (Bargas et al., 1991; Coulter et al., 1989; Gottmann et al., 1988; McCobb et al., 1989; Meyers and Barker, 1989; Thompson and Wong, 1991; Yaari et al., 1987) and then decrease with further development (Beam and Knudson, 1988; Gu and Spitzer, 1993; Kostyuk, 1989; McCobb et al., 1989). However, in some cases the T current appears in a relatively late stage of development, as in rat cerebellar Purkinje neurons (Gruol et al., 1992).

Na^+ Currents

During the course of early differentiation, sodium currents may undergo a substantial increase in density. This change is often accompanied by small changes in kinetics, as currents inactivate more rapidly (Huguenard et al., 1988; McCobb et al., 1990; O'Dowd et al., 1988; Skaliora et al., 1993). These sodium currents are thought to contribute to depolarization and activation of HVA calcium currents, since their threshold can lie between that of LVA and HVA channels (Gu and Spitzer, 1993; see below). The TTX (tetrodotoxin) resistance of many sodium currents at early stages of maturation, while in itself not of normal functional importance, appears to be characteristic of current with slower activation and inactivation kinetics and more depolarized voltage of half inactivation (Ogata and Tatebayashi, 1992; Roy and Narahashi, 1992). It thus promotes longer depolarization and potentially provides greater opportunity for stimulation of calcium influx. Of particular interest are proton-activated sodium currents which appear prior to voltage-gated calcium and sodium currents in chick dorsal root ganglion neurons and in neuronal precursor cells from rat brain (Gottmann et al., 1989; Grantyn et al., 1989). The functions of these currents at these early stages of development are still be defined, but their activation by pH imbalances could provoke depolarization and abnormal electrical discharges in the immature nervous system. Since these channels are also permeant to calcium ions, they may allow calcium entry during the acidification accompanying excessive electrical activity or tissue ischemia (Kovalchuk et al., 1990). A persistent voltage-dependent sodium current, which develops postnatally in pyramidal neurons from rat cortex, may well increase excitability at this age (Alzheimer et al., 1993).

K^+ Currents

Important for their regulation of the functional expression of early forms of excitability are potassium currents. Early in development, calcium-dependent action potentials are facilitated in some cells as a consequence of rather modest expression of potassium currents; these potassium currents are often slowly activated, thus allowing the prolonged activation of sustained inward calcium currents. The duration of the action potential is a result of the balance between these two major players. As potassium currents increase during neuronal differentiation, they suppress inward calcium currents by promoting repolarization of the neurons. In contrast, action potentials are relatively brief at the time of their first appearance in other cells, when potassium currents are large with respect to calcium currents at early stages of development. This scenario leads to short sodium-dependent spikes from the outset.

The type of potassium current exerting this early regulatory influence is different from one system to the next. In some cases sustained delayed rectifier potassium currents dominate (Krieger and Sears, 1988; McCobb et al., 1990; Nerbonne and Gurney, 1989; Ribera and Spitzer, 1989, 1990). In others the transient potassium A current precedes the expression of the delayed rectifier (Aguayo, 1989; Bader et al., 1985; Beck et al., 1992), and calcium-activated potassium currents may be involved. There is as yet no discernible logic driving the selection of one potassium current over another in any particular system. The order of maturation of potassium currents is not correlated with the extent of calcium dependence of action potentials at early stages of development. Late differentiation of delayed rectifier potassium current can be associated with long-duration calcium-dependent action potentials (O'Dowd et al., 1988) or with brief sodium-dependent impulses (Bader et al., 1985).

The changes in whole-cell potassium currents are the consequence of changes in single channels. In *Xenopus* spinal neurons, two classes of channels, with 15 and 30 picosiemens (pS) conductance, underlie the macroscopic delayed rectifier current (Harris et al., 1988). Increases in the density of both channels account for the increase in whole-cell current density, while the increase in rate of activation of the whole-cell current is accounted for by a change in the 30-pS class alone. The channels that give rise to the whole-cell calcium-dependent potassium current initially lack sensitivity to intracellular calcium, a sensitivity which is acquired during further development (Blair and Dionne, 1985). Increases in size of whole-cell potassium currents are due to increases in mean channel open time in other systems (Bregestovski et al., 1988; Yool et al., 1988).

The importance of potassium currents in the maturation of action potentials of amphibian spinal neurons has been evaluated quantitatively by computer reconstruction of action potentials from voltage-clamped currents (Barish, 1986; Gu and Spitzer, 1993; Lockery and Spitzer, 1992). These studies demonstrate that the overall waveform of the action potential is well accounted for by the currents discussed thus far. They do not exclude, however, roles for additional currents in determining further important aspects of excitability, such as action potential threshold or refractory period. Chloride currents could, in principle, contribute to repolarization of cells following impulse activity but have been little studied. Two calcium-activated chloride currents are expressed in amphibian spinal neurons during development. One of these is prominent at early stages and appears to decrease in both incidence and density during maturation; it may contribute to repolarization of long calcium-dependent action potentials at a time when potassium currents are small (Hussy, 1991). Large-conductance calcium-activated chloride channels exhibit persistent activation even after removal of calcium ions. This current could act not only to assist in repolarizing neurons but to prevent repetitive firing following repolarization (Hussy, 1992).

Developmental Changes in Ion Concentrations

Regulation of either intracellular or extracellular ion concentrations is another potential point of developmental control. Magnitudes of ionic currents depend upon the sizes of ion concentration gradients, since current is the product of conductance and driving force; the latter is determined in part by ion concentrations inside and outside the cell. This opportunity for developmental regulation appears to be one of which the nervous system has also taken advantage. Such regulation is perhaps surprising, since the effects of modulating extracellular ion concentrations might be expected to be global, not regulated with the cell-to-cell specificity that is an important characteristic of many aspects of neuronal function. However, the mechanisms that alter ion concentrations appear to be local, and diffusion is sufficiently restricted to allow specificity to be maintained for brief periods.

With respect to developmental changes in intracellular ion concentrations, reduction in intracellular sodium ion concentration, as a consequence of increase in Na/K ATPase (sodium pump) activity, appears to accompany morphological and physiological differentiation of amphibian spinal neurons (Warner, 1985). Increases in Na/K ATPase during postnatal development of rat hippocampal pyramidal neurons lead to increases in glutamate-stimulated afterhyperpolarizations due to increases in intracellular potassium ions (Fukuda and Prince, 1992). Changes in intracellular chloride ion concentration allow $GABA_A$ receptors to function in an excitatory role early in the development of the mammalian central nervous system, in contrast to their classical inhibitory function at later stages (Ben-Ari et al., 1989; Cherubini et al., 1990; Conner et al., 1987; Janigro and Schwartzkroin, 1988; Wu et al., 1992; Yuste and Katz, 1991). In principle, ion-selective intracellular microelectrodes should be useful experimentally, but the small and fragile character of neurons at early stages of development, coupled with difficulties of accurate calibration, make this a challenging approach. An alternative indirect technique—measurement of reversal potentials for voltage-gated currents—reveals developmental constancy or change, consistent with the stability or shift of intracellular ion concentrations.

Glia also play an important role in regulating ion concentrations, at least for potassium (Kuffler, 1967; Somjen, 1978). With regard to developmental changes in extracellular ion concentrations, glia appear to become more effective in stabilizing potassium ion concentrations during maturation of the neonatal rat optic nerve and spinal cord (Connors et al., 1982; Jendelova and Sykova, 1991), even though potassium currents and activity-dependent potassium efflux are likely to be increasing during this time. Na/K ATPase activity also regulates the extracellular concentration of potassium ions (Haglund and Schwartzkroin, 1990), and developmental increases in pump activity may also be expected to enhance the stability of extracellular potassium ion concentrations.

Regional Differences in Ion Channel Properties

Clear differences in the functional expression of particular classes of voltage-gated ion channels in different brain regions and in different cell types are gradually becoming apparent. It is already possible, with in situ hybridization for GABA and glutamate ligand-gated channel transcripts, to define sectors of the brain in which different specific channel receptor subunits are expressed, and similar results are now available for voltage-gated channels. Potassium channel transcripts have been shown to possess specific tissue distributions and developmental regulation (Beckh and Pongs, 1990; Drewe et al., 1992; Hwang et al., 1992; Perney et al., 1992; Ribera and Nguyen, 1993; Rudy et al., 1992; Swanson et al., 1990; Tsaur et al., 1992). Similar studies demonstrate region-specific and developmentally regulated expression of calcium and sodium channel transcripts (Brysch et al., 1991; Chin et al., 1992; Furuyama et al., 1993; Snutch et al., 1991; Westenbroek et al., 1992). Localization of specific molecular components in the brain is, however, an easy task compared to the identification of the functional consequences of positioning these molecules in particular regions, for ligand-gated as well as voltage-activated channels.

The specific localization of sodium channels within single cells at early stages of development has been known for some time (Catterall, 1981), and the developmental appearance of α subunits has now been identified (Scheinman et al., 1989). Moreover, in the few instances in which the issue has been examined, neurites appear to become electrically excitable before the cell body of developing neurons (Goodman and Spitzer, 1979, 1981; Willard, 1980). Calcium channels have been shown to be localized to growth cones or more mature nerve terminals and dendrites as well as to cell bodies of neurons, but they are often excluded from axons (Anglister et al., 1982; Mourre et al,. 1987; Streit and Lux, 1989; Westenbroek et al., 1990). These observations are consistent with some of the unusual patterns of electrical activity during development, producing unusual neurotransmitter release at the synapse on the one hand and transcriptional activation of genes in the nucleus on the other. The distribution of ion channels in single neurons can change with further differentiation. The lateral mobility and the ultimate localization and clustering of sodium channels have been extensively studied (Angelides et al., 1988; Kocsis et al., 1983; Ritchie, 1982; Waxman and Foster, 1980) but the implications of this movement for developmental function are unclear.

Activity-Dependent Regulation of Ion Channel Expression

A striking feature of recent work on the development of excitability in the central nervous system has been the observation of spontaneous transient elevations of calcium prior to the time of appearance of recognized ligand-gated channels. These studies have taken advantage of optical imaging techniques to assess intracellular calcium concentrations in differentiating neurons. Embryonic amphibian spinal neurons produce spontaneous transient elevations of intracellular calcium both in culture and in the intact spinal cord. These events appear to be cell-autonomous, since they occur in neurons differentiating in isolation in dissociated cell culture as well as in neurons in normal contact with neighbors in the spinal cord. Calcium indicators fura-2 and fluo-3 have been used to detect elevations of fluorescence and thus the increases in intracellular calcium that occur in the neuronal cell body during substantial periods of development (Gu and Spitzer, 1993; Gu et al., 1994; Holliday and Spitzer, 1990). These transient elevations are largely abolished upon removal of extracellular calcium or by agents that reduce influx through voltage-activated calcium channels. Furthermore, calcium influx triggers calcium-induced calcium release from calcium stores within the differentiating neurons. Depletion of calcium stores either with ditertbenzohydroquinone or with caffeine suppresses the elevation of intracellular calcium produced by depolarization-stimulated calcium influx (Gu et al., 1994; Holliday et al., 1991). The function of intracellular calcium stores appears to be developmentally regulated, since calcium release is highly sensitive to calcium influx at early stages of development, becoming less sensitive with further maturation. Moreover, the amplitude of elevation of intracellular calcium achieved through calcium influx-stimulated calcium release is greatest at early stages and declines thereafter. Despite this developmentally regulated change in calcium-induced calcium release, steady-state levels of intracellular calcium are relatively constant during this period of early neuronal maturation (Holliday and Spitzer, 1990). Low voltage–activated current is the immediate stimulus for spontaneous elevations of intracellular calcium, since these transients are blocked by concentrations of nickel or amiloride, which specifically suppress LVA current without significantly affecting HVA currents (Gu and Spitzer, 1993).

The natural frequency of calcium transients has been evaluated in neurons both in culture and in the intact spinal cord over periods of 1 hour, capturing images once every 5 seconds to minimize photodynamic damage and allow normal differentiation. This time-lapse approach reveals two classes of spontaneous calcium transients: rapid events, termed calcium spikes, and slow events, termed calcium waves (Fig. 6-1; Gu et al., 1994). Calcium spikes rise in several hundred milliseconds, achieving on average a fourfold elevation of intracellular calcium above baseline followed by a double exponential decay with time constants of 10 seconds and 3 minutes. Spikes raise intracellular calcium from 50 nM to more than 500 nM

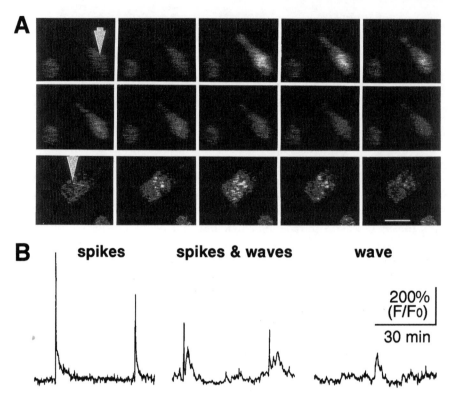

Figure 6-1. Spontaneous transient elevations of $[Ca^{2+}]_i$ at 6–8 hours in vitro. (A) Fast spike (*top*) and slow wave (*bottom*) in two spinal neurons (arrows). The nonneuronal cells are inactive. Images acquired at 0.2 Hz and displayed at 5-second and 2.5-minute intervals (*top* and *bottom;* left to right). Fluo-3 fluorescence is indicated in shades of gray; the lightest regions reflect changes of 400–600 percent of baseline. Scale (all panels), 25 μm. (B) Elevation of $[Ca^{2+}]_i$ in spikes, spikes followed by waves, and waves (left to right) in three neurons, digitized at 0.2 Hz. Spikes and waves may originate by a common mechanism. Fast and slow time constants for the two spikes at left are 9.1 seconds, 3.5 minutes, and 20 seconds, 2.0 minutes, respectively. (From Gu et al., 1994.)

(Fig. 6-2). In contrast, calcium waves rise more slowly, requiring 30 seconds or more to peak and declining over periods of minutes. The calcium elevation is smaller than that achieved by spikes and is typically less than a doubling of steady-state levels. Spikes stimulate a prominent elevation of nuclear calcium that is not achieved by waves. (Note that the terms "spike" and "wave," as used here, refer to intracellular changes in calcium and are quite different from the EEG-related spike and wave.)

In culture, one-third of neurons exhibit spikes, one-third generate waves, and one-third remain silent during a 1-hour period of observation. Cells that are contiguous may be coactive and exhibit spikes or waves that are coincident. Patterns of spike activity vary widely among different cells, raising

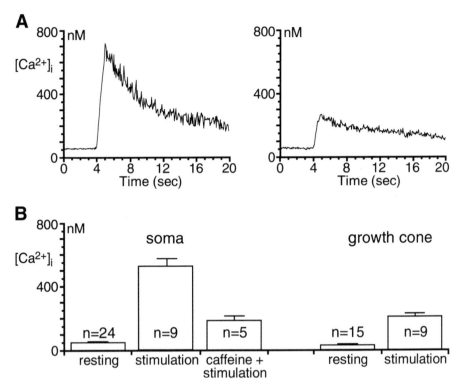

Figure 6-2. Intracellular calcium levels achieved during elicited spikes, estimated from fura-2 fluorescence. (A) *Left:* Spike elicited by electrical stimulation shows an elevation of calcium in the soma from 50 to 700 nM. *Right:* Depletion of stores with caffeine reduces the elevation of calcium following stimulation of a spike to 250 nM in the same neuron. Data acquired and displayed at 12.5 Hz. 7 hours in vitro. (B) Mean baseline and peak values of $[Ca^{2+}]_i$ in the soma ± caffeine and in the growth cone. 6–8 hours in vitro. Growth cones were not sufficiently stable to allow assessment of stores with caffeine. (From Gu et al., 1994.)

the possibility that this patterned activity is associated with particular aspects of differentiation since the cultures include sensory, motor and interneurons. Interestingly, spikes occur with a substantially higher incidence and a greater frequency in the intact spinal cord than in neurons in dissociated cell culture. Half the neurons exhibit spikes during a 1-hour period of observation at the neural tube stage, at an average frequency of 10 per hour; however, more than 10 spikes have been observed in a single neuron over a 10-minute period (Fig. 6-3). Both in culture and in the spinal cord, the incidence of spikes is developmentally regulated and decreases as neurons mature.

The mechanisms of production of calcium spikes and waves have been studied and the basis of calcium spikes is now well understood. Several lines

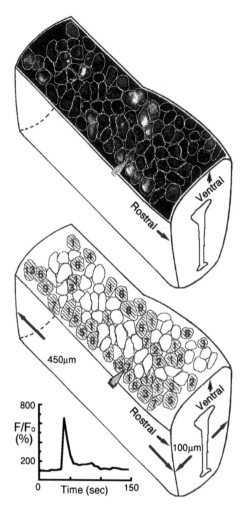

Figure 6-3. Spontaneous transient elevations of $[Ca^{2+}]_i$ in the intact embryonic spinal cord (Nieuwkoop and Faber stage 19), imaged at 0.2 Hz for 1 hour. *Top:* Single image displays 84 cells visualized on the ventral aspect of the cord, 41 of which exhibited spikes during a 10-minute period. *Middle:* Aggregate spontaneous activity; cells are represented by circles and the number in each indicates the spikes produced in that cell (1–13). *Bottom:* Time course of a calcium spike in the active cell indicated by the arrow, digitized at 0.2 Hz; rapid rate of rise and double exponential decay of fluorescence are characteristic of neurons. Scale, 25 μm. (From Gu et al., 1994.)

of evidence indicate that these spikes are generated by spontaneous calcium-dependent action potentials that trigger release of calcium from intracellular stores. First, these spikes are mimicked by stimulation of action potentials with extracellular electrodes. Second, spikes are propagated with a velocity consistent with the conduction of action potentials, as demonstrated by the rapid travel of spikes between the soma and growth cone in culture. Third, pharmacologic elimination of LVA calcium current or sodium current, which raises the threshold for initiation of calcium-dependent action potentials, suppresses the incidence of spikes in a predictable manner. Finally, calcium channel blockers, which block calcium-dependent action potentials, completely abolish these spikes. The involvement of calcium-induced calcium release is indicated by reduction of spike amplitude by caffeine (Fig. 6-2). In contrast, waves are not blocked by any of these agents, suggesting that waves may be mediated by a novel process. Spikes can be followed closely by waves, and suppression of spikes increases the incidence of waves, raising the possibility that the two events are somehow linked.

The functions of spikes and waves are now becoming apparent as well. On the one hand, spikes exert their effects in the cell body, where they produce an increase in the ratio of nuclear to cytosolic calcium indicator fluorescence that is not generated by waves. Spikes seem to regulate the normal appearance of GABA in a population of interneurons, as well as the increase in rate of activation of the delayed rectifier current; both GABA and delayed rectifier maturation are blocked by Ni^{2+}, which also blocks spikes (Fig. 6-4; Desarmenien and Spitzer, 1991; Spitzer et al,. 1993). Spontaneous calcium influx may stimulate calcium-regulated transcription (Bading et al., 1993; Dash et al., 1991; Lerea and McNamara, 1993; Sheng et al., 1990) since inhibitors of RNA synthesis have an effect on these neurons similar to that of blocking calcium influx (Desarmenien and Spitzer, 1991; Ribera and Spitzer, 1989).

On the other hand, calcium waves appear to be important in regulating the length of outgrowing neurites, and they seem to exert their effects in the growth cone (Fig. 6-5). Waves are initiated in growth cones at higher frequencies than in the cell body but typically do not invade the soma. As a result, local waves occur independently at separate growth cones of the same neuron. Only large waves originating in the soma can invade growth cones, with a velocity consistent with the diffusion of calcium (Albritton et al., 1992). Long neurites are formed in culture when calcium influx during waves is prevented by removal of extracellular calcium. Neurites are short in the presence of extracellular calcium, even when spikes are eliminated. Thus the length of each neurite can be independently regulated and the developmental persistence of waves is consistent with the continued sensitivity of growth cones to extracellular calcium (Holliday and Spitzer, 1990).

These findings demonstrate a developmental signal transduction cascade in these amphibian spinal neurons which involves slow signaling by calcium transients, some of which (calcium spikes) are mechanistically related to the generation of rapid action potentials. Spontaneous elevations of intracellular calcium have also been investigated in slice preparations of mammalian tissue. Imaging of neonatal rat cortex has shown distinct domains of spontaneously coactive neurons (Yuste et al., 1992). Spontaneous calcium transients have also been revealed in dendrites of Purkinje cells in the mature cerebellum (Sugimori and Llinas, 1990; Tank et al., 1988). In culture, cell bodies of postnatally isolated Purkinje cells exhibit spontaneous elevations

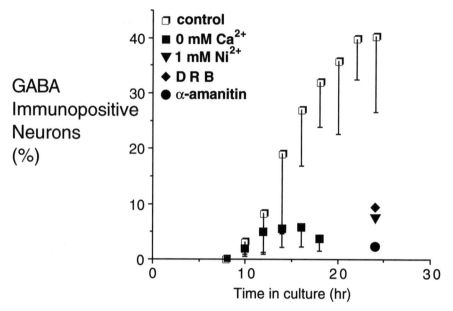

Figure 6-4. Regulation of development of GABA immunoreactivity by calcium spikes in cultured spinal neurons. Forty percent of neurons acquire GABA immunoreactivity during the first day in culture in the presence of extracellular calcium. Acquisition of immunoreactivity is suppressed by growth in calcium-free medium (■) in comparison with controls (❑). Similar results are achieved by application of 1 mM nickel in the presence of calcium, which blocks spikes but not waves. Immunoreactivity is also suppressed by RNA synthesis inhibitors dichlororibobenzimidazole (DRB) and α-amanitin. Values are mean ± SEM for 100 or more neurons from three or more cultures. (From Spitzer et al., 1993.)

of intracellular calcium involving voltage-dependent calcium and sodium channels (Sorimachi, Morita, and Kuramoto, 1990; Sorimachi, Morita, and Nakamura, 1990). Recordings from embryonic chick brainstem using voltage-sensitive dyes reveal spontaneous electrical activity occurring at a low frequency (Komuro et al., 1993). Calcium transients are generated in motor neurons in the spinal cord of chick embryos during bursting episodes driven by spontaneous synaptic activity (O'Donovan et al., 1993). Chronic treatment with calcium channel blockers can reduce the functional expression of L-type HVA current in muscle cells (Kano et al., 1992), while electrical stimulation can increase both the number and function of these channels (Freud-Silverberg and Shainberg, 1993), consistent with a role of spontaneous calcium channel activation in their regulation.

Spontaneous electrical activity in the nervous system is also prominent at later stages of development (Corner and Crain, 1972; Hamburger et al., 1966) and has been implicated in specifying patterns of motor innervation (O'Brien et al., 1990; O'Donovan and Landmesser, 1987) as well as the connections in the visual system and the cerebral cortex (Blanton and Krieg-

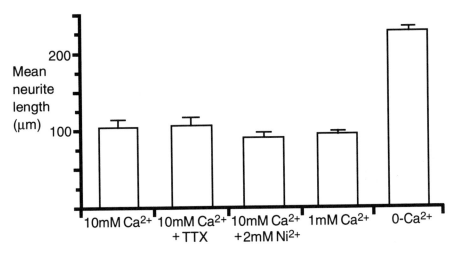

Figure 6-5. Regulation of neurite length by calcium waves. Suppression of spikes with 1 µg/ml TTX or 2 mM Ni^{2+} has no effect relative to control ($P > .16$, t test), while elimination of waves by removal of extracellular calcium promotes neurite extension ($P < .001$). Values are means for the longest neurite of over 50 mature neurons from three or more cultures. (From Gu et al., 1994.)

stein, 1991; Meister et al., 1991). While sodium-dependent action potentials clearly play a number of important roles (Harris, 1981), these impulses can trigger voltage-dependent calcium entry (Chen et al., 1990; Jaffe et al., 1992; Lev-Ram et al., 1992; Sorimachi, Morita, and Kuramoto, 1990; Sorimachi, Morita, and Nakamura, 1990), which may be the effector of developmental changes. Even mature neurons may maintain their patterns of electrical activity by regulating conductances by intracellular concentrations of calcium (LeMasson et al., 1993).

Modulation of Development of Excitability by Extrinsic Factors or Targets

In a number of cases it has been possible to clearly define the roles of specific extracellular factors in regulating the developmental expression of ion channels. These studies are relevant to an understanding of the pathophysiology of epilepsy since alterations in expression of growth factors can affect patterns of maturation of excitability. Nerve growth factor (NGF) and basic fibroblast growth factor (bFGF) can increase calcium current in rat hippocampal neurons (Cheng et al., 1993); bFGF augments calcium current in rat hypothalamic neurons as well (Koike et al., 1993). Insulinlike growth factor I increases calcium currents in a neuroblastoma cell line (Kleppisch et al., 1992). NGF also stimulates both morphologic differentiation and increases in expression and densities of sodium and LVA calcium channels in PC12 cells (Baev et al., 1992; Garber et al., 1989; Pollock et al., 1990; Reuter et al., 1992). Dexamethasone increases the incidence but not the densities of these inward currents. The action of NGF on sodium channels is mediated by cAMP-dependent protein kinase (Ginty et al., 1992; Kalman et al., 1990; Pollack et al., 1990). Basic fibroblast growth factor stimulates increases in sodium current much like NGF, while the increase stimulated by epidermal growth factor is smaller (Ginty et al., 1992; Pollack et al., 1990). Similar expression of sodium current in newborn rat dorsal root ganglion neurons is stimulated by NGF (Omri and Meiri, 1990). Interestingly the expression of potassium currents is not affected by these agents (Garber et al., 1989). Differentiation of potassium currents of neonatal superior cervical ganglion neurons is not affected by innervation but appears to require an extrinsic factor that is absent in culture (McFarlane and Cooper, 1992). The development of potassium current of chick ciliary neurons may be similarly controlled (Dourado and Dryer, 1992). Hippocampal progenitor cell lines stimulated by specific cytokines involved in the differentiation of the hematopoietic system express TTX-insensitive or TTX-sensitive action potentials (Mehler et al., 1993). The present evidence suggests that developmental modulation of ion channel expression is due to soluble factors rather than to interactions with target cell surfaces or matrix components.

Effects of Early "Seizures" on Maturational Programs

Abnormal elevation of electrical activity may have profound effects on the development of the nervous system. In recent years, there has been increasing interest in the analysis of expression of immediate early genes (IEGs), which are rapidly transcribed following such stimuli without prerequisite protein synthesis, producing messenger RNA levels that are transiently elevated. Most of these are protooncogenes, cellular genes involved in transmission of information within and between cells. Since these IEGs encode transcription factors, they are likely to be involved in expression of other gene products initiated by the electrical activity. Pentylenetetrazole, kainic acid, and electrical stimulation are only a few of the stimuli that cause the induction of c-fos, a particularly well-studied protooncogene (Greenberg et al., 1986; Lanaud et al., 1993; see Morgan and Curran, 1991, for review). Of particular interest are observations that kindling afterdischarges can provoke elevations of IEGs (Simonato et al., 1991) or increase the efficacy of electroconvulsive seizures in stimulating the levels of these transcription factors (Duman et al., 1992; Labiner et al., 1993). The expression of c-fos is governed by specific DNA promoter sequences, such as the serum response element (SRE) and the calcium or cAMP regulatory element (CRE; Montminy et al., 1986; Treisman, 1986), which appear to be activated by calcium influx. Phosphorylation of the CRE binding protein by calcium-calmodulin kinase seems to enhance its ability to stimulate transcription (Sheng et al.,

1990), while the SRE is activated by signals stimulated by protein kinase C (Gilman, 1988).

Although these studies have focused principally on the mature nervous system, it seems likely that the plasticity evident in the adult is manifest at a higher level in the immature CNS. In immature neurons, stimulation of patterned neural activity activates c-*fos* in cultured mouse dorsal root ganglion cells (Sheng et al., 1993), calcium influx by L-type calcium channels induces c-*fos* (Bading et al., 1993), and different types of ionotropic glutamate receptors activate c-*fos* transcription by different routes (Lerea and McNamara, 1993). Further studies will establish the direct linkages between IEG expression and activation of downstream genes that lead to the alteration of various aspects of neuronal function.

In other studies the effects of abnormal electrical activity have already been directly related to changes in receptor and channel properties or to alterations in neurotransmitter expression. The generation of electrographic seizures is enhanced by the greater natural calcium conductance of NMDA receptors in the immature hipppocampus (Brady et al., 1991), and sensitivity to NMDA is enhanced in the hippocampus of kindled rats (Morrisett et al., 1989). Moreover, kindling produced by periodic electrical stimulation of the brain can promote delayed upregulation of NMDA receptors, assessed by binding of specific ligands (Yeh et al., 1989). Chemical kindling, the development of seizures in response to doses of an agent initially insufficient to stimulate convulsive activity, can produce a decrease in function of GABA-activated chloride channels (Lewin et al., 1989). Stimulation of cortical seizures induces changes in responsiveness to iontophoresis of acetylcholine (Solis et al., 1992). Decreased receptor and transmitter levels are sometimes associated with neuronal loss (Johnson et al., 1992; Robbins et al., 1991) rather than modulation in intact cells. Although these effects are secondary to excitotoxicity, they are likely to be of great functional importance.

These studies parallel similar findings in the immature nervous system, showing that calcium influx can provide developmental stabilization of neurotransmitter phenotype (Nishi and Berg, 1981; Walicke and Patterson, 1981). More specifically, spontaneous electrical activity of cultured embryonic mouse spinal cord neurons drives expression of transcripts encoding enkephalin (Agoston et al., 1991). Although suppressible by TTX, the blockade can be overridden by selective activation of L-type calcium channels, consistent with a role of calcium influx stimulated by sodium-dependent action potentials. Electrical stimulation slows or arrests the extent of neurite outgrowth in culture (Cohan, 1992; Cohan and Kater, 1986; Fields et al., 1990), and this electrical activity, which can be suppressed by TTX, elevates intracellular calcium, which influences growth cone behavior (Kater et al., 1988; Kater and Mills, 1991). Blockade of spontaneous calcium influx suppresses neuronal migration in formation of the cerebellar cortex (Komuro and Rakic, 1992, 1993) and disrupts formation of patterns of neuronal connections in the visual tectum and visual cortex (Constantine-Paton et al., 1990; Shatz, 1990).

Conclusion

Several mechanisms by which early, immature forms of excitability promote epilepsy can be identified. The first of these is the acute effect of sustained depolarization and prolonged release of neurotransmitter, provoked by enhancement of calcium currents and elevation of intracellular calcium. When motor tracts are affected, the impact is to generate seizure activity. Since inhibitory pathways may also be affected, a quiescence or absence of CNS activity is expected in some cases. The second mechanism stimulating epileptiform activity at early stages of development is the chronic effect of unusual patterns of electrical activity and elevation of intracellular calcium. In this case, differentiation of neuronal properties as diverse as migration, neurite outgrowth, neurotransmitter synthesis, and channel maturation may be altered.

The developing nervous system rests in a meta-stable state and can be relatively easily pushed out of alignment. Features of early excitability are apparently important for normal specification of the process of differentiation. The maturation of the nervous system establishes a more rigorous set of checks and balances and enhances its stability. Much of this maturation involves the appearance of tighter methods of control of intracellular calcium. As the nervous system becomes fully differentiated, plasticity is reduced but stable function is assured.

Acknowledgments

I thank my colleagues for stimulating discussions. My work is supported by NIH grants NS 15918 and NS 25916.

References

Agoston, D. V., Eiden, L. E., and Brenneman, D. E. (1991) Calcium-dependent regulation of the enkephalin phenotype by neuronal activity during early ontogeny. *J. Neurosci. Res. 28:*140–148.

Aguayo, L. G. (1989) Post-natal development of K^+ currents studied in isolated rat pineal cells. *J. Physiol. 414:*283–300.

Ahmed, Z., Walker, P. S., and Fellows, R. E. (1983) Properties of neurons from dissociated fetal rat brain in serum-free culture. *J. Neurosci. 3:*2448–2462.

Albritton, N. L., Meyer, T., and Stryer, L. (1992) Range of messenger action of calcium ion and inositol 1,4,5-trisphosphate. *Science 258:*1812–1815.

Alzheimer, C., Schwindt, P. C., and Crill, W. E. (1993) Postnatal development of a persistent Na^+ current in pyramidal neurons from rat sensorimotor cortex. *J. Neurophysiol. 69:*290–292.

Angelides, K. J., Elmer, L. W., Loftus, D., and Elson, E. (1988) Distribution and lateral mobility of voltage-dependent sodium channels in neurons. *J. Cell Biol. 106*:1911–1925.

Anglister, L., Farber, I. C., Shahar, A., and Grinvald, A. (1982) Localization of voltage-sensitive calcium channels along developing neurites: Their possible role in regulating neurite elongation. *Dev. Biol. 94*:351–365.

Baccaglini, P. I. (1978) Action potentials of embryonic dorsal root ganglion neurones in *Xenopus* tadpoles. *J. Physiol. 283*:585–604.

Baccaglini, P. I., and Spitzer, N. C. (1977) Developmental changes in the inward current of the action potential of Rohon-Beard neurones. *J. Physiol. 271*:93–117.

Bader, C. R., Bertrand, D., and Dupin, E. (1985) Voltage-dependent potassium currents in developing neurones from quail mesencephalic neural crest. *J. Physiol. 366*:129–151.

Bader, C. R., Bertrand, D., Dupin, E., and Kato, A. C. (1983) Development of electrical properties of cultured avian neural crest. *Nature 305*:808–810.

Bader, C. R., Bertrand, D., and Kato, A. C. (1983) Membrane currents in a developing parasympathetic ganglion. *Dev. Biol. 98*:515–519.

Bading, H., Ginty, D. D., and Greenberg, M. E. (1993) Regulation of gene expression in hippocampal neurons by distinct calcium signaling pathways. *Science 260*:181–186.

Baev, K. V., Beresovskii, V. K., Kalunov, V. N., Luschitskaya, N. I., Rusin, K. I., Vilner, B. Y., and Zavadskaya, T. V. (1992) Potential- and acetylcholine-activated ionic currents of pheochromocytoma PC12 cells during incubation with nerve growth factor. *Neuroscience 46*:925–930.

Bargas, J., Surmeier, D. J., and Kitai, S. T. (1991) High- and low-voltage activated calcium currents are expressed by neurons cultured from embryonic rat neostriatum. *Brain Res. 541*:70–74.

Barish, M. E. (1986) Differentiation of voltage-gated potassium current and modulation of excitability in cultured amphibian spinal neurones. *J. Physiol. 375*:229–250.

Beam, K. G., and Knudson, C. M. (1988) Effect of postnatal development on calcium currents and slow charge movement in mammalian skeletal muscle. *J. Gen. Physiol. 91*:799–815.

Beck, H., Ficker, E., and Heinemann, U. (1992) Properties of two voltage-activated potassium currents in acutely isolated juvenile rat dentate gyrus granule cells. *J. Neurophysiol. 68*:2086–2099.

Beckh, S., and Pongs, O. (1990) Members of the RCK potassium channel family are differentially expressed in the rat nervous system. *EMBO J. 9*:777–782.

Ben-Ari, Y., Cherubini, E., Corradetti, R., and Gaiarsa, J. L. (1989) Giant synaptic potentials in immature rat CA3 hippocampal neurones. *J. Physiol. 416*:303–325.

Blair, L. A. C., and Dionne, V. E. (1985) Developmental acquisition of Ca^{2+}-sensitivity by K^+ channels in spinal neurones. *Nature 315*:329–331.

Blanton, M. G., and Kriegstein, A. R. (1991) Spontaneous action potential activity and synaptic currents in the embryonic turtle cerebral cortex. *J. Neurosci. 11*:3907–3923.

Blanton, M. G., Lo Turco, J. J., and Kriegstein, A. R. (1989) Whole cell recording from neurons in slices of reptilian and mammalian cerebral cortex. *J. Neurosci. Meth. 30*:203–210.

Bode-Greuel, K. M., and Singer, W. (1991) Developmental changes of calcium currents in the visual cortex of the cat. *Exp. Brain Res. 84:*311–318.

Brady, R. J., Smith, K. L., and Swann, J. W. (1991) Calcium mobilization of the *N*-methyl-D-aspartate (NMDA) response and electrographic seizures in immature hippocampus. *Neurosci. Lett. 124:*92–96.

Bregestovski, P. D., Printseva, O. Y., Serebryakov, V., Stinnakre, J., Turmin, A., and Zamoyski, V. (1988) Comparison of Ca^{2+}-dependent K^+ channels in the membrane of smooth muscle cells isolated from adult and foetal human aorta. *Pflügers Arch. 413:*8–13.

Brysch, W., Creutzfeldt, O. D., Luno, K., Schlingensiepen, R., and Schlingensiepen, K. H. (1991) Regional and temporal expression of sodium channel messenger RNAs in the rat brain during development. *Exp. Brain Res. 86:*562–567.

Catterall, W. A. (1981) Localization of sodium channels in cultured neural cells. *J. Neurosci. 1:*777–783.

Chen, C., Zhang, J., Vincent, J. D., and Israel, J. M. (1990) Sodium and calcium currents in action potentials of rat somatotrophs: Their possible functions in growth hormone secretion. *Life Sci. 46:*983–989.

Cheng, B., McMahon, D. G., and Mattson, M. P. (1993) Modulation of calcium current, intracellular calcium levels and cell survival by glucose deprivation and growth factors in hippocampal neurons. *Brain Res. 607:*275–285.

Cherubini, E., Ben-Ari, Y., and Krnjevic, K. (1990) Periodic inward currents triggered by NMDA in immature CA3 hippocampal neurones. *Adv. Exp. Med. Biol. 268:*147–150.

Chin, H., Smith, M. A., Kim, H. L., and Kim, H. (1992) Expression of dihydropyridine-sensitive brain calcium channels in the rat central nervous system. *FEBS Lett. 299:*69–74.

Cohan, C. S. (1992) Depolarization-induced changes in neurite elongation and intracellular Ca^{2+} in isolated *Helisoma* neurons. *J. Neurobiol. 23:*983–986.

Cohan, C. S., and Kater, S. B. (1986) Suppression of neurite elongation and growth cone motility by electrical activity. *Science 232:*1638–1640.

Connor, J. A., Tseng, H. Y., and Hockberger, P. E. (1987) Depolarization- and transmitter-induced changes in intracellular Ca^{2+} of rat cerebellar granule cells in explant cultures. *J. Neurosci. 7:*1384–1400.

Connors, B. W., Ransom, B. R., Kunis, D. M., and Gutnick, M. J. (1982) Activity-dependent K^+ accumulation in the developing rat optic nerve. *Science 216:*1341–1343.

Constantine-Paton, M., Cline, H. T., and Debski, E. (1990) Patterned activity, synaptic convergence, and the NMDA receptor in developing visual pathways. *Ann. Rev. Neurosci. 13:*129–154.

Corner, M. A., and Crain, S. M. (1972) Patterns of spontaneous bioelectric activity during maturation in culture of fetal rodent medulla and spinal cord tissues. *J. Neurobiol. 3:*25–45.

Coulter, D. A., Huguenard, J. R., and Prince, D. A. (1989) Calcium currents in rat thalamocortical relay neurones: Kinetic properties of the transient, low-threshold current. *J. Physiol. 414:*587–604.

Dash, P. K., Karl, K. A., Colicos, M. A., Prywes, R., and Kandel, E. R. (1991) cAMP response element-binding protein is activated by Ca^{2+}/calmodulin—as well as cAMP-dependent protein kinase. *Proc. Natl. Acad. Sci. 88:*5061–5065.

Desarmenien, M. G., Clendening, B., and Spitzer, N. C. (1993) *In vivo* development of voltage-dependent ionic currents in embryonic *Xenopus* spinal neurons. *J. Neurosci. 13:*2575–2581.

Desarmenien, M. G., and Spitzer, N. C. (1991) Determinant role of calcium and protein kinase C in development of the delayed rectifier potassium current in *Xenopus* spinal neurons. *Neuron 7:*797–805.

Dichter, M. A., Tischler, A. S., and Greene, L. A. (1977) Nerve growth factor–induced increase in electrical excitability and acetylcholine sensitivity of a rat pheochromocytoma cell line. *Nature 268:*501–504.

Dietzel, I. D. (1994) Excitability in embryogenesis. *Perspect. Dev. Neurobiol.*, in press.

Dourado, M. M., and Dryer, S. E. (1992) Changes in the electrical properties of chick ciliary ganglion neurones during embryonic development. *J. Physiol. 449:*411–428.

Drewe, J. A., Verma, S., Frech, G., and Joho, R. H. (1992) Distinct spatial and temporal expression patterns of K^+ channel mRNAs from different subfamilies. *J. Neurosci. 12:*538–548.

Duman, R. S., Craig, J. S., Winston, S. M., Deutch, A. Y., and Hernandez, T. D. (1992) Amygdala kindling potentiates seizure-stimulated immediate-early gene expression in rat cerebral cortex. *J. Neurochem. 59:*1753–1760.

Fields, R. D., Neale, E. A., and Nelson, P. G. (1990) Effects of patterned electrical activity on neurite outgrowth from mouse sensory neurons. *J. Neurosci. 10:*2950–2964.

Freud-Silverberg, M., and Shainberg, A. (1993) Electric stimulation regulates the level of Ca-channels in chick muscle culture. *Neurosci. Lett. 151:*104–106.

Fukuda, A., and Prince, D. A. (1992) Postnatal development of electrogenic sodium pump activity in rat hippocampal pyramidal neurons. *Dev. Brain Res. 65:*101–114.

Furuyama, T., Morita, Y., Inagaki, S., and Takagi, H. (1993) Distribution of I, II and III subtypes of voltage-sensitive Na^+ channel mRNA in the rat brain. *Brain Res. Mol. Brain Res. 17:*169–173.

Garber, S. S., Hoshi, T., and Aldrich, R. W. (1989) Regulation of ionic currents in pheochromocytoma cells by nerve growth factor and dexamethasone. *J. Neurosci. 9:*3976–3987.

Gilman, M. J. (1988) The c-*fos* serum response element responds to protein kinase C-dependent and -independent signals but not to cyclic AMP. *Genes Dev. 2:*394–402.

Ginty, D. D., Fanger, G. R., Wagner, J. A., and Maue, R. A. (1992) The activity of cAMP-dependent protein kinase is required at a posttranslational level for induction of voltage-dependent sodium channels by peptide growth factors in PC12 cells. *J. Cell Biol. 116:*1465–1473.

Goodman, C. S., and Spitzer, N. C. (1979) Embryonic development of identified neurones: Differentiation from neuroblast to neurone. *Nature 280:*208–214.

Goodman, C. S., and Spitzer, N. C. (1981) The development of electrical properties of identified neurones in grasshopper embryos. *J. Physiol. 313:*385–403.

Gottmann, K., Dietzel, I. D., Lux, H. D., Huck, S., and Rohrer, H. (1988) Development of inward currents in chick sensory and autonomic neuronal precursor cells in culture. *J. Neurosci. 8:*3722–3732.

Gottmann, K., Dietzel, I. D., Lux, H. D., and Ruedel, C. (1989) Proton-induced Na^+

current develops prior to voltage-dependent Na$^+$ and Ca^{2+} currents in neuronal precursor cells from chick dorsal root ganglion. *Neurosci. Lett. 99*:90–
94.

Grantyn, R., Perouansky, M., Rodríguez-Tébar, A., and Lux, H. D. (1989) Expression of depolarizing voltage- and transmitter-activated currents in neuronal
precursor cells from the rat brain is preceded by a proton-activated sodium
current. *Dev. Brain Res. 49*:150–155.

Greenberg, M. E., Ziff, E. B., and Greene, L. A. (1986) Stimulation of neuronal
acetylcholine receptors induces rapid gene transcription. *Science 234*:80–83.

Gruol, D. L., Deal, C. R., and Yool, A. J. (1992) Developmental changes in calcium
conductances contribute to the physiological maturation of cerebellar Purkinje neurons in culture. *J. Neurosci. 12*:2838–2848.

Gu, X., Olson, E. C., and Spitzer, N. C. (1994) Spontaneous neuronal calcium spikes
and waves during early differentiation. *J. Neurosci.* 14: 6325–6335.

Gu, X., and Spitzer, N. C. (1993). Low threshold Ca^{2+} current and its role in spontaneous elevations of intracellular Ca^{2+} in developing *Xenopus* neurons. *J.
Neurosci. 13*:4936–4948.

Hagland, M. M., and Schwartzkroin, P. A. (1990) Role of Na-K pump potassium
regulation and IPSPs in seizures and spreading depression in immature rabbit
hippocampal slices. *J. Neurophysiol. 63*:225–239.

Hamburger, V., Wenger, E., and Oppenheim, R. (1966) Motility in the chick embryo
in the absence of sensory input. *J. Exp. Zool. 162*:133–160.

Harris, G. L., Henderson, L. P., and Spitzer, N. C. (1988) Changes in densities and
kinetics of delayed rectifier potassium channels during neuronal differentiation. *Neuron 1*:739–750.

Harris, W. A. (1981) Neural activity and development. *Ann. Rev. Physiol. 43*:689–
710.

Holliday, J., Adams, R. J., Sejnowski, T. J., and Spitzer, N. C. (1991) Calcium-
induced release of calcium regulates differentiation of spinal neurons. *Neuron
7*:787–796.

Holliday, J., and Spitzer, N. C. (1990) Spontaneous calcium influx and its roles in
differentiation of spinal neurons in culture. *Dev. Biol. 141*:13–23.

Huguenard, J. R., Hamill, O. P., and Prince, D. A. (1988) Developmental changes in
Na$^+$ conductances in rat neocortical neurons: Appearance of a slowly inactivating component. *J. Neurophysiol. 59*:778–795.

Hussy, N. (1991) Developmental change in calcium-activated chloride current during
the differentiation of *Xenopus* spinal neurons in culture. *Dev. Biol. 147*:225–
238.

Hussy, N. (1992) Calcium-activated chloride channels in cultured embryonic *Xenopus* spinal neurons. *J. Neurophysiol. 68*:2042–2050.

Hwang, P. M., Glatt, C. E., Bredt, D. S., Yellen, G., and Snyder, S. H. (1992) A
novel K$^+$ channel with unique localizations in mammalian brain: Molecular
cloning and characterization. *Neuron 8*:473–481.

Jaffe, D. B., Johnston, D., Lasser-Ross, N., Lisman, J. E., Miyakawa, H., and Ross,
W. N. (1992) The spread of Na$^+$ spikes determines the pattern of dendritic
Ca^{2+} entry into hippocampal neurons. *Nature 357*:244–246.

Janigro, D., and Schwartzkroin, P. A. (1988) Effects of GABA and baclofen on pyramidal cells in the developing rabbit hippocampus: An "in vitro" study. *Brain
Res. 469*:171–178.

Jendelova, P., and Sykova, E. (1991) Role of glia in K$^+$ and pH homeostasis in the neonatal rat spinal cord. *Glia 4:*56–63.

Johnson, E. W., deLanerolle, N. C., Kim, J. H., Sundaresan, S., Spencer, D. D., Mattson, R. H., Zoghbi, S. S., Baldwin, R. M., Hoffer, P. B., and Seibyl, J. P. (1992) "Central" and "peripheral" benzodiazepine receptors: Opposite changes in human epileptogenic tissue. *Neurology 42:*811–815.

Kalman, D., Wong, B., Horvai, A. E., Cline, M. J., and O'Lague, P. H. (1990) Nerve growth factor acts through cAMP-dependent protein kinase to increase the number of sodium channels in PC12 cells. *Neuron 4:*355–366.

Kano, M., Satoh, R., and Nakabayashi, Y. (1992) Calcium channels in embryonic chick skeletal muscle cells after cultivation with calcium channel blocker. *Neurosci. Lett. 144:*161–164.

Kater, S. B., Mattson, M. P., Cohan, C., and Connor, J. (1988) Calcium regulation of the neuronal growth cone. *Trends Neurosci. 11:*315–321.

Kater, S. B., and Mills, L. R. (1991) Regulation of growth cone behavior by calcium. *J. Neurosci. 11:*891–899.

Kleppisch, T., Klinz, F. J., and Hescheler, J. (1992) Insulin-like growth factor I modulates voltage-dependent Ca^{2+} channels in neuronal cells. *Brain Res. 591:*283–288.

Kocsis, J. D., Ruiz, J. A., and Waxman, S. G. (1983) Maturation of mammalian myelinated fibers: Changes in action-potential characteristics following 4-amino-pyridine application. *J. Neurophysiol. 50:*449–463.

Koike, H., Saito, H., and Matsuki, N. (1993) Effect of fibroblast growth factors on calcium currents in acutely isolated neuronal cells from rat ventromedial hypothalamus. *Neurosci. Lett. 150:*57–60.

Komuro, H., Momose-Sato, Y., Sakai, T., Hirota, A., and Kamino, K. (1993) Optical monitoring of early appearance of spontaneous membrane potential changes in the embryonic chick medulla oblongata using a voltage-sensitive dye. *Neuroscience 52:*55–62.

Komuro, H., and Rakic, P. (1992) Selective role of N-type calcium channels in neuronal migration. *Science 257:*806–809.

Komuro, H., and Rakic, P. (1993) Modulation of neuronal migration by NMDA receptors. *Science 260:*95–97.

Kostyuk, P. G. (1989) Diversity of calcium ion channels in cellular membranes. *Neuroscience 28:*253–261.

Kovalchuk, Y. N., Krishtal, O. A., and Nowycky, M. C. (1990) The proton-activated inward current of rat sensory neurons includes a calcium component. *Neurosci. Lett. 115:*237–242.

Krieger, C., and Sears, T. A. (1988) The development of voltage-dependent ionic conductances in murine spinal cord neurones in culture. *Can. J. Physiol. Pharm. 66:*1328–1336.

Kuffler, S. W. (1967) Neuroglial cells: The physiological properties and a potassium mediated effect of neuronal activity on the glial cell membrane. *Proc. R. Soc. London B 168:*1–21.

Labiner, D. M., Butler, L. S., Cao, Z., Hosford, D. A., Shin, C., and McNamara, J. O. (1993) Induction of c-*fos* mRNA by kindled seizures: Complex relationship with neuronal burst firing. *J. Neurosci. 13:*744–751.

Lanaud, P., Maggio, R., Gale, K., and Grayson, D. R. (1993) Temporal and spatial patterns of expression of c-*fos, zif/*268, c-*jun* and *jun*-B mRNAs in rat brain following seizures evoked focally from the deep prepiriform cortex. *Exp. Neurol. 119:*20–31.

LeMasson, G., Marder, E., and Abbott, L. F. (1993) Activity-dependent regulation of conductances in model neurons. *Science 259:*1915–1917.

Lerea, L. S., and McNamara, J. O. (1993) Ionotropic glutamate receptor subtypes activate c-*fos* transcription by distinct calcium-requiring intracellular signaling pathways. *Neuron 10:*31–41.

Lev-Ram, V., Miyakawa, H., Lasser-Ross, N., and Ross, W. N. (1992) Calcium transients in cerebellar Purkinje neurons evoked by intracellular stimulation. *J. Neurophysiol. 68:*1167–1177.

Lewin, E., Peris, J., Bleck, V., Zahniser, N. R., and Harris, R. A. (1989) Chemical kindling decreases GABA-activated chloride channels of mouse brain. *Eur. J. Pharmacol. 160:*101–106.

Lockery, S. R., and Spitzer, N. C. (1992) Reconstruction of action potential development from whole-cell currents of differentiating spinal neurons. *J. Neurosci. 12:*2268–2287.

Lovinger, D. M., and White, G. (1989) Post-natal development of burst firing behavior and the low-threshold transient calcium current examined using isolated neurons from rat dorsal root ganglia. *Neurosci. Lett. 102:*50–57.

Matsuda, Y., Yoshida, S., and Yonezawa, T. (1978) Tetrodotoxin sensitivity and Ca component of action potentials of mouse dorsal root ganglion cells cultured in vitro. *Brain Res. 154:*69–82.

McCobb, D. P., Best, P. M., and Beam, K. G. (1989) Development alters the expression of calcium currents in chick limb motoneurons. *Neuron 2:*1633–1643.

McCobb, D. P., Best, P. M., and Beam, K. G. (1990) The differentiation of excitability in embryonic chick limb motoneurons. *J. Neurosci. 10:*2974–2984.

McFarlane, S., and Cooper, E. (1992) Postnatal development of voltage-gated K currents on rat sympathetic neurons. *J. Neurophysiol. 67:*1291–1330.

Mehler, M. F., Rozental, R., Dougherty, M., Spray, D. C., and Kessler, J. A. (1993) Cytokine regulation of neuronal differentiation of hippocampal progenitor cells. *Nature 362:*62–65.

Meister, M., Wong, R. O., Baylor, D. A., and Shatz, C. J. (1991) Synchronous bursts of action potentials in ganglion cells of the developing mammalian retina. *Science 252:*939–943.

Meyers, D. E., and Barker, J. L. (1989) Whole-cell patch-clamp analysis of voltage-dependent calcium conductances in cultured embryonic rat hippocampal neurons. *J. Neurophysiol. 61:*467–477.

Miyake, M. (1978) The development of action potential mechanism in a mouse neuronal cell line *in vitro. Brain Res. 143:*349–354.

Montminy, M. R., Sevarino, K. A., Wagner, J. A., Mandel, G., and Goodman, R. H. (1986) Identification of a cyclic-AMP-responsive element within the rat somatostatin gene. *Proc. Natl. Acad. Sci. 83:*6682–6686.

Morgan, J. I., and Curran, T. (1991) Stimulus-transcription coupling in the nervous system: Involvement of the inducible proto-oncogenes *fos* and *jun. Ann. Rev. Neurosci. 14:*421–451.

Mori-Okamoto, J., Ashida, H., Maru, E., and Tatsuno, J. (1983) The development of action potentials in cultures of explanted cortical neurons from chick embryos. *Dev. Biol. 97:*408–416.

Morrisett, R. A., Chow, C., Nadler, J. V., and McNamara, J. O. (1989) Biochemical evidence for enhanced sensitivity to *N*-methyl-D-aspartate in the hippocampal formation of kindled rats. *Brain Res. 496:*25–28.

Mourre, C., Cervera, P., and Lazdunski, M. (1987) Autoradiographic analysis in rat brain of the postnatal ontogeny of voltage-dependent Na$^+$ channels, Ca^{2+}-dependent K$^+$ channels and slow Ca^{2+} channels identified as receptors for tetrodotoxin, apamin and (–)-desmethoxyverapamil. *Brain Res. 417:*21–32.

Mynlieff, M., and Beam, K. G. (1992) Developmental expression of voltage-dependent calcium currents in identified mouse motoneurons. *Dev. Biol. 152:*407–410.

Nerbonne, J. M., and Gurney, A. M. (1989) Development of excitable membrane properties in mammalian sympathetic neurons. *J. Neurosci. 9:*3272–3286.

Nishi, R., and Berg, D. K. (1981) Two components from eye tissue that differentially stimulate the growth and development of ciliary ganglion neurons in cell culture. *J. Neurosci. 1:*505–513.

O'Brien, M. K., Landmesser, L., and Oppenheim, R. W. (1990) Development and survival of thoracic motoneurons and hindlimb musculature following transplantation of the thoracic neural tube to the lumbar region in the chick embryo: Functional aspects. *J. Neurobiol. 21:*341–355.

O'Donovan, M. J., Ho, S., Sholomenko, G., and Yee, W. (1993) Real-time imaging of neurons retrogradely and anterogradely labelled with calcium-sensitive dyes. *J. Neurosci. Meth. 46:*91–106.

O'Donovan, M. J., and Landmesser, L. (1987) The development of hindlimb motor activity studied in the isolated spinal cord of the chick embryo. *J. Neurosci. 7:*3256–3264.

O'Dowd, D. K., Ribera, A. B., and Spitzer, N. C. (1988) Development of voltage-dependent calcium, sodium and potassium currents in *Xenopus* spinal neurons. *J. Neurosci. 8:*792–805.

Ogata, N., and Tatebayashi, H. (1992) Ontogenic development of the TTX-sensitive and TTX-insensitive Na$^+$ channels in neurons of the rat dorsal root ganglia. *Dev. Brain Res. 65:*93–100.

O'Lague, P. H., and Huttner, S. L. (1980) Physiological and morphological studies of rat pheochromocytoma cells (PC12) chemically fused and grown in culture. *Proc. Natl. Acad. Sci. 77:*1701–1705.

Omri, G., and Meiri, H. (1990) Characterization of sodium currents in mammalian sensory neurons cultured in serum-free defined medium with and without nerve growth factor. *J. Membrane Biol. 115:*13–29.

Perney, T. M., Marshall, J., Martin, K. A., Hockfield, S., and Kaczmarek, L. K. (1992) Expression of the mRNAs for the Kv3.1 potassium channel gene in the adult and developing rat brain. *J. Neurophysiol. 68:*756–766.

Pettigrew, A. G., Crepel, F., and Krupa, M. (1988) Development of ionic conductances in neurons of the inferior olive in the rat: An *in vitro* study. *Proc. R. Soc. London B 234:*199–218.

Pollock, J. D., Krempin, M., and Rudy, B. (1990) Differential effects of NGF, FGF, EGF, cAMP, and dexamethasone on neurite outgrowth and sodium channel expression in PC12 cells. *J. Neurosci. 10:*2626–2637.

Reuter, H., Bouron, A., Neuhaus, R., Becker, C., and Reber, B. F. (1992) Inhibition of protein kinases in rat pheochromocytoma (PC12) cells promotes morphological differentiation and down-regulates ion channel expression. *Proc. R. Soc. London B 249:*211–216.

Ribera, A. B., and Nguyen, D.-A. (1993) Primary sensory neurons express a *Shaker*-like potassium channel gene. *J. Neurosci. 13:*4988–4996.

Ribera, A. B., and Spitzer, N. C. (1989) A critical period of transcription required for differentiation of the action potential of spinal neurons. *Neuron 2:*1055–1062.

Ribera, A. B., and Spitzer, N. C. (1990) Differentiation of I_{KA} in amphibian spinal neurons. *J. Neurosci. 10:*1886–1991.

Ritchie, A. K. (1979) Catecholamine secretion in a rat pheochromocytoma cell line: Two pathways for calcium entry. *J. Physiol. 286:*541–561.

Ritchie, J. M. (1982) Sodium and potassium channels in regenerating and developing mammalian myelinated nerves. *Proc. R. Soc. London B 215:*273–287.

Robbins, R. J., Brines, M. L., Kim, J. H., Adrian, T., de Lanerolle, N., Welsh, W., and Spencer, D. D. (1991) A selective loss of somatostatin in the hippocampus of patients with temporal lobe epilepsy. *Ann. Neurol. 29:*325–332.

Roy, M. L., and Narahashi, T. (1992) Differential properties of tetrodotoxin-sensitive and tetrodotoxin-resistant sodium channels in rat dorsal root ganglion neurons. *J. Neurosci. 12:*2104–2111.

Rudy, B., Kentros, C., Weiser, M., Fruhling, D., Serodio, P., Vega-Saenz de Miera, E., Ellisman, M. H., Pollock, J. A., and Baker, H. (1992) Region-specific expression of a K⁺ channel gene in brain. *Proc. Natl. Acad. Sci. 89:*4603–4607.

Sakmann, B., Edwards, F., Konnerth, A., and Takahashi, T. (1989) Patch clamp techniques used for studying synaptic transmission in slices of mammalian brain. *Q. J. Exp. Physiol. 74:*1107–1118.

Scheinman, R. I., Auld, V. J., Goldin, A. L., Davidson, N., Dunn, R. J., and Catterall, W. A. (1989) Developmental regulation of sodium channel expression in the rat forebrain. *J. Biol. Chem. 264:*10660–10666.

Shatz, C. J. (1990) Impulse activity and the patterning of connections during CNS development. *Neuron 5:*745–756.

Sheng, H. Z., Fields, R. D., and Nelson, P. G. (1993) Specific regulation of immediate early genes by patterned neuronal activity. *J. Neurosci. Res. 35:*459–467.

Sheng, M., McFadden, G., and Greenberg, M. E. (1990) Membrane depolarization and calcium induce *c-fos* transcription via phosphorylation of transcription factor CREB. *Neuron 4:*571–582.

Simonato, M., Hosford, D. A., Labiner, D. M., Shin, C., Mansbach, H. H., and McNamara, J. O. (1991) Differential expression of immediate early genes in the hippocampus in the kindling model of epilepsy. *Brain Res. Mol. Brain Res. 11:*115–124.

Skaliora, I., Scobey, R. P., and Chalupa, L. M. (1993) Prenatal development of excitability in cat retinal ganglion cells: Action potentials and sodium currents. *J. Neurosci. 13:*313–323.

Snutch, T. P., Tomlinson, W. J., Leonard, J. P., and Gilbert, M. M. (1991) Distinct calcium channels are generated by alternative splicing and are differentially expressed in the mammalian CNS. *Neuron 7:*45–57.

Solis, H., Bravo, J., and Galindo-Morales, J. A. (1992) Rapidly recurring cortical seizures induce changes in neuronal responsiveness to acetylcholine. *Boll. Estud. Med. Biol. 40:*49–56.

Somjen, G. G. (1978) Extracellular potassium in the mammalian nervous system. *Ann. Rev. Physiol. 41:*159–178.

Sorimachi, M., Morita, Y., and Kuramoto, K. (1990) Regulation of the cytosolic free calcium concentration by Na^+ spikes in immature cerebellar neurons with *N*-methyl-D-aspartate receptors. *Br. Res. 527:*155–158.

Sorimachi, M., Morita, Y., and Nakamura, H. (1990) Possible regulation of the cytosolic-free calcium concentration by Na^+ spikes in immature cerebellar Purkinje cells. *Neurosci. Lett. 111:*333–338.

Spitzer, N. C. (1979) Ion channels in development. *Ann. Rev. Neurosci. 2:*363–397.

Spitzer, N. C. (1985) The control of development of neuronal excitability. In G. M. Edelman, W. E. Gall, and W. M. Cowan (eds.), *Molecular Bases of Neural Development*. New York: Wiley, pp. 67–88.

Spitzer, N. C. (1991) A developmental handshake: Neuronal control of ionic currents and their control of neuronal differentiation. *J. Neurobiol. 22:*659–673.

Spitzer, N. C., deBaca, R. C., Allen, K., and Holliday, J. (1993) Calcium dependence of differentiation of GABA immunoreactivity in spinal neurons. *J. Comp. Neurol. 337:*168–175.

Spitzer, N. C., and Lamborghini, J. E. (1976) The development of the action potential mechanism of amphibian neurons isolated in cell culture. *Proc. Natl. Acad. Sci. 73:*1641–1645.

Streit, J., and Lux, H. D. (1989) Distribution of calcium currents in sprouting PC12 cells. *J. Neurosci. 9:*4190–4199.

Sugimori, M., and Llinás, R. R. (1990) Real-time imaging of calcium influx in mammalian cerebellar Purkinje cells *in vitro*. *Proc. Natl. Acad. Sci. 87:*5084–5088.

Swanson, R., Marshall, J., Smith, J. S., Williams, J. B., Boyle, M. B., Folander, K., Luneau, C. J., Antanavage, J., Oliva, C., and Buhrow, S. A. (1990) Cloning and expression of cDNA and genomic clones encoding three delayed rectifier potassium channels in rat brain. *Neuron 4:*929–939.

Tank, D. W., Sugimori, M., Connor, J. A., and Llinás, R. R. (1988) Spatially resolved calcium dynamics of mammalian Purkinje cells in cerebellar slice. *Science 242:*773–777.

Thompson, S. M., and Wong, R. K. (1991) Development of calcium current subtypes in isolated rat hippocampal pyramidal cells. *J. Physiol. 439:*671–689.

Treisman, R. (1986) Identification of a protein-binding site that mediates transcriptional response of the *c-fos* gene to serum factors. *Cell 46:*567–574.

Tsaur, M. L., Sheng, M., Lowenstein, D. H., Jan, Y. N., and Jan, L. Y. (1992) Differential expression of K^+ channel mRNAs in the rat brain and down-regulation in the hippocampus following seizures. *Neuron 8:*1055–1067.

Walicke, P. A., and Patterson, P. H. (1981) On the role of Ca^{2+} in the transmitter choice made by cultured sympathetic neurons. *J. Neurosci. 1:*343–350.

Walton, K., and Fulton, B. P. (1986) Ionic mechanisms underlying the firing properties of rat neonatal motoneurons studied *in vitro*. *Neuroscience 19:*669–683.

Warner, A. E. (1985) Factors controlling the early development of the nervous system. In G. M. Edelman, W. E. Gall, and W. M. Cowan (eds.), *Molecular Bases of Neural Development*. New York: Wiley, pp. 11–34.

Waxman, S. G., and Foster, R. E. (1980) Development of the axon membrane during differentiation of myelinated fibres in spinal nerve roots. *Proc. R. Soc. London B 209:*441–446.

Westenbroek, R. E., Ahlijanian, M. K., and Catterall, W. A. (1990) Clustering of L-type Ca^{2+} channels at the base of major dendrites in hippocampal pyramidal neurons. *Nature 347:*281–284.

Westenbroek, R. E., Hell, J. W., Warner, C., Dubel, S. J., Snutch, T. P., and

Catterall, W. A. (1992) Biochemical properties and subcellular distribution of an N-type calcium channel alpha 1 subunit. *Neuron 9:*1099–1115.

Willard, A. L. (1980) Electrical excitability of ougrowing neurites of embryonic neurones in cultures of dissociated neural plate of *Xenopus laevis. J. Physiol. 301:*115–128.

Wu, W. L., Ziskind-Conhaim, L., and Sweet, M. A. (1992) Early development of glycine- and GABA-mediated synapses in rat spinal cord. *J. Neurosci. 12:*3935–3945.

Yaari, Y., Hamon, B., and Lux, H. D. (1987) Development of two types of calcium channels in cultured mammalian hippocampal neurons. *Science 235:*680–682.

Yeh, G. C., Bonhaus, D. W., Nadler, J. V., and McNamara, J. O. (1989) N-methyl-D-aspartate receptor plasticity in kindling: Quantitative and qualitative alterations in the N-methyl-D-aspartate receptor-channel complex. *Proc. Natl. Acad. Sci. 86:*8157–8160.

Yool, A. J., Dionne, V. E., and Gruol, D. L. (1988) Developmental changes in K^+-selective channel activity during differentiation of the Purkinje neuron in culture. *J. Neurosci. 8:*1971–1980.

Yuste, R., and Katz, L. C. (1991) Control of postsynaptic Ca^{2+} influx in developing neocortex by excitatory and inhibitory neurotransmitters. *Neuron 6:*333–344.

Yuste, R., Peinado, A., and Katz, L. C. (1992) Neuronal domains in developing neocortex. *Science 257:*665–669.

Ziskind-Conhaim, L. (1988) Electrical properties of motoneurons in the spinal cord of rat embryos. *Dev. Biol. 128:*21–29.

7

Candidate Genes in the Childhood Epilepsies: Molecular Biology of Channels and Receptors

BRUCE L TEMPEL

Preceding chapters have emphasized the diversity of the childhood epilepsies with respect to both etiology and clinical presentation. The molecular mechanisms that underlie these motor disturbances are probably equally diverse. This chapter summarizes, from the viewpoint of a molecular geneticist, our current understanding of both the molecular causes of epilepsy and the consequences of epileptic hyperexcitability on gene expression. Particular emphasis will be placed on ionic channels and their genes as candidates for causing epilepsy and on our progress toward understanding the epilepsies that are genetically heritable.

Nominally spontaneous seizure episodes are the clinical hallmark of epilepsy. In an attempt to understand the molecular basis of this susceptibility to hyperexcitability, it is important to recognize that the cause of a specific epilepsy may be quite subtle and difficult to detect at the molecular level. This difficulty is due not only to the transient nature of the phenotype but also to the likelihood that minor changes in the DNA sequence, like single base-pair alterations, may have significant consequences. For example, in two different forms of dominant human periodic paralysis, hyperkalemic periodic paralysis (HYPP) and paramyotonia congenita (PC), four different *single* amino acid residues are mutated in the adult skeletal muscle sodium channel (Ptacek et al., 1991, 1992; Rojas et al., 1991). The physiological consequences of these mutations is a slowing or failure of channel inactivation. Even when only a percentage of the Na channel population fails to inactivate, for instance when the mutation is carried in a heterozygous individual, the membrane does not repolarize fully after an action potential. Subsequent action potentials can fail because Na channels are not available for reactivation. Paralysis is the result (Cannon and Strittmatter, 1993). Alternatively, temporal or spatial misexpression of a gene during development might have long-lasting effects, including epilepsy (Gall et al., 1991). Thus in attempting to understand epilepsy, the basic scientist must consider as candidates a wide variety of gene products thought to be involved in determining excitability in the nervous system. One must also consider examples of chronic hyperexcitability in animal models because they can provide important clues to the types of gene products that may be more subtly altered in humans to give rise to motor phenotypes with spontaneous onset, characteristic of epilepsy.

Here we will consider several different ionic channel types, reviewing the diversity of their respective gene families and their subunit structures as well as asking how the expression of specific members might change during development and/or be correlated or causally related to epilepsy. Finally, human and animal models of genetically determined excitability disturbances will be summarized.

Ionic Channels as Candidates for Causing Epilepsy

Ionic current flux provides the basis for electrical excitability in all cell types. Here we will consider voltage-gated ionic channels and amino acid neurotransmitter receptors that contain ionic channels as part of their structure. In either instance, ionic flux through the channel pore is passive, being driven by the electrochemical gradient of the ion (Hille, 1991). As first described for voltage-gated channels in the squid giant axon, the opening of Na channels allows Na^+ ions to flow down their concentration gradient, into the cell, thereby depolarizing the membrane. Repolarization of the action potential occurs because the Na channels spontaneously inactivate (close) and because potassium (K) channels open, driving the membrane potential toward K^+ equilibrium, usually about -80 mV. Calcium (Ca^{2+}) influx depolarizes the cell, being particularly important at synapses where Ca^{2+} is directly involved in vesicular release of neurotransmitter as well as in soma/dendritic compartments where Ca^{2+} may underlie burst generation (Stewart and Wong, 1993) and/or synaptic potentiation (Madison et al., 1991). Activated by voltage or by the neurotransmitters GABA or glycine, chloride (Cl^-) channel opening is usually inhibitory, since its reversal potential is variable but quite negative (-50 to -80 mV). Because of their direct effect on membrane excitability, mutation or misexpression of any one of the ionic channel genes could lead to epilepsy.

Voltage-Gated Ionic Channels

The general structure of voltage-gated Na, Ca, and K channels is quite similar. Four protein domains, each containing several hydrophobic transmembrane segments, surround an aqueous pore that is selective for the specific ion. Critical differences in amino acid sequences of the pore-lining segments determine the channel's ion selectivity (Imoto, 1993). Na and Ca channels are composed of a single large polypeptide containing the four domains, while K channels are formed by assembling four subunits (Fig. 7-1). Integral to each subunit or domain is a transmembrane sequence called S4 that contains a number of positively charged residues (arginine or lysine). These charged residues, by virtue of their location in the transmembrane region, can sense voltage changes across the membrane, thereby endowing the channels with their defining characteristic of voltage-responsiveness. Site-directed mutagenesis of these charged residues causes an alteration in the voltage sensitivity of both Na and K channels (Papazian et al., 1991; Stuhmer and Parekh, 1992). These types of functional studies are usually carried out by expressing the cloned gene of interest (normal or mutagenized in vitro) in a heterologous expression system where the endogenous currents are thought not to interfere with analysis of the expressed gene product. Transformed mammalian cell lines or the frog *(Xenopus)* oocyte expression system is often used.

Potassium Channels

Given that the general function of K channels is to inhibit or curtail excitation in the nervous system, and given that most mutations are deleterious to

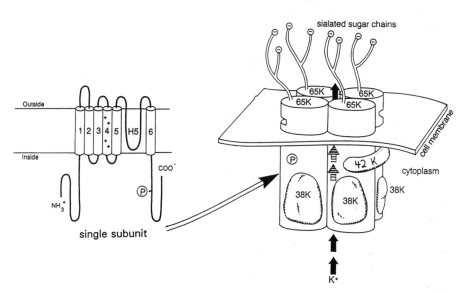

Figure 7-1. Proposed structure of a voltage-gated potassium channel. The proposed transmembrane topography of a single subunit is predicted from a Shaker-like gene sequence. Four subunits from within the *Shaker* family (Kv1.X) come together to form a K^+-selective pore. The charged S4 segment provides voltage-sensitivity. The H5 region is thought to line the pore. Associated subunits of molecular weights 38,000 and 42,000 are also shown, although their function is not known.

the gene's normal function, one might logically argue that alterations in the K channel would result in increased excitability. This hypothesis is supported by findings in the fruit fly, *Drosophila,* where mutations in various K channel genes have been found in three hyperactive mutants, *Shaker, slowpoke,* and *ether-a-go-go.* Although molecularly defined K channel mutants (diseases) have not yet been identified in mammals, it makes sense to regard K channels as candidate genes whose mutation might cause sensory or cognitive impairment or motor dysfunction, as is found in the epilepsies. In this section, as in those that follow, the diversity of the gene family will first be reviewed, specific characteristics of the gene products that might contribute to hyperexcitability will be discussed, and finally specific examples of changes in gene expression during development or in response to epilepsy will be presented.

K channels are by far the largest family of voltage-gated ionic channels. Physiologic studies have identified K^+ currents that are activated (gated) by voltage, calcium, nucleotides, and mechanical forces (Hille, 1991). At the molecular level, the voltage-gated family has been characterized most extensively. The first potassium channel gene was isolated from the *Shaker* locus of *Drosophila* using a positional cloning approach that required no knowledge of the channel sequence or structure. In brief, the *Shaker* mutant, displaying a hyperexcitable, shaking phenotype, was localized by classical genetic studies to a specific region of the X chromosome. Genomic DNA from the region was cloned and cDNAs were isolated and analyzed in order to identify the K channel coding sequences (Tempel, 1990). When expressed in *Xenopus* oocytes, cRNA from individual *Shaker* cDNA clones gave rise to fast, transient K^+ currents, similar to those affected by the *Shaker* mutation in vivo. Mutagenesis and expression studies carried out by a number of investigators have revealed specific regions of the K channel that are involved in determining rates of inactivation, pharmacologic sensitivity, and toxin binding and in forming the channel pore (reviewed in Miller, 1991).

Using probes from the *Shaker* locus, three other K channel genes (Shab, Shal, and Shaw) were isolated from *Drosophila* (Butler et al., 1990). In both rats and mice, 16 different genes that give rise to voltage-gated K^+ currents have been isolated (Table 7-1). These genes can be classified into four different subfamilies based on their sequence-relatedness (including their similarity to the *Drosophila* genes) and on the functionally important observation that, at least in *Xenopus* oocytes, heteromultimeric channels can form within, but not between, these subfamilies (Covarrubias et al., 1991). Within the *Shaker*-like subfamily, heteromultimer formation is directed by conserved sequences in the *N*-terminal region of the channel subunits (Hopkins et al., 1994; Li et al., 1992; Shen et al., 1993). This ability to mix subunits can give rise to a potentially staggering complexity of channel types given multiple members of each subfamily. It also suggests that a defect in the expression or function of one gene product may deleteriously affect the normal physiology of a number of other genes. While the number of heteromeric channels formed in vivo is limited by the fact that not all K channel genes are expressed in every cell, two recent reports have shown that different

TABLE 7-1.   Ionic Channels

Channel Gene	Characteristics
Potassium	
Kv1.1–1.8	Shaker-like, rapid V-activation, slow to fast inactivation
Kv2.1–2.2	Shab-like, sustained currents
Kv3.1–3.4	Shaw-like, high threshold, slow to fast inactivation
Kv4.1–4.2	Shal-like, rapid transient currents
mSlo	Ca^{2+}-activated, complex alternative splicing
IRK1	Inward rectifying, Mg^{2+} blocked
GIRK1	G-protein activated, inward rectifying
Sodium	
Na I–III	TTX-sensitive, type I in adult brain and spinal cord, type II in adult spinal cord, type III neonatal
SkM 1–2	Skeletal muscle, TTX-sensitive, developmental switch from SkM 2 (neonatal) to SkM 1 (day 10–adult rat)
Calcium	
Ca 1	Skeletal muscle, L type (i.e., high threshold, dihydropyridine-sensitive, sustained current)
Ca 2 (C)	Cardiac L type, also expressed in brain, other tissues
Ca 3 (D)	Neuronal, endocrine L type
Ca 4 (A)	Neuronal (especially cerebellum), P type(?), high threshold
Ca 5 (B)	Neuronal, physiological properties unknown

members of the Shaker-like subfamily can form heteromultimers in vivo and are colocalized in specific regions of the hippocampus and cerebellum that are involved in control of motor activity. Wang et al. (1993) showed that Kv1.1 and Kv1.2 are colocalized to the terminal plexus of cerebellar basket cells and to juxtaparanodal regions of nodes of Ranvier in many axons of the mouse brain. In the basket cell plexus, these K channels may help control GABA release, thereby regulating the motor output from cerebellar Purkinje cells. The paranodal distribution of Kv1.1 and Kv1.2 is likely to be important for conducting action potentials in myelinated axons. Sheng et al. (1993) showed that Kv1.2 and Kv1.4 are colocalized to what appears to be mossy fiber terminals in the rat hippocampus. Since the rapid inactivation kinetics of Kv1.4 can dominate over the very slowly inactivating Kv1.2, the authors suggest that Kv1.2-1.4 heteromultimers contribute a transient, A-type current to the mossy fiber ending. Each of these examples is particularly relevant when considering the role defective K channels might play in movement disorders, including epilepsy.

Using various expression systems, a number of biophysical parameters have been described for each of the cloned K channels. One functional parameter of particular importance to their potential role in epilepsy is the sensitivity of some K^+ currents to changes in extracellular K^+ concentration (Heinemann et al., 1986). At K^+ concentrations likely to be reached during repetitive neuronal firing (5–15 mM), expression studies have shown that the conductance of Kv1.4 increases dramatically (Fig. 7-2). The increase is due to a change in the number of available channels, not to a change in single-channel conductance. A single lysine residue near the extracellular

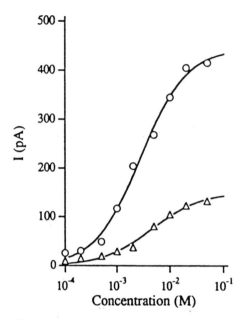

Figure 7-2. Dose-dependence of the K^+ current (I) observed in frog oocytes expressing Kv1.4 when stimulated by pulse depolarizations to $+40$ mV from a holding potential of -100 mV, plotted as a function of $[K^+]_o$ (O) and $[Cs^+]_o$ ($\triangle$). All currents were measured in the same outside-out patch with 100 mM KCl/1.8 mM CaCl$_2$/10 mM hepes-KOH, pH 7.2, in the pipette. The fits through the data points are Bolzmann distributions with the following parameters: $K_d = 2.8$ mM, slope $= 1.00$ for K^+; $K_d = 4.6$ mM, slope $= 0.92$ for Cs^+. (Reproduced with permission from Pardo et al., 1992.)

mouth of the pore is responsible for this K^+ sensitivity (Pardo et al., 1992). Heteromultimers containing Kv1.1 and Kv1.4 are also sensitive to the external K^+ concentration, although Kv1.1 alone is not. If the K^+ sensitivity of Kv1.4 dominates in all heteromultimeric situations, the Kv1.4-1.2 heteromultimers hypothesized by Sheng et al. (1993) to form the transient current in mossy fiber terminals would be sensitive to changes in external K^+. Mutations affecting this region of Kv1.4 or mutations that alter its normal level of expression may therefore alter the sensitivity of these neurons to activity of surrounding neurons.

Because alterations in the normal timing of developmentally programmed switches in gene expression may lead to miswiring or hyperexcitability, it is important to recognize that the patterns and levels of expression of several different K channel genes change during development (reviewed in Ribera and Spitzer, 1992). In the frog *Xenopus leavis*, voltage-gated Ca^{2+}, K^+, and Na^+ currents appear sequentially during electrogenesis in the developing tadpole (Spitzer, Chapter 6). In *Xenopus*, K channel gene expression is turned on early in the differentiation of the nervous system, preceding the appearance of the presumed corresponding functional K^+ currents by only a few hours (Ribera, 1990). The precise timing and rapid rise in functional expression of this K^+ current may be important developmentally for first permitting, then limiting the Ca^{2+} currents already expressed in these neurons. By limiting Ca^{2+} flux, K channel expression may prevent the deleterious effects that Ca^{2+} is thought to have on neuronal survival. In rats, comparable examples of developmental changes in K channel expression have been reported, although the complexities of subunit mixing, discussed earlier, make it difficult to establish a correlation to a specific current. Perney et al. (1992) have shown that the Kv3.1 gene is strongly upregulated perinatally, especially in Purkinje and granule cell layers of the cerebellum (Fig. 7-3). Alterations in these normal developmental expression patterns may cause inappropriate neuronal activity at critical developmental time points, leading in turn to abnormalities in neuronal routing, synapse formation, or intercellular signaling. These considerations must be taken into account when evaluating the role that any gene product may play in causing epilepsy in childhood.

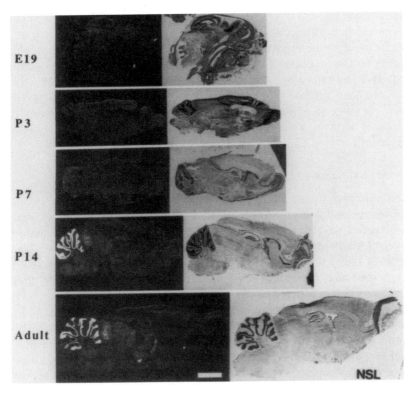

Figure 7-3. Developmental expression of Kv3.1 in the rat brain, studied by in situ hybridization. Dark field micrographs of audioradiographs (left column) reveal that expression increases markedly in the cerebellum of postnatal day 14 (P14) animals. To the right are shown Nissl-stained, light-field micrographs of the same sections. (Reproduced with permission from Perney et al., 1992.)

That a change in K channel gene expression is correlated with hyperactivity has been established. From the *Shaker* phenotype it is clear that mutation or deletion of a voltage-gated K channel can lead to hyperactivity. Reciprocally, when generalized seizure activity was induced in rats by a single intraperitoneal injection of the convulsant drug pentylenetetrazole (Metrazole), the expression of two different K channel genes, Kv1.2 and Kv4.2, was decreased in the hippocampus as measured by quantitative in situ hybridization and polymerase chain reaction (PCR) techniques (Tsuar et al., 1992). The maximal decrease in expression levels (to ~30 percent of normal) was at 3–6 hours postinjection for both K channel mRNAs; normal expression levels were reestablished by 12 hours. While this correlation of seizure activity with a decrease in K channel expression is quite interesting, it does not answer the question of whether misexpression of K channels can <u>cause</u> epilepsy in mammals. Direct manipulation of K channel expression in vivo, presumably by targeted gene disruption techniques available in mouse, will be required to establish this causal link.

We have used examples from the K channel literature to explore several issues that should be kept in mind when considering each of the other ionic channels as candidates for causing epilepsy. When multiple subunits are involved in forming a functional channel, alterations in any one subunit might have effects on the function of other gene products with which it coassembles. Therefore, an important goal is to define the identities and cellular localization of those heteromultimeric combinations that occur in vivo. Finally, changes in gene expression during development and in response to experimentally induced epilepsy may provide important clues to possible mechanisms underlying clinically observed epilepsy.

Other Potassium Channel Genes

Parallel in approach to the isolation of the *Shaker* gene, positional cloning of the *slowpoke* and the *ether-a-go-go* loci from *Drosophila* have yielded calcium-activated and presumed cyclic nucleotide–gated K channel genes, respectively (Atkinson et al., 1991; Warmke et al., 1991). A mammalian homologue of the *slowpoke* gene gives rise to Ca^{2+}-activated K^+ currents when expressed and shows a remarkable number of different cDNAs that result from alternative splicing of the primary transcript (Butler et al., 1993). Inwardly rectifying K channels have also been cloned recently (Kubo et al., 1993). While structurally unique, each of these K channels retains a surprising amount of homology in its pore-lining sequences, supporting the proposal that ionic selectivity is determined in this region. While these K channels are not voltage-gated, they too may be involved in the etiology of epilepsy.

Sodium, Calcium, and Chloride Channel Genes

The structure and function of Na and Ca channels have been reviewed extensively (Catterall, 1991; Snutch and Reiner, 1992; Stuhmer and Parekh,

1992; Tsien et al., 1991). One function, distinct to Na channels and relevant to the regulation of neuronal excitability, is rapid channel inactivation and its modulation by phosphorylation. Catterall and colleagues have shown that rapid inactivation is dependent on a few amino acid residues predicted to lie in the cytoplasmic loop between the third and fourth domains of the Na channel. As shown in Figure 7-4, they suggest that this region acts as a "hinged lid" that can rapidly close the channel pore (West et al., 1992). Nearby in the primary sequence is a site where phosphorylation by protein kinase C leads to a reduction in the peak amplitude of the Na^+ current as well as a slowing of the inactivation rate (Numann et al., 1991; West et al., 1991). The functional consequences of this modulation in vivo are not well understood. Tissue-specific and developmental regulation of various Na channel types has also been reported (Mandel, 1992).

Chloride (Cl^-) flux accounts for approximately 70 percent of the resting membrane current in skeletal muscle, therefore contributing to the repolarization and stability of the muscle membrane. As with K^+ currents, one would suspect that mutation of these inhibitory channels might lead to hyperexcitability. The first voltage-gated Cl channel gene was cloned by expression (Jentsch et al., 1990). The rat homologous gene was shown to be expressed primarily in muscle, with strong, tissue-specific developmental upregulation occurring at 3–4 weeks after birth (Steinmeyer, Ortland et al., 1991). The structure of the cloned voltage-gated Cl channel genes is predicted to include 12 hydrophobic transmembrane regions. Among these transmembrane regions are dispersed several charged amino acid residues, although there is no single segment that is clearly homologous to the charged

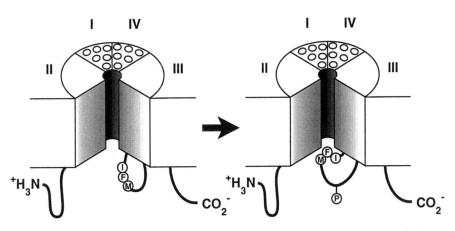

Figure 7-4. A "hinged-lid" model for Na channel inactivation. The cytoplasmic loop region between domain III and IV is depicted as a hinged lid that occludes the transmembrane pore of the Na channel during inactivation. Phenylalanine 1489 is illustrated in a pore-blocking position in the inactivated state. Phosphorylation (*) of the loop region can affect the speed of inactivation. (Adapted from West et al., 1992, with permission.)

S4 voltage sensor of Na, Ca, and K channels. Recent studies have shown that the sequences involved in detecting voltage are located in the amino terminus of the Cl channel (Gründer et al., 1992). Further studies are needed to define the Cl channel gene family and to understand more clearly the structural domains of these Cl channels. This work is of particular importance because myotonic mutants of both mouse and man have been found to be causally related to mutations in specific Cl channel genes (Koch et al., 1992; Steinmeyer, Klocke et al., 1991). These mutations result in repetitive firing of action potentials in muscle membrane, causing stiffness and impaired relaxation of the skeletal muscle.

Ligand-Gated Ionic Channels

The ligand-gated ionic channel superfamily includes receptors for the amino acid neurotransmitters: acetylcholine (AChR), glutamate (GluR), γ-aminobutyric acid ($GABA_A$ receptors), and glycine (GlyR). The receptors can be distinguished not only by their agonists but also by the selectivity of their channels: $GABA_R$ and GlyR are selective for Cl^- and are therefore generally inhibitory, while GluR and AChR allow inward cation flux (predominantly Na^+) and are therefore excitatory. Here we will discuss only the ionic channel forms of these receptors. G-protein coupled, seven-transmembrane-motif receptors for glutamate (metabotropic, or mGluR), acetylcholine (muscarine, or mAChR), and GABA ($GABA_B$ receptors) have been discussed elsewhere (Baskys, 1992; Jones, 1993; Schoepp and Conn, 1993).

The AChR is composed of five subunits, two α and one each of β, γ, and δ. Each of the subunits contributes to formation of the pore since residues in the second transmembrane segment (TM2) of each subunit are involved in determining the ion flux characteristics (Changeux et al., 1992). This basic structure is thought to be common to all ligand-gated ionic channels of the superfamily, although direct evidence of subunit stoichiometries and domain functions are not available for each receptor type. Nonetheless, each subunit cloned to date from the $GABA_A$, GlyR, and GluR families has a similar predicted primary structure, including a signal sequence that places the amino terminus extracellularly, four predicted transmembrane segments, and a relatively large cytoplasmic loop between TM3 and TM4 (see Fig. 7-5; reviewed in Betz, 1990; Olsen and Tobin, 1990). Variations in subunit diversity, rules for functional assembly, and tissue-specific expression during development will be highlighted for each receptor family.

$GABA_A$ Receptors

$GABA_A$ receptors are generally inhibitory since their channels conduct Cl^- ions. As argued for voltage-gated K and Cl channels, an alteration in the function or expression of inhibitory GABA receptors may lead to hyperexcitability. The molecular characteristics of the $GABA_A$ receptor family have been reviewed recently (Olsen and Tobin, 1990; Seeburg et al., 1990; Wisden

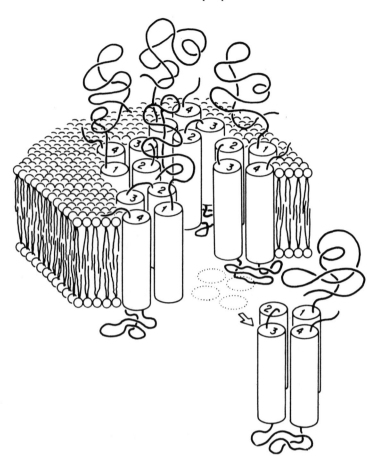

Figure 7-5. Model of the GABA$_A$ receptor–chloride channel protein complex. The ligand-gated ionic channel is proposed to be a heterooligomer composed of five subunits, each with four membrane-spanning domains (cylinders numbered 1–4). Transmembrane domain 2 is depicted as lining the pore. The subunit composition and stoichiometry of the receptor is likely to vary in different cells and at different developmental times. The structure is generally similar among other members of the ligand-gated receptor superfamily. (Reproduced with permission from Olsen and Tobin, 1990.)

and Seeburg, 1992). In rodents, the subunit classes include six α, three β, and three γ genes. Expression studies on cloned subunits show that homomultimers do not express well and that GABA receptors composed of $\alpha\beta\gamma$ subunits appear to form preferentially if allowed (Angelotti et al., 1993). The presence of at least one γ_2 subunit (i.e., $\alpha\beta\gamma_2$ receptors) appears to contribute to the ubiquitous high-affinity benzodiazepine binding observed in vivo, with the γ subunit imparting an increase in conductance as well as reduced desensitization rates and increased mean open times (see Dulac, Macdonald, and Kelly (Chapter 11) for a more detailed pharmacologic profile of the GABA receptor). A novel subunit class, containing only one isoform (ρ_1), is expressed primarily in the retina (Cutting et al., 1991). This subunit has the unique property of assembling into functional, homomultimeric, GABA-activated channels in *Xenopus* oocytes.

An important determinant of the $GABA_A$-type receptors likely to form in vivo is the tissue-specific expression pattern of each subunit. Studied by in situ hybridization of specific probes to expressed mRNAs, each of the α subunits shows a unique expression pattern; β subunits overlap in some areas, including the hippocampus, although their relative level of expression differs and some β's are unique to certain brain regions; γ subunits, especially γ_2, are ubiquitously distributed in the central nervous system (Laurie et al., 1992). These findings are corroborated at the protein level using subunit-specific antibodies which suggest that many receptors in vivo contain a single α type as well as a β and a γ_2 subunit (McKernan et al., 1991). Further immunocytochemical localization and coprecipitation studies will help clarify the subcellular localization, composition, and subunit stoichiometry of the pharmacologically distinct $GABA_A$ receptor subforms observed in vivo.

During development the various GABA subunit genes are differentially expressed in the hippocampus (Killisch et al., 1991). For example, α_1 expression is detected first postnatally, while α_5 is expressed continuously from the early stages of hippocampal development (embryonic day 17) through adult. These patterns may be of particular interest because of the suggestion that activation of $GABA_A$ receptors in embryonic and early postnatal life may result in depolarization due to a difference in the reversal potential for Cl^- in young neurons (Cherubini et al., 1991). The role that specific GABA receptors may play in determining the development of neuronal circuitry deserves further attention, although the apparent functional interchangeability of some subunit types may complicate the analysis because of inherent functional redundancy in this receptor system.

Glycine Receptors

Inhibitory glycine receptors are expressed strongly in brainstem and spinal cord. They are selective for Cl^- ion flow and are composed of α and β subunits in what is assumed to be a pentameric channel structure (Betz, 1990, 1992). The general transmembrane topology of GlyR subunits is predicted to be similar to other members of the amino acid ligand receptors, with an extracellular among terminus and four transmembrane segments. Cysteines, thought to form disulfide bridges important for the structure of the ligand-binding site in ACh and $GABA_A$ receptors, are present in the amino terminal region of the GlyR α subunits. Four different α subunits have been described. The function of the single β subunit described to date is not clear as functional GlyR arise from the expression of α subunits alone. Further, the β subunit gene is highly expressed in cerebellum and cortex, regions that do not display comparably high levels of any of the known α subunit genes. It therefore seems likely that other GlyR subunits are yet to be identified.

Our understanding of the developmental regulation of GlyR has been greatly aided by an elegant analysis of the recessive *spastic (spa)* mutant mouse (Becker et al., 1992). Mice homozygous for *spa* develop severe muscle rigidity, tremor, and myoclonic jerks in the second postnatal week, corresponding to a failure in the development of the high-affinity strychnine binding, which characterizes the adult form of GlyR. The subunit responsible for high-affinity strychnine binding in the adult GlyR is primarily α_1, whose expression is upregulated perinatally, even in the *spa* mutant. Thus although both mRNA blot and oocyte expression data show that α_1 transcript is normal in *spa,* adult GlyR do not develop. The molecular basis for this developmental defect is not yet clear; adult GlyR may fail to assemble because of instability of the α_1 protein, because other GlyR subunits are required for assembly, or because of metabolic influences on receptor assembly that are specific to the perinatal period. Further analysis of *spa,* including coincidence studies aimed at correlating GlyR subunit gene loci with the known location of *spa* on mouse chromosome 3, should help define whether *spa* directly affects a specific GlyR subunit gene or whether it is a mutation in a processing enzyme that alters GlyR assembly during development, causing motor dysfunction in this mouse model. (See *Note Added in Proof.*)

Glutamate Receptors

Excitatory glutamate receptors have been extensively studied electrophysiologically and categorized pharmacologically into three main groups depending on their sensitivity to the agonists *N*-methyl-D-aspartate (NMDA), L-α-amino-3-hydroxy-5-methyl-4-isoxazole propionate (AMPA), and kainic acid. Their role in the regulation of excitability in the CNS is emphasized by the fact that kainate injections induce seizures (Mathis and Ungerer, 1992) and the NMDA receptors play an activity-dependent role in the synaptic plasticity underlying long-term potentiation in the hippocampus (Stevens, 1993). The unique ability of GluRs to regulate Ca^{2+} influx is central to their role in synaptic plasticity and can now be explained in molecular terms. Recent findings on the structure and function of receptor family are reviewed in greater detail elsewhere (Sommer and Seeburg, 1992; Sprengel and Seeburg, 1993).

The first glutamate receptor to be cloned was isolated by selection screening of a cDNA library whose member clones were expressed in *Xenopus* oocytes and assayed for their response to kainate (Hollmann et al., 1989). Now recognized as a member of the AMPA subfamily, $GluR_1$ was used to isolate several related genes sensitive to AMPA and kainate (Table 7-2). AMPA-sensitive GluR are assembled from $GluR_1$ through $GluR_4$ subunits, although in order to achieve the fast kinetics and low divalent cation permeability characteristic of AMPA receptors in vivo, heteromultimers must include $GluR_2$. The gating kinetics and conductance properties of heteromultimers are dominated by $GluR_2$, which displays linear current–voltage relations and low Ca^{2+} permeability. The finding that $GluR_2$ is widely expressed in most neurons of the CNS suggests that it, in large part, deter-

TABLE 7-2. Receptors with Channel-forming Domains

Receptor Genes	Assembly Rules	Functional Characteristics
GABA$_A$		
α_1–α_6	Homomultimers give low expression, $\alpha\beta$ allowed,	α and β variants have distinct expression patterns, γ confers
β_1–β_3	$\alpha\beta\gamma$ preferred	benzodiazepine sensitivity
γ_1–γ_3	γ_2 is ubiquitous	
ρ_1	Forms only homomultimers	Nondesensitizing, expressed in retina
GlycineR		
α_1–α_3	α homomultimers	α provides high-affinity glycine
β	expression, $\alpha\beta$ are copurified (spinal cord)	binding, β may be structural component of channel
GlutamateR		
AMPA/kainate		
GluR$_1$–GluR$_4$	Homomultimers or heteromultimers	Low Ca^{2+} permeability, rapid kinetics, nondesensitizing current with kainate
Kainate		
GluR$_5$–GluR$_7$	Homomultimers or heteromultimers	Rapid kinetics, rapid desensitization with kainate
KA$_1$–KA$_2$	Forms heteromultimers with GluR$_5$–GluR$_7$	
NMDA		
NR$_1$	Heteromultimer between NR$_1$ and NR$_2$ gives	High Ca^{2+} permeability, slow kinetics, little desensitization,
NR$_{2A}$–NR$_{2D}$	robust current	blocked by Mg^{2+}

mines the characteristics of glutamate-activated AMPA receptors. Potentially relevant to the epileptogenic effects of kainate, these AMPA receptors are also sensitive to kainate (though with low affinity), leading some scientists to refer to this subfamily as the AMPA–kainate subfamily. The effect of kainate binding to AMPA receptors is to activate a nondesensitizing excitatory current, in contrast to the desensitizing current activated by glutamate in vivo.

During development, alternatively spliced variants of each of GluR$_1$ through GluR$_4$ are differentially expressed (Monyer et al., 1991). The alternatively spliced exons, called Flip and Flop, are located in the cytoplasmic loop immediately preceding the last transmembrane region. In general, the Flip versions are expressed prominently in the embryo and during postnatal brain development. Although many specific exceptions exist (e.g., Flop forms are never expressed in CA$_3$ pyramidal neurons), the Flop forms increase around postnatal day 8, reaching adult levels by day 14. This developmental switching may be particularly important if the larger conductances observed for the Flip variants (when expressed in *Xenopus* oocytes) are useful at early stages of neural development. At later stages of synaptic maturation, the lower conductances of the Flop versions may allow for finer control of excitability and the avoidance of excitotoxicity. In some neurons both forms are expressed, presumably leading to Flip-Flop heteromultimers with unique conductance properties. During development, failure to make appropriately timed switches in the expression of specific splice forms may lead to altered synaptic efficacy and aberrant development.

Two high-affinity kainate-binding GluR subfamilies have been isolated (Table 7-2; Sprengel and Seeburg, 1993). The function of these receptors in vivo is not clear, although emerging evidence suggests that they may be located exclusively in dendrites. Members of the $GluR_5$ through $GluR_7$ subfamily can form functional homomultimers if expressed alone or heteromultimers if coexpressed with each other or with members of the other subfamily, KA_1 and KA_2. The KA subunits fail to form homomultimers or heteromultimers with each other, being limited to heteromultimer formation with the $GluR_5$–$GluR_7$ subfamily.

Similar in approach to the isolation of $GluR_1$, the first NMDA glutamate receptor (NR_1) was isolated by expression cloning (Moriyoshi et al., 1991). When expressed alone, NR_1 gives rise to a glutamate-activated current with many characteristics of NMDA receptors in vivo, including modulatory effects of glycine, voltage-dependent Mg^{2+} block, and pronounced Ca^{2+} permeability. When coexpressed with one of the four known β subunits (NR_{2A} through NR_{2D}), channel conductance is enhanced and different pharmacologic and Mg^{2+} block properties are observed. Like the $GluR_2$ AMPA subunit, the NR_1 subunit is ubiquitously expressed in virtually every neuron, with the various NR_2 subunits displaying differential tissue-specific expression patterns. Thus for both the AMPA and the NMDA GluR subfamilies, a single subunit ($GluR_2$ and NR_1, respectively) dominates in terms of both its anatomical distribution and its role in determining the physiologic properties of heteromultimeric channels.

A unique characteristic of the GluR family is its ability to regulate Ca^{2+} influx—physiologically by means of the voltage-dependent Mg^{2+} block characteristic of NMDA receptors and, in the AMPA–kainate subfamilies, by molecular modification of the subunit sequence. Both these functions can be traced primarily to variations at a single amino acid residue position, called the Q/R site in the pore region of the AMPA subfamily. In $GluR_2$ cDNA this site is occupied by the charged amino acid arginine (R), while in the other three AMPA receptors the site is occupied by uncharged glutamine (Q). Comparing their conductances, R-containing subunit(s) dominate the channel properties by preventing Ca^{2+} permeation while Q allows Ca^{2+} to pass (Hume et al., 1991). At a comparable site in the NMDA receptor NR_1 subunit, an uncharged asparagine residue (N) determines both high Ca^{2+} permeability and voltage-dependent Mg^{2+} block.

The final surprise in GluR regulation of Ca^{2+} flux is the mechanism by which changes in the Q/R site are brought about. Seeburg and colleagues discovered that, in its genomic DNA sequence, the $GluR_2$ gene predicts Q at the Q/R site, while cDNA derived from $GluR_2$ mRNA predicts R. The change apparently occurs by RNA editing, a process that involves a site-specific change in the sequence of the newly synthesized RNA transcript (Higuchi et al., 1993). The editing of the RNA sequence at the Q/R site is directed by specific sequence information in the adjacent intron, so it must occur before these intronic sequences are removed by splicing (Fig. 7-6). This modification of the RNA occurs in more than 99 percent of the GluR$_2$ transcripts while intermediate percentages of the other subunits are edited. More recently, RNA editing has been described for two other sites in the transmembrane regions of the high-affinity kainate receptor GluR$_6$, which also affect Ca^{2+} permeability (Kohler et al., 1993). A defect in this editing machinery would have devastating effects on excitability since Ca^{2+} entry would be elevated in many neurons. This final example points clearly to the

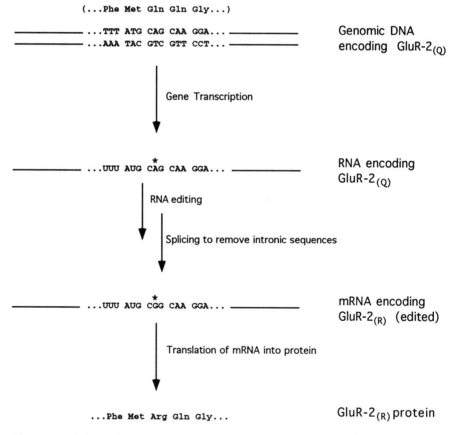

Figure 7-6. Schematic representation of the steps involved in expression of GluR$_2$, focusing on the Q/R (Gln/Arg) site where changes in sequence determine Ca^{2+} permeability. Editing of the RNA occurs soon after transcription, before introns are removed during processing of the RNA into mature messenger RNA that is ready for translation into protein. Standard single-letter nucleotide and three-letter amino acid abbreviations are used.

fact that genetic defects that might result in hyperexcitability are considerably broader than those that directly alter ionic channel genes themselves.

Heritable Epilepsies and Motor Dysfunction

Recent advances in molecular genetic techniques have made possible the undertaking of a project as large as the sequencing of the entire human genome. Important steps in this project will be to establish the linear alignment of genes along the chromosomes, then to determine the structure of each gene and to identify alterations in those genes that lead to disease. One especially promising development in this area is the identification of anonymous, highly polymorphic (i.e., variable in the population), simple sequence repeats (e.g., . . . CACACA . . .) that are scattered throughout the genome. These variable number tandem repeat (VNTR) or simple sequence length polymorphism (SSLP) markers have unique flanking sequences that allow each to be recognized specifically and placed on the chromosome map (reviewed in Leppert, 1990).

Anonymous markers provide landmarks in the genome so that specific diseases or candidate genes can be mapped. For those with an interest in a specific gene or disease, the first step in linking one with the other is to identify the chromosomal locus of the gene or disease. At the clinical level, such mapping requires special attention to familial patterns of disease, inherited in the patient population. A multigeneration pedigree with multiple affected individuals is an invaluable genetic tool. Once the disease locus is established by analyzing VNTRs in the diseased family pedigree, one can ask if any reasonable candidate genes have been mapped to the region. This disease-mapping approach has been successful in localizing the chromosomal regions that contain mutations causing several human neurological diseases, including benign familial neonatal convulsion (BFNC), juvenile myoclonic epilepsy (JME), progressive myoclonic epilepsy (PME) of the Unverricht-Lundborg type, and one locus for autosomal dominant cerebellar ataxia (SCA2) (Table 7-3). In mice, several genetic models of epilepsy have been identified and mapped (reviewed by Noebels in Chapter 3 of this volume). These include the single gene mutants *tottering (tg)* (Noebels, 1984) and *stargazer (stg)* (Noebels et al., 1990), each of which is characterized electrophysiologically by altered EEG records and behaviorally by seizures. The epilepsylike (El) mouse strain has a predisposition to develop seizures, precipitated by several forms of vestibular stimulation. At least two different loci contribute to the El phenotype (Rise et al., 1991). The specific gene defect has not been identified for any of these epileptic syndromes or animal models.

In the pursuit of genes that might be causally related to a disease phenotype, specific genes or gene families can be mapped to their chromosomal loci, and coincident diseases or mutant models can be investigated. In this way, virtually all the known voltage-gated K channel genes in the mouse

TABLE 7-3. Movement Disorders and Genetic Loci

Disease or Mutation	Gene Defect; Locus	Phenotype
Human		
JME	Unknown; hChr. 6p	Juvenile myoclonus
SCA1	Unknown; hChr. 6p	Cerebellar ataxia
BFNC	Unknown; hChr. 20q13	Benign convulsions
PME (Unverricht-Lundborg type)	Unknown; hChr. 21q22.3	Progressive myoclonus
HYPP	Na^+ channel; hChr. 17q	Periodic paralysis
SCA2	Unknown; hChr. 12q23	Cerebellar ataxia
Generalized myotonia	Cl^- channel; hChr. 7q	Progressive stiffness
Mus musculus		
adr mouse	Cl^- channel; mChr. 6	Progressive myotonia
pink-eyed cleft palate	$GABA_A$ Rs; mChr. 7	Hypopigmentation, tremor
tottering	Unknown; mChr. 8	Ataxia, focal myoclonus
Epilepsylike	Unknown; multigenic	Predisposed to tonic-clonic seizures
opisthotonus	Unknown; mChr. 6	Generalized seizures
quivering	Unknown; mChr. 7	Deaf, shaking
stargazer	Unknown; mChr. 15	Ataxia, focal myoclonus
Drosophila		
Shaker	Voltage-gated K channel	Shaking
ether-a-go-go	Nucleotide-gated K channel	Hyperexcitable, shaking
slowpoke	Ca^{2+}-activated K channel	Sluggish, shaking

(Lock et al., 1994) and several in the human genome have been mapped. We are currently investigating the potential causal relationship between the K channels and three coincident mouse mutants, *opisthotonus, deafwaddler,* and *quivering,* each of which shows chronic motor hyperexcitability that is phenotypically analogous to that seen in the various known K channel mutants of *Drosophila* (Table 7-3). It is also interesting to note that based on our mouse mapping data, Kv2.1 (KCNB1) is predicted to be encoded in a region of human chromosome 20q that is roughly coincident with the BFNC locus (Leppert et al., 1989); in addition, Kv3.2 (KCNC2) is predicted to be localized to human chromosome 12q in the region of SCA2 (Gispert et al., 1993).

Are there any examples of epilepsy, or other forms of neurologic hyperexcitability, wherein the gene defect that causes the disease is known? There are at least four examples (see Table 7-3). First, as mentioned in the introduction, two different single-base mutations in the adult skeletal muscle Na channel have been shown to cause hyperkalemic periodic paralysis (HYPP); two other mutations in the same gene cause paramyotonia congenita (PC). Second, the skeletal muscle myotonias are caused by defects in Cl channel genes. Third, the maternal inheritance pattern observed in myoclonic epilepsy and ragged-red fibers syndrome (MERRF) has been traced to the mitochondrial genome where an A-to-G substitution occurs in the gene that encodes the transfer RNA (tRNA) used by ribosomes to add the amino acid lysine to growing proteins during the process of translation (Shoffner et al., 1990). The wide variability in penetrance observed in MERRF is likely explained by the peculiarities of mitochondrial inheritance and the fact that the disruption of a tRNA gene would be expected to have pleotropic effects since all proteins containing the amino acid lysine would be affected. Fourth, Nakatsu et al. (1993) have shown that a cluster of three GABA$_A$ receptor subunits (α_5, β_3, and γ_3) are disrupted or deleted in the recessive mouse mutant *pink-eyed cleft-palate (p^{cp})*, whose phenotype includes tremor and a jerky gait in those rare mutant individuals that survive beyond the first few perinatal days. Additional genes whose identity and function are not known may also be affected by the p^{cp} deletion, precluding assignment of a direct causal role of the affected GABA subunits in the developmental and motor dysfunction displayed by the mutant. This question can be addressed using transgenic techniques that are available in mice to replace individually each of the affected genes in the p^{cp} mutant. Analysis of the p^{cp} mutation may also help explain Angelman syndrome, a complex human neurologic disorder characterized by mental retardation, seizures, ataxia, and hypopigmentation (Reis et al., 1993). The syndrome maps to the homologous human chromosomal region and is associated with deletions that affect expression of at least GABA$_A$ β_3 as well as some critical genes likely to be outside the p^{cp} deletion.

The molecular basis for two additional neurological disorders have been recently identified. Hereditary hyperekplexia, or familial startle disease (STHE), has been shown to be caused by different point mutations, all at the same base pair in the α_1 subunit of the glycine receptor in four different families (Shiang et al., 1993). Episodic ataxia, or myokymia syndrome has been shown to be associated with various point mutations in transmembrane regions of a potassium channel gene, KCNA1 (Kv1.1), in two different families (Litt et al., 1994). In both cases, motor dysfunction has been shown to be causally linked to candidate genes.

Conclusion

Rapid progress is being made toward a molecular understanding of the structure and function of some of the genes and gene products that are involved in determining electrical excitability of the nervous system. In parallel, many heritable diseases of hyperexcitability, including some of the classically defined childhood epilepsy syndromes, are being mapped to their chromosomal sites of origin. In the coming years, these areas of knowledge will converge as the causal bases for complex neurological disorders are discovered.

Note Added in Proof

The *spa* mutation has recently been identified as an insertional mutation in the glycine receptor β subunit gene (Kingsmore et al., 1994).

References

Angelotti, T. P., Uhler, M. D., and Macdonald, R. L. (1993) Assembly of GABA$_A$ receptor subunits: Analysis of transient single-cell expression utilizing a fluorescent substrate/marker gene technique. *J. Neurosci. 13:*1418–1428.

Atkinson, N. S., Robertson, G. A., and Ganetzky, B. (1991) A component of calcium-activated potassium channels encoded by the *Drosophila slo* locus. *Science 253:*551–555.

Baskys, A. (1992) Metabotropic receptors and "slow" excitatory actions of glutamate agonist in the hippocampus. *Trends Neurosci. 15:*92–96.

Becker, C.-M., Schmieden, V., Tarroni, P., Strasser, U., and Betz, H. (1992) Isoform-selective deficit of glycine receptors in the mouse mutant *spastic. Neuron 8:*283–289.

Betz, H. (1990) Ligand-gated ion channels in the brain: The amino acid receptor superfamily. *Neuron 5:*383–392.

Betz, H. (1992) Structure and function of inhibitory glycine receptors. *Q. Rev. Biophys. 25:*381–394.

Butler, A., Tsunoda, S., McCobb, D. P., Wei, A., and Salkoff, L. (1993) *mSlo,* a complex mouse gene encoding "maxi" calcium-activated potassium channels. *Science 261:*221–224.

Butler, A., Wei, A., and Salkoff, L. (1990) Shal, Shab, and Shaw: Three genes encoding potassium channels in *Drosophila. Nucleic Acids Res. 18:*2173–2174.

Cannon, S. C., and Strittmatter, S. M. (1993) Functional expression of sodium channel mutations identified in families with periodic paralysis. *Neuron 10:*317–326.

Catterall, W. A. (1991) Structure and function of voltage-gated sodium and calcium channels. *Curr. Opin. Neurobiol. 1:*5–13.

Changeux, J.-P., Galzi, J.-L., Devillers-Thiery, A., and Bertrand, D. (1992) The functional architecture of the acetylcholine nicotinic receptor explored by affinity labelling and site-directed mutagenesis. *Q. Rev. Biophys. 25:*395–432.

Cherubini, E., Gaiarsa, J. L., and Ben-Ari, Y. (1991) GABA: An excitatory transmitter in early postnatal life. *Trends Neurosci. 14:*515–519.

Covarrubias, M., Wei, A., and Salkoff, L. (1991) Shaker, Shal, Shab, and Shaw express independent K$^+$ current systems. *Neuron 7:*763–773.

Cutting, G. R., Luo, L., O'Hara, B. F., Kasch, L. M., Montrose-Rafizadeh, C., et al. (1991) Cloning of the γ-aminobutyric acid (GABA) ρl cDNA: A GABA receptor subunit highly expressed in the retina. *Proc. Natl. Acad. Sci. 88:*2673–2677.

Gall, C., Lauterborn, J., Bundman, M., Murray, K., and Isackson, P. (1991) Seizures and the regulation of neurotrophic factor and neuropeptide gene expression in brain. *Epilepsy Res. 4* (Suppl.):225–245.

Gispert, S., Twells, R., Orozco, G., Brice, A., Weber, J., et al. (1993) Chromosomal assignment of the second locus for autosomal dominant cerebellar ataxia (SCA2) to chromosome 12q23–24.1. *Nature Genetics 4:*295–299.

Gründer, S., Thiemann, A., Pusch, M., and Jentsch, T. J. (1992) Regions involved in the opening of ClC-2 chloride channel by voltage and volume. *Nature 360*:759–762.

Heinemann, U., Konnerth, A., Pumain, R., and Wadman, W. J. (1986) Extracellular calcium and potassium concentration changes in chronic epileptic brain tissue. *Adv. Neurol. 44*:641–661.

Higuchi, M., Single, F. N., Kohler, M., Sommer, B., Sprengel, R., and Seeburg, P. H. (1993) RNA editing of AMPA receptor subunit GluR-B: A base-paired intron-exon structure determines position and efficiency. *Cell 75*:1361–1370.

Hille, B. (1992) *Ionic Channels of Excitable Membranes.* 2nd ed. Sunderland, Mass.: Sinauer.

Hollmann, M., O'Shea-Greenfield, A., Rogers, S. W., and Heinemann, S. (1989) Cloning by functional expression of a member of the glutamate receptor family. *Nature 342*:643–648.

Hopkins, W. F., Demas, V., and Tempel, B. L. (1994) Both *N*- and *C*-terminal regions contribute to the assembly and functional expression of homo- and hetero-multimeric voltage-gated K channels. *J. Neurosci. 14*:1385–1393.

Hume, R. I., Dingledine, R., and Heinemann, S. (1991) Identification of a site in glutamate receptor subunits that controls calcium permeability. *Science 253*:1028–1031.

Imoto, K. (1993) Ion channels: Molecular basis of ion selectivity. *FEBS Lett. 325*:100–103.

Jentsch, T. J., Steinmeyer, K., and Schwarz, G. (1990) Primary structure of *Torpedo marmorata* chloride channel isolated by expression cloning in *Xenopus* oocytes. *Nature 348*:510–514.

Jones, S. V. (1993) Muscarinic receptor subtypes: Modulation of ion channels. *Life Sci. 52*:457–464.

Killisch, I., Dotti, C. G., Laurie, D. J., Luddens, H., and Seeburg, P. H. (1991) Expression patterns of GABA$_A$ receptor subtypes in developing hippocampal neurons. *Neuron 7*:927–936.

Kingsmore, S. F., Giros, B., Suh, D., Bieniarz, M., Caron, M. G., and Seldin, M. F. (1994) Glycine receptor beta-subunit gene mutation in *spastic* mouse associated with LINE-1 element insertion. *Nature Genetics 7*:136–141.

Koch, M. C., Steinmeyer, K., Lorenz, C., Ricker, K., Wolf, F., et al. (1992) The skeletal muscle chloride channel in dominant and recessive human myotonia. *Science 257*:797–800.

Kohler, M., Burnashev, N., Sakmann, B., and Seeburg, P. H. (1993) Determinants of Ca^{2+} permeability in both TM1 and TM2 of high affinity kainate receptor channels: Diversity by RNA editing. *Neuron 10*:491–500.

Kubo, Y., Baldwin, T. J., Jan, Y. N., and Jan, L. Y. (1993) Primary structure and functional expression of a mouse inward rectifier potassium channel. *Nature 362*:127–133.

Laurie, D. J., Seeburg, P. H., and Wisden, W. (1992) The distribution of 13 GABA$_A$ receptor subunit mRNAs in the rat brain: II. Olfactory bulb and cerebellum. *J. Neurosci. 12*:1063–1076.

Leppert, M., Anderson, V. E., Quattlebaum, T., Stauffer, D., O'Connell, P., et al. (1989) Benign familial neonatal convulsions linked to genetic markers on chromosome 20. *Nature 337*:647–648.

Leppert, M. F. (1990) Gene mapping and other tools for discovery. *Epilepsia 31* (Suppl.):S11–S18.

Li, M., Jan, Y. N., and Jan, L. Y. (1992) Specification of subunit assembly by the hydrophilic amino-terminal domain of the Shaker potassium channel. *Science 257:*1225–1230.

Litt, M., Browne, D. L., Gancher, S. T., Nutt, J. G., Brunt, E. R. P., and Smith, E. A. (1994) Episodic ataxia/myokymia syndrome is associated with point mutations in the human potassium channel gene KCNA1 (Kv1.1). *J. Gen. Physiol. 104:*10a.

Lock, L. F., Gilbert, D. J., Street, V. A., Migeon, M. B., Jenkins, N. A., et al. (1994) Voltage-gated potassium channel genes are clustered in paralogous regions of the mouse genome. *Genomics. 20:*354–362.

Madison, D. V., Malenka, R. C., and Nicoll, R. A. (1991) Mechanisms underlying long-term potentiation of synaptic transmission. *Ann. Rev. Neurosci. 14:*379–397.

Mandel, G. (1992) Tissue-specific expression of the voltage-gated sodium channel. *J. Membrane Biol. 125:*193–205.

Mathis, C., and Ungerer, A. (1992) Comparative analysis of seizures induced by intracerebroventricular administration of NMDA, kainate, and quisqualate in mice. *Exp. Brain Res. 88:*277–282.

McKernan, R. M., Quirk, K., Prince, R., Cox, P. A., Fillard, N. P., et al. (1991) GABA$_A$ receptor subtypes immunopurified from rat brain with α subunit-specific antibodies have unique pharmacological properties. *Neuron 7:*667–676.

Miller, C. (1991) 1990: Annus mirabilis of potassium channels. *Science 252:*1092–1096.

Monyer, H., Seeburg, P. H., and Wisden, W. (1991) Glutamate-operated channels: Developmentally early and mature forms arise by alternative splicing. *Neuron 6:*799–810.

Moriyoshi, K., Masu, M., Ishii, T., Shgemoto, R., Mizuno, N., et al. (1991) Molecular cloning and characterization of the rat NMDA receptor. *Nature 354:* 31–37.

Nakatsu, Y., Tyndale, R. F., DeLorey, T. M., Durham-Pierre, D., Gardner, J. M., et al. (1993) A cluster of three GABA$_A$ receptor subunit genes is deleted in a neurological mutant of the mouse p locus. *Nature 364:*448–450.

Noebels, J. L. (1984) A single gene error of noradrenergic axon growth synchronizes central neurons. *Nature 310:*409–411.

Noebels, J. L., Qiao, X., Bronson, R., Spencer, C., and Davisson, M. (1990) *Stargazer,* a new neurological mutation on chromosome 15 in the mouse with prolonged cortical seizures. *Epilepsy Res. 7:*129–135.

Numann, R., Catterall, W. A., and Scheuer, T. (1991) Functional modulation of brain sodium channels by protein kinase C phosphorylation. *Science 254:*115–118.

Olsen, R. W., and Tobin, A. J. (1990) Molecular biology of GABA$_A$ receptors. *FASEB J. 4:*1469–1480.

Papazian, D. M., Timpe, L. C., Jan, Y. N., and Jan, L. Y. (1991) Alteration of voltage-dependence of *Shaker* potassium channel by mutations in the S4 sequence. *Nature 349:*305–310.

Pardo, L. A., Heinemann, S. H., Terlau, H., Ludewig, U., Lorra, C., et al. (1992) Extracellular K$^+$ specifically modulates a rat brain K$^+$ channel. *Proc. Natl. Acad. Sci. 89:*2466–2470.

Perney, T. M., Marshall, J., Martin, K. A., Hockfield, S., and Kaczmarek, L. K. (1992) Expression of the mRNAs for the Kv3.1 potassium channel gene in the adult and developing rat brain. *J. Neurophysiol. 68:*756–766.

Ptacek, L. J., George, A. L., Barchi, R. L., Griggs, R. C., Riggs, J. E., et al. (1992) Mutations in an S4 segment of the adult skeletal muscle sodium channel cause parmyotonia congenita. *Neuron 8:*891–897.

Ptacek, L. J., George, A. L., Griggs, R. C., Tawil, R., Kallen, R. G., et al. (1991) Identification of a mutation in the gene causing hyperkalemic periodic paralysis. *Cell 67:*1021–1027.

Reis, A., Kunze, J., Ladanyi, L., Enders, H., Klein-Vogler, U., and Niemann, G. (1993) Exclusion of the GABA$_A$ receptor beta 3 subunit gene as the Angelman's syndrome gene. *Lancet 341:*122–123.

Ribera, A. B. (1990) A potassium channel gene is expressed at neural induction. *Neuron 5:*691–701.

Ribera, A. B., and Spitzer, N. C. (1992) Developmental regulation of potassium channels and their impact on neuronal differentiation. *Ion Channels 3:*1–38.

Rise, M., Frankel, W., Coffin, J., and Seyfried, T. (1991) Genes for epilepsy mapped in the mouse. *Science 253:*669–673.

Rojas, C. V., Wang, J., Schwartz, L. S., Hoffmann, E. P., Powell, B. R., et al. (1991) A val-to-met mutation in the skeletal muscle Na channel alpha-subunit in hyperkalemic periodic paralysis. *Nature 354:*387–389.

Schoepp, D. D., and Conn, P. J. (1993) Metabotropic glutamate receptors in brain function and pathology. *Trends Pharm. Sci. 14:*13–20.

Seeburg, P. H., Wisden, W., Verdoorn, T. A., Pritchet, D. B., Werner, P., et al. (1990) The GABA$_A$ receptor family: Molecular and functional diversity. *Cold Spring Harbor Symp. Quant. Biol. 55:*29–40.

Shen, N. V., Chen, X., Boyer, M. M., and Pfaffinger, P. J. (1993) Deletion analysis of K$^+$ channel assembly. *Neuron 11:*67–76.

Sheng, M., Liao, Y. J., Jan, Y. N., and Jan, L. Y. (1993) Presynaptic A-current based on heteromultimeric K$^+$ channels detected *in vivo*. *Nature 365:*72–75.

Shiang, R., Ryan, S. G., Zhu, Y.-Z., Hahn, A. F., O'Connell, P., and Wasmuth, J. J. (1993) Mutations in the alpha 1 subunit of the inhibitory glycine receptor cause the dominant neurologic disorder, hyperekplexia. *Nature Genetics 5:*351–357.

Shoffner, J. M., Lott, M. T., Lezza, A. M. S., Seibel, P., Ballinger, S. W., et al. (1990) Myoclonic epilepsy and ragged-red fiber disease (MERRF) is associated with a mitochondrial DNA tRNA^{Lys} mutation. *Cell 61:*931–937.

Snutch, T. P., and Reiner, P. B. (1992) Ca^{++} channels: Diversity of form and function. *Curr. Opin. Neurobiol. 2:*247–253.

Sommer, B., and Seeburg, P. H. (1992) Glutamate receptor channels: Novel properties and new clones. *Trends Pharm. Sci. 13:*291–296.

Sprengel, R., and Seeburg, P. H. (1993) The unique properties of glutamate receptor channels. *FEBS Lett. 325:*90–94.

Steinmeyer, K., Klocke, R., Ortland, C., Gronemeier, M., Jockusch, H., et al. (1991) Inactivation of muscle chloride channel by transposon insertion in myotonic mice. *Nature 354:*304–308.

Steinmeyer, K., Ortland, C., and Jentsch, T. J. (1991) Primary structure and functional expression of a developmentally regulated skeletal muscle chloride channel. *Nature 354:*301–304.

Stevens, C. F. (1993) Quantal release of neurotransmitter and long-term potentiation. *Cell/Neuron 72/10:*55–63.

Stewart, M., and Wong, R. K. (1993) Intrinsic properties and evoked responses of guinea pig subicular neurons *in vitro. J. Neurophysiol. 70:*232–245.

Stuhmer, W., and Parekh, A. B. (1992) The structure and function of Na⁺ channels. *Curr. Opin. Neurobiol. 2:*243–246.

Tempel, B. L. (1990) Potassium channel genes and genetics in flies, mice and man. *Semin. Neurosci. 2:*197–205.

Tsien, R. W., Ellinor, P. T., and Horne, W. A. (1991) Molecular diversity of voltage-dependent Ca⁺⁺ channels. *Trends Pharm. Sci. 12:*349–354.

Tsuar, M.-L., Sheng, M., Lowenstein, D. H., Jan, Y. N., and Jan, L. Y. (1992) Differential expression of K⁺ channel mRNAs in the rat brain and down-regulation in the hippocampus following seizures. *Neuron 8:*1055–1067.

Wang, H., Kunkel, D. D., Martin, T. M., Schwartzkroin, P. A., and Tempel, B. L. (1993) Heteromultimeric K⁺ channels in terminal and juxtaparanodal regions of neurons. *Nature 365:*75–79.

Warmke, J., Drysdale, R., and Ganetzky, B. (1991) A distinct potassium channel polypeptide encoded by the *Drosophila eag* locus. *Science 252:*1560–1562.

West, J. W., Numann, R., Murphy, B. J., Scheuer, T., and Catterall, W. A. (1991) A phosphorylation site in the Na⁺ channel required for modulation by protein kinase C. *Science 254:*866–868.

West, J. W., Patton, D. E., Scheuer, T., Wang, Y., Goldin, A. L., et al. (1992) A cluster of hydrophobic amino acid residues required for fast Na⁺-channel inactivation. *Proc. Natl. Acad. Sci. 89:*10910–10914.

Wisden, W., and Seeburg, P. H. (1992) GABA$_A$ receptor channels: From subunits to functional entities. *Curr. Opin. Neurobiol. 2:*263–269.

8

Synaptogenesis and Epileptogenesis in Developing Neural Networks

JOHN W. SWANN

Proper functioning of the central nervous system relies on highly stereotyped patterns of neuronal connectivity. During brain development millions of neurons send out axons, some of which grow over remarkably long distances to their proper target cells. Along the way these axons bypass many other nerve cells. Only after reaching their destination do the axons branch to form a plexus of nerve terminal arbors. Synapses are formed with many cells in the group of neurons located at this final destination. As the brain matures, these synaptic connections are refined or remodeled. Some axons are pruned while others continue to grow to a selected subset of neurons in the target area. Synaptic remodeling leads eventually to adult patterning of connectivity.

For the most part, the first phase in the formation of neuronal connections is believed to take place independent of neuronal activity. That is, action potential generation is not thought to be required for axonal outgrowth, growth cone guidance, or the elaboration of the initial patterns of neuronal connections. These processes appear to rely largely on the molecular cues that are distributed along the pathway of axonal outgrowth. In contrast, experiments over the last decade have shown that the second phase in the formation of neuronal connections, axonal and synaptic remodeling, is largely activity-dependent.

This chapter will consider current knowledge about the formation of synapses. Particular attention will be given to (1) the ontogeny of inhibitory and excitatory synaptic connections in cortical areas that are thought to be involved in the generation of seizure discharges of focal origin; (2) the contribution that a late formation of inhibitory relative to excitatory synapses makes to enhanced seizure susceptibility in early life; (3) the possibility that local circuit axon collaterals may be remodeled during postnatal life; (4) the contribution that this process may make to changes in seizure susceptibility; and (5) whether the abnormal physiologic activity that accompanies seizures in early life alters the normal course of age-dependent network remodeling.

The Ontogeny of Recurrent Inhibition

Synaptic Inhibition in Cortical Networks

Studies in the mature hippocampus and neocortex have shown that local circuit inhibition plays a major role in regulating neuronal excitability and preventing the generation of seizures. In this regard, interneurons that use GABA as a neurotransmitter play a pivotal role. Studies over the last decade using in vitro slices have been particularly informative in furthering an understanding of how GABA-containing inhibitory interneurons regulate the excitability of hippocampal and neocortical neural networks (Connors, 1984; Miles and Wong, 1987).

Mature CA_3 hippocampal pyramidal cells communicate with each other via recurrent excitatory connections (Ishizuka et al., 1990; Miles and Wong, 1986, 1987). In addition, pyramidal cells synaptically activate local circuit inhibitory interneurons such as basket cells (Miles, 1990). In so doing they initiate recurrent or feedback inhibition in hundreds of nearby pyramidal cells. It is well known that interneurons produce a large, short-duration (50–100 ms) inhibitory postsynaptic potential (IPSP) in pyramidal cells (Miles and Wong, 1984). This IPSP produces inhibition not only by transiently hyperpolarizing the membrane potential of pyramidal cells but also by diminishing the effectiveness of any coincident excitatory postsynaptic potentials (EPSPs) via a large decrease in the pyramidal cell membrane resistance. Recurrent inhibitory synapses are strategically localized to the soma of the pyramidal cells. This localization permits them to limit action potential generation and thus control the excitability of networks of mutually excitatory neurons.

Based on the importance of local circuit inhibition in preventing seizure generation, a number of researchers have focused their attention on understanding the ontogeny of GABA systems in hippocampus and neocortex. Particular attention has been given to the hypothesis that GABA synapses develop relatively late in postnatal life and that a mismatch in terms of the development of excitation versus inhibition is responsible for enhanced seizure susceptibility in early postnatal life.

In rat hippocampus, GABA interneurons are born around gestational day 14 (Amaral and Kurz, 1985). However, biochemical markers for GABA neurons are low at early postnatal ages. For instance, at birth the activity of the synthetic enzyme for GABA, glutamic acid decarboxylase, is only a fraction of that measured in the adult. GABA levels themselves are low, although a substantial quantity of this neurotransmitter is present perinatally (Coyle and Enna, 1976; Swann et al., 1989).

Anatomic studies have also shown that during the first postnatal week the number of synapses that are immunoreactive for GABA or glutamic acid decarboxylase (GAD) is less than in adults (Kunkel, 1966; Seress and Ribak, 1988). Nonetheless, some GABA-containing neurons and synapses are present at these early ages. Ultrastructural studies have shown that these GAD- and GABA-containing presynaptic nerve terminals are quite different from their mature counterparts. Nerve terminals have been reported to be small and to contain few synaptic vesicles (Seress et al., 1989). Other synaptic specializations have also been reported not to be fully formed or to be absent (Kunkel, 1966).

Other histochemical methods have been used to monitor the maturation of hippocampal interneurons. Among these are Golgi/EM (Lang and Frotscher, 1990) and immunocytochemistry for parvalbumin (Bergmann et al., 1991). Results obtained from these procedures also suggest that hippocampal GABA interneurons are quite immature at birth. Golgi studies suggest that most interneurons have very short dendritic arbors. Axon terminal arbors first appear on day 10. In keeping with neurophysiologic results discussed later, interneurons appear to develop differently in hippocampal areas CA_3 and CA_1. CA_3 interneurons are more mature during week 1 and 2 than their counterparts in area CA_1. Interneurons in the dentate gyrus are the last to show anatomic features like those described in adults.

GABA Receptors: Molecular Biology

Results from $GABA_A$ receptor binding studies are in keeping with measures of biochemical and anatomic markers for GABA in presynaptic nerve terminals. At birth, binding of GABA and muscimol, a $GABA_A$ receptor agonist, is only a fraction of that seen in the adult CNS (e.g., Skerritt and Johnston, 1982). Moreover, the pharmacologic properties of these binding sites appear to change with neuronal maturation. For instance, type II benzodiazepine receptors are thought to predominate in early life and evolve into type I receptors in adulthood (Chisholm et al., 1983; Reichelt et al., 1991).

The first subunit of the $GABA_A$ receptor was cloned and sequenced in the late 1980s (Schofield et al., 1987). At this writing, thirteen separate subunits have been identified. There are six α, three β, three γ, and one δ (for review see Wisden and Seeburg, 1992). In situ hybridization studies have shown that gene expression of these subunits varies among brain regions (Persohn et al., 1992; Wisden et al., 1992). For instance, in adult neocortex α_1–α_4 are present in varying degrees in neocortical layers II–VI. However, α_5 is present in very small quantities and only in layer VI, and α_6 is absent. By comparison, α_5 mRNA is abundant in all areas of the hippocampus and dentate gyrus. Also present are α_1, α_2, and α_4, but α_3 is in low amounts. Further, α_6 is also absent in the hippocampal formation. For the β subunits,

β_1 mRNA is highly expressed in hippocampus but absent in neocortex; β_2 and β_3 and γ_2 are present in large quantities in both neocortex and hippocampus.

Expression of $GABA_A$ subunits in *Xenopus* oocytes and cultured cells have shown that receptors comprised of different subunit combinations have different electrophysiologic and pharmacologic properties (Angelotti and Macdonald, 1993; Pritchett, Luddens et al., 1989). For instance, results show that the γ_2 subunit imparts benzodiazepine sensitivity to the $GABA_A$ receptor (Pritchett et al., 1989). Recombinant receptors comprised of β_1 and γ_2 that are in combination with α_1, α_2, or α_3 have distinctly different sensitivities to benzodiazepines (Pritchett, Southeimer et al., 1989). Thus whether type I or type II benzodiazepine receptors are present in a given brain region is likely to be dictated by which α subunit is expressed.

In the developing CNS the profiles of $GABA_A$ receptor subunits vary with age (Bovolin et al., 1992; Laurie et al., 1992; MacLennan et al., 1991). Figure 8-1 summarizes some of these changes. In neocortex considerable changes occur in subunit expression between birth and adulthood. For example, α_5, which is absent in the adult neocortex, undergoes a marked transient expression around postnatal day 6. Similarly, α_3 and β_3 mRNA levels peak in early postnatal life. Indeed, of the α subunits, α_3 is the most prominent perinatally. In contrast, the γ_2 subunit is present at adult levels as early as embryonic day 17 (E17) and maintains that level until adulthood.

Developmental changes of GABA subunits occur during hippocampal development (Laurie et al., 1992). However, these are less dramatic than those in neocortex. α_2 and α_5 subunits reach adult levels as early as E17. α_1, α_3, and α_4 are present at birth. β_3 and γ_2 are present in significant quantities in late embryonic life and increase to adult levels during early postnatal life. γ_1 and γ_3 undergo transient expression between postnatal day 0 and 12.

Based on these recent molecular biological observations, one would predict that substantial changes in the electrophysiologic and pharmacologic properties of GABA-mediated IPSPs would occur during brain maturation. If this were so, such changes would be expected to directly influence epileptogenic processes at various developmental periods.

GABA Inhibition: Electrophysiology

Indeed, a number of electrophysiological studies have been undertaken that address this issue. When a mature CA_1 pyramidal cell responds to an orthodromic electrical stimulus, it undergoes a brief EPSP, which is followed by a large prolonged hyperpolarization. Nicoll and his colleagues (Alger and Nicoll, 1982a; Alger and Nicoll, 1982b; Newberry and Nicoll, 1985) showed that this afterhyperpolarization actually consists of two separate IPSPs. The first component is produced by the $GABA_A$ postsynaptic receptor. As discussed earlier, this mediates an increase in membrane permeability to Cl^-. The second component is produced by the $GABA_B$ receptor. It activates a

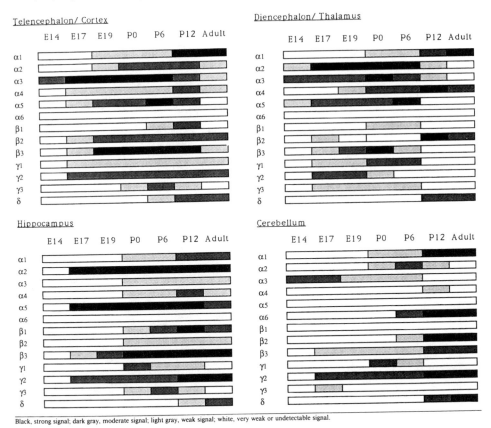

Figure 8-1. Schematic illustration of the developmental changes in the expression of GABA$_A$ receptor subunit mRNAs in selected brain regions. Based on results from in situ hybridization studies. The shading of bars signifies the following: black, strong signal; dark gray, moderate signal; light gray, weak signal; white, very weak or undetectable signal. (Modified with permission from Laurie et al., 1992.)

K$^+$ conductance increase mechanism. Remarkably similar recordings have been reported in pyramidal cells in mature neocortex (Connors et al., 1988).

Synaptic inhibition is quite different in area CA$_1$ of developing hippocampus and neocortex than in adult brain. During the first postnatal week orthodromic stimuli do not produce hyperpolarizing IPSPs, producing instead large prolonged depolarizing responses (Dunwiddie, 1981; Harris and Teyler, 1983; Kriegstein et al., 1987; Schwartzkroin, 1982; Schwartzkroin and Altschuler, 1977; Swann et al., 1989). The lower panel of Figure 8-2 illustrates these developmental changes. In some instances these prolonged depolarizations result in the generation of action potentials, and thus these events might be classified as excitatory. In some instances the application of GABA$_A$ receptor antagonists has been reported to attenuate these prolonged depolarizations in the immature CNS (Cherubini, Ben-Ari, et al., 1991). This

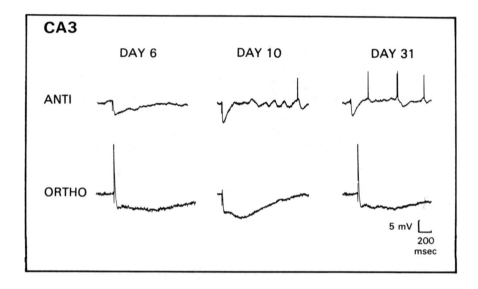

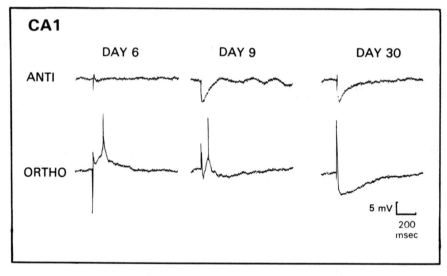

Figure 8-2. Comparison of responses of rat CA$_3$ and CA$_1$ hippocampal neurons to orthodromic (ORTHO) and antidromic (ANTI) stimulation at three different post-natal ages. Responses were elicited in each cell by two independently manipulated stimulating electrodes. Responses are averages of three events. Spontaneous action potentials were thus reduced in amplitude. (Reproduced with permission from Swann et al., 1989.)

has led investigators to propose that GABA is not an inhibitory but instead an excitatory neurotransmitter in the developing CNS (Cherubini, Gaiarsa, et al., 1991). Indeed, when GABA is applied to immature cortical or hippocampal neurons it can produce a dramatic depolarization. Depolarizing responses to GABA have also been reported in mature hippocampus and neocortex, but only when the neurotransmitter is applied to pyramidal cell dendrites (Alger and Nicoll, 1982b; Connors et al., 1988; Janigro and Schwartzkroin, 1988a). Application to cell bodies results in a membrane hyperpolarization. Some authors have suggested that depolarizing responses might be produced by extrasynaptic receptors. Thus depolarizing responses produced when GABA is applied to the cell bodies in developing CNS has been suggested to be a sign of the immaturity of GABA synapses (Mueller et al., 1983).

Recently two groups studied the responsiveness of immature hippocampal and cortical neurons to GABA. Both Zhang et al. (1990, 1991) and Luhmann and Prince (1991) concluded that age-dependent differences in GABA responsiveness are not due solely to differences in GABA receptor makeup. Instead a late development of Cl^- transport mechanisms in plasma membrane is suggested to contribute to differences in GABA-mediated IPSPs. In "mature" CA_1 neurons (e.g., postnatal day 15–20) the reversal potential for somatic GABA responses was shown to be more negative than the resting membrane potential and was highly dependent on the transmembrane Cl^- gradient. Zhang et al. (1991) also showed that normally (i.e., under resting conditions) the plasma membrane had a low permeability to Cl^-. The reversal potential of GABA responses in these cells was altered by external K^+, furosemide, and changes in temperature, suggesting that a K–Cl cotransporter regulated the concentration of Cl^- internally and thus made GABA IPSPs hyperpolarizing. In slices from 2- to 5-day-old rats, GABA responses in CA_1 neurons were also highly dependent on the Cl^- gradient. However, in these immature cells the equilibrium potential for GABA was very near the resting membrane potential; the membrane of very immature CA_1 pyramidal cells was found to be highly permeable to Cl^-; thus Cl^- homeostasis of these cells was thought to be largely dictated by passive Donnan equilibrium.

These results help to explain the lack of hyperpolarizing IPSPs in CA_1 and neocortical cells. However, they fail to explain why GABA responses and synaptic potentials are depolarizing at a very early age. If they are depolarizing and yet dependent solely on Cl^- permeability, then Cl^- must be actively accumulated by the cells. In this regard it is important to mention that Misgeld et al. (1986) suggested that a Cl^- transporter existed in hippocampal pyramidal cells that resulted in Cl^- accumulation intracellularly. The presence of such a Cl^- transporter could underlie depolarizing responses to GABA. Misgeld et al. invoked such a transport process to explain the existence of depolarizing responses to GABA in the dendrites of mature hippocampal pyramidal cells. It is commonly observed that application of GABA to dendrites will result in membrane depolarizations while applications to pyramidal cell soma produce a hyperpolarization. The presence of two transport processes, one in soma that excrudes Cl^- and one in dendrites that accumulates Cl^-, could explain the regionalized difference in GABA responsiveness. Hypothetically, the transporter that extrudes Cl^- may be absent early in life and the Cl^- transport process that pumps Cl^- into cells may be active and in both soma and dendrites this scenario would produce depolarizing responses to GABA that are mediated by an increase in Cl⁻ conductance. Alternatively, another ion may be responsible for depolarizing responses to GABA. Bicarbonate, HCO_3^-, has been suggested as a candidate. In crayfish muscle this ionic species appears to mediate GABA depolarization. However, experiments in mature hippocampal neurons have failed to support bicarbonate's role in dendritic depolarizations produced by GABA (Grover et al., 1993). Thus questions still remain regarding how GABA responses are produced early in life. In this regard it should be noted that Michelson and Wong (1991) recently reported that GABA can be the excitatory neurotransmitter on interneurons in mature CNS. These investigators proposed that at least some hippocampal inhibitory interneurons make synaptic contact with each other and form networks of mutually excitatory cells. GABA appears to excite these inhibitory cells. The ionic mechanism that underlies these responses has yet to be described.

It would appear that a late onset of GABAergic synaptic inhibition in developing cortex and hippocampus could contribute to enhanced seizure susceptibility in early life. However, in other areas of the immature CNS, even in other areas of the hippocampal formation, GABA inhibition has been shown to be present. Indeed, at these sites it plays a key role in preventing seizure generation. However, these areas still demonstrate enhanced seizure susceptibility in early life. For instance, in hippocampal area CA_3 Swann et al. (1989), Schwartzkroin (1982), and Janigro and Schwartzkroin (1988b) have shown that large hyperpolarizing IPSPs can be present as early as postnatal day 5 (see upper panel of Fig. 8-2). During postnatal week 2, when inhibition is suppressed pharmacologically in area CA_3 by $GABA_A$ receptor antagonists, prolonged electrographic seizures are routinely recorded (Brady and Swann, 1984; Swann and Brady, 1984). Under these conditions, slices from mature rats do not produce electrographic seizure discharges but instead only brief interictal events. Similarly, Hablitz (1987) has shown that neocortical slices from 1- to 2-week-old rats can produce electrographic seizures when exposed to $GABA_A$ receptor antagonists (see Moshé, Shinnar, and Swann, Chapter 2, for discussion of critical periods of enhanced seizure susceptibility). Thus attention has turned to a search for mechanisms other than a late onset of synaptic inhibition to explain the generation of seizures in developing hippocampus and neocortex.

The Ontogeny of Recurrent Excitation

Synaptic Excitation in Cortical Networks

Another major feature of cortical neural networks in mature brain is the presence of recurrent excitatory synapses. In both neocortex and hippocampus blockade of synaptic inhibition reveals the extent of excitatory interactions among principal cortical or hippocampal neurons (Connors, 1984; Miles and Wong, 1987). These excitatory synapses use an amino acid, such as glutamate, as their neurotransmitter. In hippocampus, where these connections have been studied in detail (Miles and Wong, 1986), dual intracellular recordings have demonstrated the presence of direct monosynaptic pyramidal cell–to–pyramidal cell interactions. Recurrent EPSPs recorded in CA$_3$ pyramidal cell pairs are usually 1–2 mV in amplitude. Their time course appears to be shaped by both intrinsic inward and outward currents (Miles and Wong, 1986).

When GABA$_A$-mediated synaptic inhibition is suppressed by receptor antagonists, so-called latent multisynaptic excitatory connections are revealed (Miles and Wong, 1987). Recordings in Figure 8-3 illustrate this phenomenon. During dual intracellular recordings, action potentials in one pyramidal cell typically will not produce a response in another nearby pyramidal cell. Monosynaptic interactions are seen rarely, in only 1–2 percent of pairs. However, when a GABA$_A$ receptor antagonist such as picrotoxin is applied, polysynaptic EPSPs are often produced. Thus it is thought that under normal conditions firing of a pyramidal cell activates inhibitory interneurons, leading to generation of powerful disynaptic IPSPs in many other pyramidal cells. This counters the excitation produced by the nearly simultaneous re-

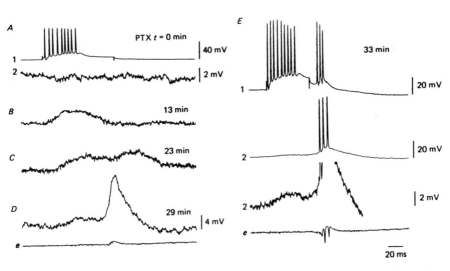

Figure 8-3. Evolution of the influence of a single CA$_3$ pyramidal cell on picrotoxin-induced CA$_3$ network discharging. Dual intracellular recordings (1 and 2) were made simultaneous with an extracellular field recording (*e*). Before picrotoxin was added (*A*) the presynaptic cell, cell 1, did not influence the activity of cell 2. However, between 13 and 29 minutes after addition of picrotoxin (5 μM) to the bath, polysynaptic EPSPs were produced in cell 2. By 29 minutes a late, large polysynaptic EPSP occurred simultaneously with a small network discharge in the field potential recordings. At 33 minutes firing of cell 1 initiated a large network burst in the CA$_3$ population (*E, e,* lower trace), which "reverberated" and resulted in a burst in both cells 1 and 2. In *E* the trace from cell 2 is shown at two amplifications. (Reproduced with permission from Miles and Wong, 1987.)

current EPSPs. When inhibition is suppressed, pyramidal cell–to–pyramidal cell excitation is unopposed by synaptic inhibition. Thus spontaneous firing of a single pyramidal cell leads to EPSPs in several other pyramidal cells. Resultant spiking in these cells will in turn excite other pyramidal cells and lead to a cascade of synaptic excitation through the CA_3 network. After picrotoxin application, polysynaptic EPSPs are recorded in 30 percent of pyramidal cell pairs. They are longer in duration and larger in amplitude than monosynaptic recurrent EPSPs. Under these conditions excitation spreads so readily through networks of mutually excitatory CA_3 pyramidal cells that action potentials in a single cell can initiate the generation of an interictal discharge (Miles and Wong, 1983). Results from numerous pharmacologic experiments also suggest that recurrent excitation plays a central role in epileptiform discharges since interictal spikes in hippocampus and neocortex are suppressed by excitatory amino acid receptor antagonists.

As discussed earlier, during critical periods in brain development both hippocampus and neocortex have an increased susceptibility for seizures (Brady and Swann, 1984; Hablitz, 1987; Swann and Brady, 1984). In in vitro slice experiments these differences can be quite dramatic. When slices from 3- to 4-week-old animals are exposed to convulsant drugs they produce brief (≈ 100 ms) synchronized discharges that closely resemble interictal spikes in EEG recordings. These are identical to those recorded from slices of fully mature animals. In 1- to 2-week-old rats, $GABA_A$ antagonists produce electrographic seizure discharges that are often 30 seconds in duration. Earlier in life (during postnatal week 1) epileptiform discharges occur much less frequently than at any other age; usually these epileptiform events occur asynchronously and are of low amplitude, if they are present at all. Electrographic seizure discharges are abolished by excitatory amino acid antagonists; thus recurrent excitation has been implicated in their generation (Brady and Swann, 1986, 1988; Lee and Hablitz, 1991). Accordingly, attention has turned to the study of excitatory amino acid synaptic transmission in developing cortical networks. The hypothesis has been developed that differences in recurrent excitation early in life could promote seizure generation and play a central role in epileptogenesis in developing brain.

Indeed, our neurophysiologic studies of local excitatory synaptic interactions in developing hippocampus appear to support the view that the basic physiologic properties of recurrent excitation in early postnatal life promote epileptogenesis. For instance, when $GABA_A$ receptor antagonists are applied to hippocampal slices taken during the second postnatal week, the majority (85 percent) of CA_3 pyramidal cells impaled were able to initiate synchronized discharging of the entire CA_3 population. The comparable study in adults reported a much smaller proportion of pyramidal cells capable of initiating epileptiform events (Miles and Wong, 1983). Thus in early life excitation easily propagates from a single pyramidal cell through a population of CA_3 neurons. Dual intracellular recordings have shown that recurrent EPSPs can be recorded in 50 percent of pairs, the majority of which are polysynaptically mediated (see Fig. 8-4; Swann, Smith, Brady, et al., 1993).

CELL 1 **CELL 2**

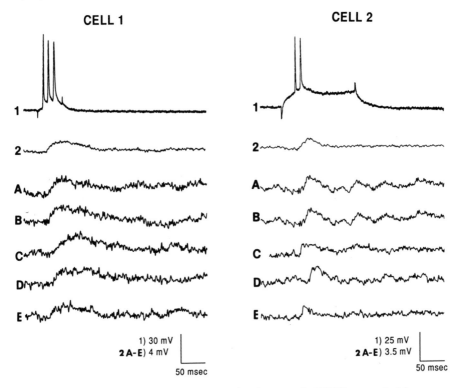

1) 30 mV
2 A–E) 4 mV

50 msec

1) 25 mV
2 A–E) 3.5 mV

50 msec

Figure 8-4. Dual intracellular recordings of polysynaptic EPSPs recorded in a mutually excitatory pair of hippocampal neurons in a minislice taken from a 1-week-old rat pup. IPSPs were blocked with penicillin. Traces 1 show action potentials produced by a brief depolarizing pulse of current injected intracellularly. Traces 2 are averaged ($n = 12$, cross-correlation variable latency averaging techniques were employed) EPSPs recorded in the other cell of the pair. Individual representative responses from the "postsynaptic" cell are shown in traces A–E. Action potentials in cell 1 produced a prolonged polysynaptically mediated EPSP in cell 2. The EPSP produced in cell 1 by discharging in cell 2 was shorter in duration. (Reproduced with permission from Swann, Smith, Brady et al., 1993.)

The frequency of transmission failure between polysynaptically coupled pairs was found to be surprisingly very low—on average only about 15 percent. In some pairs, virtually every discharge of only one action potential in the presynaptic neuron produced an EPSP in the second cell of the pair. The time to EPSP onset was 10–15 ms, supporting the view that a polysynaptic path existed between the two cells. These data indicate that excitation readily propagates through CA_3 neuronal networks early in postnatal life. Indeed, excitation appears to spread more easily during the "critical period" of seizure susceptibility than in adulthood. Thus understanding how recurrent excitatory networks form and characterizing their physiological properties in early life have become the focus of our research.

Synaptogenesis: Basic Mechanisms

Unfortunately, little information is available on the basic processes that govern the formation of local circuit synapses in cortical networks. However, results from simpler model systems and studies of projecting pathways in CNS have provided a great deal of information about factors that contribute to the growth and guidance of axons to their target sites and the formation of synapses.

Surprisingly, one factor that does not appear to contribute importantly is action potential–based neural activity. It has been shown in numerous neural systems, among which are visual pathways and neuromuscular junctions, that axons grow over remarkably long distances and make synaptic contact with correct targets in the absence of action potentials (for reviews see Goodman and Shatz, 1993; Nelson and Sur, 1992; Shatz, 1990). It is known that growth cones can correctly traverse complex pathways before the onset of electrical activity (Goodman and Spitzer, 1979, 1981). There is ample evidence that growth cones of cholinergic neurons spontaneously release acetylcholine immediately upon contact with postsynaptic cells (Evers et al., 1989; Haydon and Zoran, 1989; Xie and Poo, 1986). In other words, functional synapses appear to form immediately upon growth cone contact. This has been demonstrated in a remarkable series of experiments during which investigators followed the formation of single synapses between pairs of cells in culture with video microscopy while simultaneously recording electrophysiologic activity (Evers et al., 1989). These experiments clearly demonstrated that functional synapses can form within a few seconds to minutes of cell-to-cell contact. However, action potential generation did not correlate with the presence of spontaneous synaptic events. Indeed, synaptic events could be recorded in the presence of tetrodotoxin (TTX). These results further support the notion that at least the initial phase of synapse formation is not dependent upon action potential generation. In other experiments TTX has been used routinely to block action potential generation during neural development in vivo (for review see Goodman and Shatz, 1993; Nelson and Sur, 1992). Under these circumstances axons appear to grow and make appropriate synaptic contacts. The neural systems operate in a normal fashion as soon as the effect of the toxin has worn off.

The formation of synapses between cultured hippocampal and neocortical neurons has been studied extensively and the results suggest that synaptic activity does not play a critical role in the early stages of synapse formation. For instance, microcultures of hippocampal neurons have been grown while excitatory amino acid receptors were blocked pharmacologically (Furshpan and Potter, 1989; Segal, 1991; Segal and Furshpan, 1990). In these experiments, dissociated cultures or microcultures of only one or two hippocampal neurons were grown in media containing 1–5 mM kynurenic acid and 11 mM Mg^{2+}. Under these circumstances excitatory amino acid synaptic transmission would be expected to be greatly suppressed or abolished. After several weeks in vitro, cultures were studied electrophysiologically. As soon as kynurenate was washed from the media and Mg^{2+} lowered to normal levels, spontaneous excitatory synaptic events were recorded. This activity was so intense that seizure-like discharges were generated—even when there was only a single cell in the microculture. In these instances the discharges were thought to be mediated by autaptic synaptic contacts (that is, the cells made excitatory synapses on their own dendrites).

In related experiments, Smith and Swann (1993) recently studied explant cultures from neonatal rat hippocampus grown in media containing 3-mM kynurenate. Consistent with the prior studies in dissociated cultures, recurrent excitatory synapses appeared to form even when postsynaptic receptors were suppressed by kynurenate. Immediately upon wash out of the receptor blocker, pronounced spontaneous excitatory synaptic potentials were recorded. Application of GABA receptor antagonists to the explant cultures led to electrographic seizure discharges similar to those recorded in acute slices from 2-week-old rats. These events were abolished by excitatory amino acid receptor antagonists. Similar recordings were never observed on postnatal day 4–5 when the hippocampal slices were placed in culture. Thus excitatory synapses appear to grow and make functional contacts even when the postsynaptic receptors for these synapses are blocked.

How do neurons find their target sites? The mechanisms that underlie growth cone guidance and target recognition are a very active area of experimentation (Goodman and Shatz, 1993; Sanes, 1993) and may be divided into two general categories. The first is often referred to as differential adhesion. In these instances axons appear to be guided by the expression of cell adhesion molecules (CAMs) on growth cones and cells that are distributed along projection pathways. There are at least two large gene families of CAMs: the immunoglobulin and cadhedrin families. Growth cone integrin receptors for extracellular matrix proteins are also thought to play important roles in axon growth and guidance. Besides growth-promoting molecules it is also known that repulsive molecules exist. These are demonstrated by the collapse of growth cones and axon withdrawal when contact is made with particular cells or tissue types. Thus both differential adhesion and repulsion appear to help guide axons to their targets.

The second process involves diffusible cues that provide a "tropic" influence. Sperry first proposed the chemoaffinity hypothesis of axon guidance in the early 1960s (Sperry, 1963). He argued that growth cones were guided toward their targets by gradients of chemotaxic substances. Today the strongest support for chemotropic guidance comes from studies in tissue culture (Tessier-Lavigne, 1992). However, results from some in vivo experiments also favor this notion. For instance, O'Leary et al. (1991) showed that when fetal rats were irradiated at a critical stage in the development of the basilar pons, this brain area was often absent at birth. However, ectopic islands of pontine neurons were produced. Normally, as cortical pyramidal cells project to spinal cord, they produce collateral branches in the pons which synapse on the basilar pontine neurons. In the irradiated rats, the corticospinal axons did not send collaterals toward the missing basilar pons but instead projected directly to the misplaced islands of pontine neurons. These results implicate a chemotaxic agent produced by pontine neurons in axon pathfinding by corticospinal neurons.

Properties of EPSPs in Neonatal Hippocampus and Cortex

As mentioned, functional synaptic transmission can be observed a few seconds after presynaptic contact with a postsynaptic cell. However, neurophysiologic studies have shown that the properties of immature synapses can be different from their adult counterparts. The first intracellular recordings of excitatory postsynaptic potentials from neonatal cortex were performed in vivo in kittens. These studies suggested that the properties of EPSPs in early life differed markedly from those of adult cats (Purpura, 1969; Purpura et al., 1965, 1968). For instance, EPSPs in neonatal hippocampus and cortex were reported to be unusually prolonged. Recent studies have consistently supported this early observation. Moreover, some insights have been gained into the mechanisms underlying these long-lasting synaptic events. In vitro studies have shown that EPSPs can be several hundred milliseconds in duration. For instance, Schwartzkroin (1982) reported EPSPs in CA_1 pyramidal cells to be 150–200 ms in duration. Kriegstein et al. (1987) reported the average EPSP duration to be three times longer on postnatal days 5–7 than on postnatal days 7–14. Recently, Burgard and Hablitz (1993), using whole-cell recordings, found neonatal EPSPs to be on average 400 ms in duration on day 4. They reported a progressive daily shortening of the EPSPs through day 14. Voltage clamp recordings showed that the change in EPSP duration was mirrored by a shortening of the underlying postsynaptic currents. Thus the prolonged nature of the events in early life were not thought to be explained by a prolongation of brief EPSPs by intrinsic membrane currents. Instead, long-duration EPSPs appear to be produced by long-duration excitatory postsynaptic currents (EPSCs).

In mature neocortical and hippocampal pyramidal cells, EPSPs often consist of two components: an early, relatively brief, EPSP that is mediated by an AMPA receptor, and a longer lasting component that is produced by the NMDA receptor. Both components have been reported in EPSPs from neonatal rats. Indeed, Luhman and Prince (1990, 1991) suggest that the multicomponent EPSPs are unusually large during the second postnatal week in neocortex. Burgard and Hablitz (1993) have recorded both components as early as postnatal day 3. Dual-component miniature EPSPs have been reported for 1- to 2-week-old CA_3 hippocampal pyramidal cells as well (McBain and Dingledine, 1992).

Two whole-cell voltage clamp studies have reported that EPSPs mediated by NMDA receptors are unusually prolonged in early life. Figure 8-5 illustrates age-dependent changes in NMDA receptor-mediated excitatory postsynaptic currents. They were obtained from layer IV of visual cortex. Both evoked and spontaneous EPSCs, recorded during the second postnatal week, were found to be more prolonged than those in month-old rats. The decay rates of EPSCs at both ages were described by exponential functions.

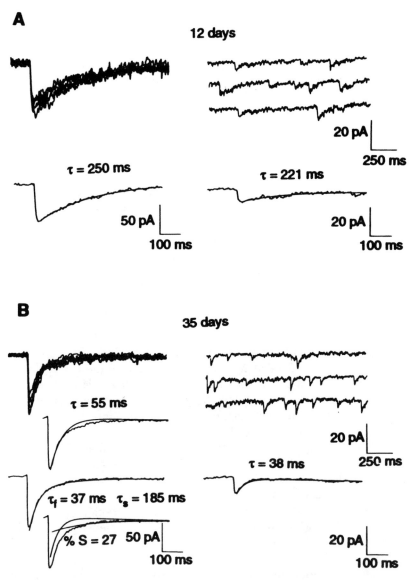

Figure 8-5. Comparison of the kinetic properties of NMDA-EPSCs recorded from layer IV cortical neurons on postnatal days 12 and 35. (A) Five superimposed EPSCs, recorded in postnatal day 12 cortical neuron in response to electrical stimulation, are shown at top left. Below is an averaged EPSC ($n = 20$). A single exponential curve is superimposed on the decay of the averaged event ($\tau = 250$ ms). To the right are spontaneous EPSCs. An average ($n = 30$) is shown below. (B) Similar recordings taken on postnatal day 35. The time constant of EPSC decay fit by a single exponential was much shorter ($\tau = 55$ ms). A better fit was obtained with a double exponential curve with a fast ($\tau = 37$ ms) and a slow ($\tau = 185$ ms) component. The slow component was estimated to be 27 percent of the entire EPSC. Spontaneous EPSCs also had fast rates of decay ($\tau = 38$ ms). (Modified with permission from Carmignoto and Vicini, 1992.)

However, a slow component comprised, on average, 90 percent of the EPSC in immature rat but less than 20 percent of its adulthood counterpart. Studies of NMDA channel currents in outside-out patches have also been conducted. These and other results have suggested that the differences in NMDA EPSPs are due to age-dependent modification of channel properties (Carmignoto and Vicini, 1992; Hestrin, 1992). Thus experimental results indicate that excitatory synapses are functional very early in postnatal life but that the properties of these synapses differ markedly from their counterparts in mature rats.

In this regard, a number of studies have reported age-dependent changes in the voltage dependency of NMDA receptors in hippocampal pyramidal cells. For instance, Ben-Ari et al. (1988) suggested that NMDA receptors on neonatal rat CA_3 pyramidal cells lack voltage dependency. Bowe and Nadler (1990) reported that the Mg^{2+} sensitivity of NMDA receptors in 2-week-old rat hippocampus is less than that in adults. Kleckner and Dingledine (1991) came to similar conclusions when they compared NMDA receptors expressed in *Xenopus* oocytes that were derived from mRNA extracts of neonatal and adult rat brain. Results of Brady et al. (1991) suggested that the Mg^{2+} sensitivity of NMDA receptors on 1- to 2-week-old rat CA_3 pyramidal cells is diminished. However, these authors also reported that NMDA ion channels were voltage-dependent at this time. In immature tissue Ca^{2+} appears to play a role similar to magnesium's role in the adult with respect to NMDA receptor voltage dependency. Indeed, decreasing the extracellular Ca^{2+} concentration dramatically reduced NMDA voltage dependency in cells from 1- to 2-week-old rats. Interestingly, this same experimental maneuver enhanced electrographic seizure discharges in hippocampal slices taken from 1- to 2-week-old rats but not from adult rats.

Taken together these results suggest that during maturation, changes occur in the biophysical properties of hippocampal NMDA receptor channel complex, especially in its sensitivity to divalent cations. Such alterations would be expected to promote excitatory synaptic transmission and thus could be important to epileptogenic mechanisms in the developing brain. In contrast to these findings are reports of NMDA receptor-mediated events in developing neocortex. Uniformly, these reports suggest that in embryonic and newborn rats, NMDA receptors display a voltage dependency that is Mg^{2+}-dependent and not unlike that observed in adults (Blanton et al., 1990; Burgard and Hablitz, 1993; Lo Turco et al., 1991). Thus it would appear that there are major differences between the NMDA receptor on developing neocortical and hippocampal pyramidal cells. It would seem likely that such differences will eventually be explained by variations in receptor subunit expression in these two brain areas.

Ontogeny of Excitatory Amino Acid Receptors

Based on electrophysiologic findings reviewed earlier one would predict that the binding sites for both NMDA and AMPA receptors would be present in neonatal brain. Indeed, many neurochemical studies describe the ontogeny of these receptors in some detail (for review see McDonald and Johnston, 1990). Results of these studies also suggest that major ontogenic alterations occur in excitatory amino acid synapses. During critical periods of development in both neocortex and hippocampus there is a transient increase in density of excitatory amino acid receptors. In rat hippocampus this change occurs during the second and third postnatal week. In other brain regions, such as globus pallidus, the AMPA receptor population is only transiently expressed and disappears as an animal matures. A number of studies suggest that the pharmacologic properties of the receptor are distinctly different at various stages in brain development (for review see McDonald and Johnston, 1990). For instance, in hippocampus the ontogenic profiles for components of the NMDA receptors are quite different. Patterns of strychnine-insensitive glycine binding and TCP (N-[1-(thienyl)cyclohexyl]piperidine) binding to PCP (phencyclidine) receptors in the NMDA channel are delayed relative to NMDA binding. These developmental differences lead investigators to suggest that there are multiple forms of the NMDA receptor.

Such observations were made well before subunits of the NMDA receptor were cloned. In the early 1990s numerous subunits for both NMDA and AMPA receptors were described molecularly (for review see Seeburg, 1993). Among the 16 different subunits for ionotropic excitatory amino acid receptors recently cloned, there are (1) AMPA receptor subunits, $GluR_1$ to $GluR_4$, (2) kainic acid receptor subunits, $GluR_5$ to $GluR_7$, KA_1 and KA_2, and (3) NMDA receptor subunits NR_1 and NR_{2A} to NR_{2D}. Most recently, two new subunits, δ_1 and δ_2, have been reported whose function is unknown at this time (Lomeli et al., 1993). Finally, five metabotropic glutamate receptor subunits, $mGluR_1$ to $mGluR_5$, have been described (Schoepp and Conn, 1993; Tanabe et al., 1992). Splice variants for many of these excitatory amino acid receptor subunits have also been reported. Indeed, NR_1 has been shown to have as many as eight splice variants (Hollmann et al., 1993; Sugihara et al., 1992). When expressed in oocytes or cultured cells, heteromeric configurations of various subunits and/or splice variants have been shown to have different biophysical properties (Seeburg, 1993).

As described earlier for the $GABA_A$ receptor subunits, a number of in situ hybridization studies have shown that subunit mRNAs are expressed in different amounts in different areas of CNS. Particularly striking are in situ hybridization studies that localized KA_1 receptor subunits to CA_3 hippocampal neurons (Werner et al., 1991); message for this subunit is virtually absent in CA_1 pyramidal cells. Moreover, the expression of some receptor subunits appears to change during brain development (Williams et al., 1993). One study has reported that $GluR_1$ and $GluR_3$ mRNAs were transiently elevated in early life compared to adult levels (Pellegrini-Giampietro et al., 1991). This finding is reminiscent of results from receptor binding studies mentioned previously (McDonald and Johnston, 1990). Expression of $GluR_1$ and $GluR_3$ mRNA peaked at day 14 in hippocampus and neocortex at approximately 200 percent of the adult level. In contrast, $GluR_2$, mRNA levels were near adult levels throughout postnatal life. Alternative splice variants for excitatory amino acid receptor subunits have also been reported to vary in regional expression during postnatal development (Monyer et al., 1991). At the present time a comprehensive review of the distribution of all excitatory amino acid receptor subunits is not possible, since many of these subunits have only recently been cloned. However, it should be safe to predict that continuing studies will show that excitatory amino acid receptors undergo substantial alterations at the molecular level during brain development.

Experience-Dependent Remodeling of Circuits During Early Life

In the mammalian CNS the development of neuronal networks extends well into postnatal life. However, maturation is not simply characterized by an increase in the complexity of connectivity with age. Often pathways are overrepresented perinatally. "Exuberant" projections of axons to their targets are commonly observed. In brain, the use of retrograde and anterograde tracers has shown that early "aberrant" projections take place. Commonly, adult patterns of innervation evolve, not via the death of parent neurons (O'Leary and Koester, 1993), but instead via the elimination of aberrant axon branches (for review see Constantine-Paton et al., 1990; Goodman and Shatz, 1993). For example, quantitative ultrastructural studies in primates have shown that there are three to four times as many axons in the corpus callosum at birth than in adults; axons are eliminated at rates as high as 4 million per day (LaMantia and Rakic, 1990). Following axon elimination, adult patterns of connectivity generally result from the further elaboration of axons and synapses at the selected target sites. Such remodeling of connectivity has been best demonstrated at the neuromuscular junction and within visual pathways. In both instances experimental evidence strongly favors the notion that the remodeling process is dependent upon neuronal activity (for reviews see Goodman and Shatz, 1993; O'Leary and Koester, 1993; Shatz, 1990).

The sequence of axon elimination and synapse remodeling is illustrated by studies of the neuromuscular junction. All mammalian muscle fibers are thought to receive polyneuronal innervation prior to birth. However, during early postnatal life, many motor axons retract and eventually muscle fibers become innervated by only one axon. Axon loss and synapse elimination have been shown to be dependent upon motoneuron activity (Thompson et al., 1979). A number of recent studies have employed time-lapse imaging techniques of living neuromuscular junctions to follow the time course of synapse and axon elimination. Results show that acetylcholine receptors at a given synapse are lost prior to nerve terminal elimination (Balice-Gordon and Lichtman, 1993; Colman and Lichtman, 1993). This finding suggests that a postsynaptic mechanism plays an important role in the remodeling process at developing nerve muscle synapses. How activity-dependent processes mediate elimination of neuromuscular synapses has been studied recently in tissue culture preparations (Dan and Poo, 1992; Harish and Poo, 1992; Lo and Poo, 1991). In these experiments, where single muscle cells were innervated by two motoneurons, repetitive activation of one neuron led to a long-lasting suppression of synaptic potentials produced by the other neuron. Results also suggested that the postsynaptic changes induced by stimulation were in turn followed by presynaptic alterations (perhaps mediated by a transynaptic retrograde messenger). This long-lasting depression of excitatory junction potential is presumably the forerunner of synapse elimination and axon withdrawal.

Much like results from studies at the neuromuscular junction, the visual systems in mammals and lower vertebrates appear to undergo dramatic remodeling of connectivity that is dependent upon neural activity. For instance, at birth the left and right eye projections to layer IV of visual cortex (from the lateral geniculate nucleus) are intermixed. However, during a critical period in early postnatal life, the lateral geniculate axons from the eyes segregate into separate eye-specific patches in layer IV. These alternating left and right eye patches are the anatomical basis for the ocular dominance columns (LeVay et al., 1978, 1980).

The first results that indicated that remodeling of these layer IV afferents was dependent on neural activity came from the laboratories of Hubel and Wiesel (1970). They showed that when the lids of one eye of a kitten were closed, the formation of ocular dominance columns was dramatically altered. Following lid closure, the closed eye activated cortical neurons in a much smaller area of layer IV. The open eye was overrepresented. The physiological recordings showed that the deprived eye had lost its ability to drive cortical units, whereas most cortical neurons responded to stimulation of the open eye. This phenomenon is referred to as an ocular dominance shift.

Experiments from many laboratories have expanded on these initial observations and have shown that activity-dependent synaptic competition between axons representing the left and right eye is the basis for ocular dominance column formation. For instance, in one study TTX was injected into both eyes of an experimental animal, thus abolishing neural activity arising from visual stimulus. Under these circumstances the segregation of axons in layer IV did not occur (Stryker and Harris, 1986). However, while these results show that the segregation is activity-dependent, they do not clarify how electrical activity mediated the segregation. Other studies showed that it is not the *level* of activity but instead the *pattern* of activity arising from the two eyes that is important in axon segregation and synaptic competition. To show the importance of patterned activity, TTX was injected into both eyes and stimulating electrodes were placed in the optic nerves (Stryker and Strickland, 1984). When both nerves were stimulated at the same time ocular dominance columns did not form, but when the nerves were stimulated asynchronously the ocular dominance columns developed. Thus it would appear that the temporal patterning of a neural activity is important for segregation of afferents in layer IV of visual cortex.

These results are reminiscent of those obtained in fish where optic nerve regeneration was studied. After optic nerves are cut in these lower vertebrates, axons grow back to their appropriate target sites in tectum. However, if TTX is applied, fine-tuning or segregation of these projections is prevented. Moreover, if the fish are raised in strobe light so that all retinal cells fire synchronously, refined patterns of tectal innervation fail to develop (Schmidt and Eisele, 1985). Thus, much like in lateral geniculate innervation of layer IV in mammalian cortex, patterning of electrical activity appears to be all-important in the phenomena of synapse selection and normal circuit formation.

Results such as these have led to specific hypotheses on how axon segregation and synaptic remodeling take place during normal development. For instance, retinal ganglion cells that are near each other would be activated by the same visual stimuli and discharge together, but ganglion cells located in the opposite eye should discharge asynchronously with these cells. These firing patterns should lead to regional strengthening (and selection) of correlated or synchronized inputs and a weakening (or elimination) of asynchronous inputs, and thus to the segregation of axons into ocular dominance patches in layer IV.

Experience-Dependent Remodeling: Underlying Mechanisms

The prevailing view of how neuronal connections are remodeled during maturation is often summarized by the "correlated activity rule." It simply states that coincident activity in afferents leads to the preferential stabilization of their synaptic connections. In contrast, noncoincidentally activated synapses are eliminated. Based on these ideas, one would predict that developing neurons in some way have the capacity to detect coincident activity and as a consequence modify neuronal connections (Constantine-Paton et al., 1987). Recent studies have identified one such physiologic "detector" of temporally correlated synaptic events—the NMDA receptor.

The role the NMDA receptor plays in synaptic plasticity in the mature CNS, especially in the hippocampal formation, is well established. Long-term potentiation (LTP) in both hippocampus and neocortex have been shown to be selectively blocked by NMDA receptor antagonists, such as APV (2-amino-5-phosphonovalerate; e.g., Wigstrom and Gustafsson, 1985). The voltage dependency of the NMDA receptor produced by Mg^{2+} blockade of the receptor-associated ion channel is thought to play a central role in its ability to detect synchronized activity. EPSPs, elicited by afferents, depolarize the postsynaptic cells, thereby reducing channel blockade. Upon arrival of a second coincident EPSP, a greater depolarization occurs, leading to an increase in Ca^{2+} intracellularly. The rise in intracellular Ca^{2+} triggers a cascade of metabolic events in the postsynaptic cell. Finally, a retrograde messenger is thought to signal the presynaptic terminals which leads to the consolidation of the two activated synaptic terminals (O'Dell et al., 1991; for reviews of LTP see Colley and Routtenberg, 1993; Malenka and Nicoll, 1993; McNaughton, 1993).

A number of laboratories have provided data that suggest that the same mechanisms responsible for LTP may contribute importantly to synapse consolidation during development. For instance, chronic application of NMDA receptor antagonists, such as APV and ketamine, prevent ocular dominance shifts in monocularly deprived kittens (Bear et al., 1990; Kleinschmidt et al., 1987; Rauschecker and Hahn, 1987). Segregation of inputs from "normal" and supernumerary eyes in tadpoles have also been shown to be blocked by APV and enhanced by NMDA itself (Cline et al., 1987). NMDA receptors have been implicated in the formation of binocular maps in the tectum of *Xenopus* (Scherer and Udin, 1989). However, some investigators have raised a cautionary note concerning the role NMDA receptors may play in synapse selection in early life, at least in developing mammals (Goodman and Shatz, 1993; see also Fox and Daw, 1993). One argument that has been raised is that NMDA receptors play an unusually important role in excitatory synaptic transmission in the developing brain. As discussed previously, both neurophysiological recordings and neurochemical studies have suggested that NMDA receptors contribute importantly to EPSPs, especially in developing neocortex. Therefore, APV treatment might block consolidation simply by a general silencing of neocortical electrical activity (e.g., like TTX) and not by specifically blocking NMDA receptor-mediated consolidation processes (Goodman and Shatz, 1993).

Recently several studies have suggested that some neural networks produce endogenous synchronized activity of one form or another and that this activity may play an important role in synapse selection and the fine-tuning of neuronal connectivity. It has been shown that afferents from retina to lateral geniculate nucleus segregate into eye-specific layers before eye opening. In this instance, it would be easy to conclude that segregation of inputs to the geniculate does not follow the rules of activity-dependent remodeling described for neocortical layer IV. However, Meister et al. (1991) recorded from the retina of fetal cats and neonatal ferrets and found that retinal ganglion cells spontaneously discharge in synchronized bursts very early in life. Cells that were near each other fired together; waves of excitation, several hundred micrometers in width, traveled from one side of the retina to the other at approximately 100 μm/s. Since the two eyes discharge independently, the investigators postulated that this spontaneous activity mediated the formation of eye-specific layers in the lateral geniculate in an activity-dependent manner.

In other studies Yuste et al. (1992) described a different form of spontaneous synchronized neuronal activity arising from neuronal networks in the developing neocortex. In their experiments, slices of neocortex were stained with the Ca^{2+}-sensitive indicator fura-2. Large areas of the slices, 50–120 μm in diameter, were shown to spontaneously increase the level of cytoplasmic Ca^{2+}. These so-called neuronal domains spanned several cortical layers and likely consist of networks of neurons coupled through gap junctions, since separate studies have shown extensive dye coupling in fetal and neonatal neocortex (Connors et al., 1983; Peinado et al., 1993). The Ca^{2+} transients were prolonged (e.g., 20 seconds) and were not dependent upon Na^+ action potential generation since they were observed in the presence of

TTX. Thus it is interesting to consider how these large networks of coupled cells influence the course of cortical development. It is possible that such forms of cellular communication permit a temporal coordination of electrical and metabolic activity within local networks. Whether there is an interplay between this type of neuronal communication and use-dependent remodeling of connectivity is unknown.

Experience-Dependent Remodeling: Local Circuits

Only a few studies have been directed at understanding how axons develop within local cortical networks (for review see Katz and Callaway, 1992). Currently, the view is that some intracortical connections are at first exuberant and random in their direction of outgrowth. Later, axon arbors are sculpted by pruning of branches, which leads to a mature pattern of innervation. However, other local axon arbors appear to project to very specific areas, even at the earliest stages of axon outgrowth. In this instance, little or no remodeling of connectivity is thought to take place. Examples of this latter type of growth are some intracortical vertical connections. For example, in early stages of development, as in adults, axons from layer II/III cells arborize only in layer II/III and layer V; they do not send collaterals into layer IV (Katz, 1991). Similarly, spiny stellate cells of layer IV appear to follow a pattern of directed vertical axon growth and show no evidence of collateral remodeling during development (Callaway and Katz, 1992).

On the other hand, patterns of growth of horizontal projections appear to be remodeled with maturation. For instance, in human neonatal brain, horizontal projections within layers IV and V of visual cortex are at first diffuse; only later in life do patchy innervated patterns develop through collateral pruning (Burkhalter et al., 1993). Similar remodeling has been reported for axons which emanate from layer II/III cells in kitten cortex and project to other layer II/III cells with similar visual receptive field properties (Callaway and Katz, 1990). In these instances, the adult pattern of selective connectivity is derived from an initial diffuse one. Figure 8-6 shows results of an experiment in which red and green fluorescent latex microspheres were separately injected into kitten visual cortex. The injection site that was produced was quite small, around 100–400 μm in diameter (unlabeled area in center of figure). Red microspheres were injected on day 15 while green microspheres were injected at the same site on day 29. Retrograde labeling in nearby cells was examined on day 31. Results show a diffuse pattern of labeling of beads injected on day 15 (small dots). Labeling produced by the day 29 injection was more localized, with clusters of distinct groups of cells (large squares). These cells were labeled with both the red and green microspheres. Results suggest that early in life many cells throughout the nearby cortex project to the injection site, but with maturation most of these cells prune axons projecting to this site. The axons that are maintained do not originate from random locations in cortex. The clusters of neurons likely represent cortical columns with similar visual receptive fields, interconnected in mature cortex.

P15,29,31

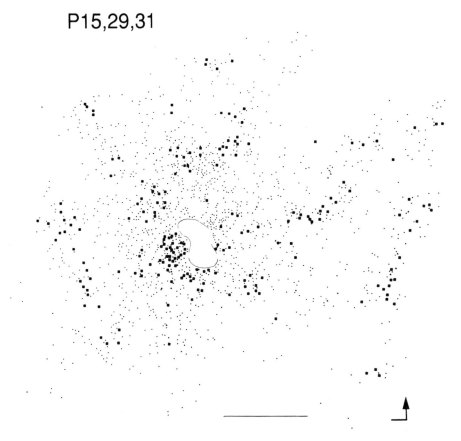

Figure 8-6. Retrograde labeling of cortical neurons following injection of fluorescent latex microspheres. Red microspheres were injected on day 15 while green microspheres were injected at the same site on day 29. This figure depicts labeling observed in superficial cortical layers on day 31. Dots mark the location of cells labeled after the day 15 injection. Large squares mark cells labeled from both injections. Arrowheads point anteriorly, and perpendicular lines extend medially from the base of the arrow. Scale bar, 1 mm. (Reproduced with permission from Callaway and Katz, 1990.)

Both binocular lid closure (Callaway and Katz, 1991) and surgically induced strabismus (Lowel and Singer, 1992) have been reported to disrupt the refinement of these intracortical connections. Thus at least this type of local circuit remodeling appears to be dependent on visual input. Results also suggest that the remodeling is dependent on patterned neuronal activity. In this regard, it would be of some interest to investigate the consequences focal seizure discharges have on such neocortical axon remodeling. Indeed, studies reported more than 10 years ago suggest that in penicillin foci of developing visual cortex the receptive field properties of single units were dramatically altered (Crabtree et al., 1981). Unfortunately, possible anatomical substrates for these changes have never been explored.

Experience-Dependent Remodeling of Circuitry and Early-Onset Epilepsy

Based on the currently held view of how neural activity contributes to refining connectivity during brain maturation it is conceivable that abnormal patterns of neural activity in early life may lead to abnormalities in network remodeling that could enhance seizure susceptibility and even lead to chronic epileptic conditions (see also Swann Smith, Brady, et al. 1993). Although this area of investigation is still in its infancy, recent results from several animal models suggest that this might be the case. One such model involves audiogenic seizures produced by auditory deprivation in early postnatal life.

Audiogenic Seizures

Since 1967 it has been known that auditory deprivation during a critical period of development can induce audiogenic susceptibility in seizure-resistant mouse strains. This deprivation can be induced by ear-plugging (Chen et al., 1973; McGinn et al., 1973) or the administration of low doses of cochleotoxic drugs such as kanamycin (Chen and Aberdeen, 1981; Norris et al., 1977; Pierson and Swann, 1988; Tepper and Schlesinger, 1980), or it may simply involve a single exposure to intense high-frequency sound (Henry, 1967; Iturrian and Fink, 1969; Pierson and Swann, 1991). In Wistar rats intense noise exposure induces chronic audiogenic seizure susceptibility if the noise is administered between postnatal days 14 and 32, with days 15–18 being the most sensitive development period (Pierson and Swann, 1991). Auditory deprivation during this critical period, a time when projections from the cochlea to the central auditory pathway are forming, appears to be the necessary condition for this experience-induced audiogenic seizure susceptibility.

Studies of c-fos-like immunoreactivity induced in inferior colliculus by pure-tone auditory stimuli suggest that the segregation of ascending auditory afferent fibers that normally takes place in postnatal life is disrupted by experimentally induced auditory deprivation. This abnormal maturation of connectivity appears to play a pivotal role in sound-triggered seizures. Pierson and Snyder-Keller (1994) recently reported that when adult rats are exposed to pure-tone stimuli, varying in frequency from 5,000 to 50,000 Hz, the inferior colliculus demonstrates c-fos immunopositivity that is arranged in discrete bands that traverse the central nucleus and dorsal cortex of this midbrain structure. In immature rats, 12 days of age, high-frequency pure tones do not produce discrete bands but instead generate diffuse immunoreactive patterns. The authors suggested that this developmental difference likely reflects exuberant projections of ascending fibers, some of which are eliminated as auditory pathways become tonotopically arranged. Adult rats that had been exposed to an intense noise on day 14, and were thus susceptible to audiogenic seizures, were found to have a diffuse pattern of fos immunoreactivity very similar to that observed in 12-day-old rat pups (Fig. 8-7). The segregation of afferents into tonotopic bands, which occurs in the inferior colliculus during postnatal life, is reminiscent of the formation of ocular dominance patches in visual pathways. As in the visual system, auditory deprivation appears to disrupt the segregation of innervating fibers, leaving an immature pattern of innervation in adulthood. This aberrant pattern of innervation likely plays a role in sound-triggered seizures in these animals.

Hippocampus

In a recent in vitro slice study of local recurrent axon collaterals emanating from single CA_3 hippocampal pyramidal cells, Swann and Gomez-DiCesare (1994) labeled neurons with biocytin day 4-5, day 10-15, and day 45-70. Axon arbors of single neurons were reconstructed by computer-assisted camera lucida drawings. The length of axon arbors and their branching patterns were quantified and the distribution of axon fiber swellings (or varicosities) was examined. Previous ultrastructural studies showed that each of these varicosities is a site of local circuit synaptic contact (Deitch et al., 1991).

The results show that on day 5 very few axon collaterals emanate from individual pyramidal cells. However, by day 10 an exuberant outgrowth of axons from pyramidal cells takes place. In contrast, axon collaterals from the adult CA_3 pyramidal cell are less dense and appear to be reduced in complexity compared to the cell observed on day 10.

When axons at each of these ages are viewed at high magnification, fiber swellings or varicosities are seen along the length of the axon arbor. The density of varicosities on the axon are similar at the two older ages. In younger rats, varicosity density is significantly lower, only half that observed later in life. Figure 8-8 summarizes data obtained from nine reconstructions. To promote direct comparisons axons were analyzed in a defined but geographically limited area of the CA_3 subfield in the slices. This area, measuring 600 μm along the cell body layer, was centered on the soma of the reconstructed neuron and included both apical and basilar dendritic layers. By analyzing axons within the same volume of tissue comparison of age-dependent changes in the density of local axon arbors was possible. Results support the notion that there is an exuberant outgrowth of axons between day 5 and 10 and that there is a dramatic decrease in the density of axon arbors with maturation. Three parameters of axon morphology were compared: axon length, varicosity number, and number of axon branch points. In axons from the first postnatal week, measures of all three parameters were between 15 and 35 percent of adult values. However, during the second postnatal week they increased dramatically and were 175–225 percent of their mature counterparts.

These results show clearly that there is a large increase in density of local recurrent collaterals and varicosities in area CA_3 during the second postnatal week. This overshoot is reminiscent of results from many other studies which have reported exuberant outgrowth of axons and overshoots in measurements of synaptic density. An increased synaptic density could play a

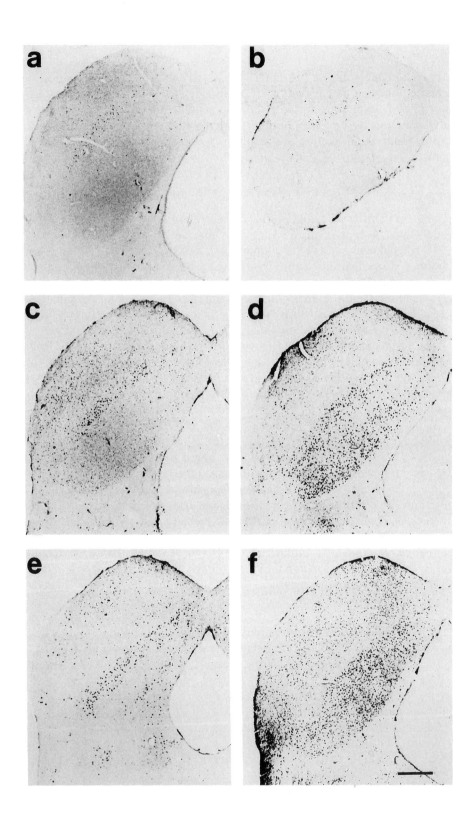

role in enhanced seizure susceptibility in early life. For instance, it has been reported by several laboratories that in immature hippocampus and neocortex epileptic discharges are accompanied by extremely large changes in extracellular K^+ (see Hablitz and Heinemann, 1987; Swann et al., 1986; Moshé, Shinnar, and Swann, Chapter 2). Since potassium is released from neurons in response to activation of excitatory amino acid receptors, these large changes in extracellular K^+ might be explained, at least in part, by a greater density of excitatory synapses.

These measurements of axon and varicosity density indicate that an excess in recurrent excitatory synapses exists during the critical period of enhanced seizure susceptibility. However, between birth and adulthood the hippocampus becomes considerably larger in volume. Since hippocampal pyramidal cells are born prenatally, and since there is no evidence of CA_3 pyramidal cell death during the postnatal period, the number of CA_3 pyramidal neurons likely remains unchanged between birth and adulthood. Thus as the hippocampus grows and expands in volume, the density of neurons should decrease significantly with age. If an overabundance of recurrent excitatory contacts was actually to exist, then, on average, the number of synaptic contacts made per neuron in the local network should be greater early in life. However, if age-dependent alterations in neuron density are comparable to alterations in the varicosity density, then the network of CA_3 neurons might actually be comparable at the two different ages. That is, it is conceivable that the differences between 10- to 14-day-old rats and 52-day old rats shown in Figure 8-8 do not show that there is an excess in network connectivity early in life but rather reflect only a difference in neuronal density. To address this concern, the density of neurons in the CA_3 cell body layer were estimated at each age of interest. Between days 11 and 60 there was a 33 percent decrease in neuronal density. Based on these results the data were reanalyzed so differences in neuronal densities could be taken into account. Segments of different sizes of the CA_3 subfield were analyzed and the sizes of the areas analyzed were adjusted to contain the same number of CA_3 neurons. Results of this analysis showed that there is a dramatic 50 percent decrease in the number of axon branch points between the second postnatal week and adulthood; however, there is little or no difference in axon length or varicosity number per cell. Thus these latter results do not lend support to the idea that an excess in recurrent collateral connectivity

---

Figure 8-7. Unusually broad bands of *fos* immunoactivity are induced by high-frequency pure tones in inferior colliculi of (ICs) of audiogenic seizure–prone rats compared to normal rats. Panels a, c, and e (left column): responses in ICs of untreated rats to pure tones 7,500 Hz, 15,000 Hz, and 30,000 Hz, respectively. Panels b, d, and f (right column): corresponding frequency responses in ICs of rats which were noise-exposed on day 14 and consequently were audiogenic seizure–prone. Ages of rats (in days) were as follows: (a) 28, (b) 28, (c) 36, (d) 36, (e) 24, (f) 28. (Reproduced with permission from Pierson and Snyder-Keller, 1994.)

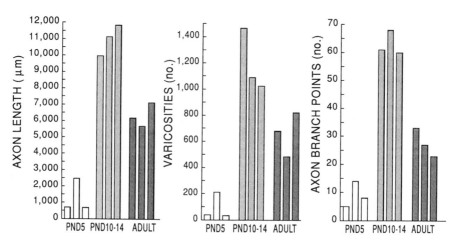

Figure 8-8. Age-dependent alterations in the density of three different measures of recurrent excitatory axon collaterals in the hippocampal CA₃ subfield. Analyses were performed on sectors of the CA₃ subfield centered on the cell body of biocytin-labeled neurons. Sections were 600 μm as measured along stratum pyramidale. Bar graphs show developmental changes in the length of axons, number of axon branch points, and number of varicosities or axon swellings (which were used to estimate the number of potential synapses) within sectors. Axons from three pyramidal cells were examined at each age. Results show that these measures of local recurrent collaterals increased dramatically between postnatal week 1 and 2 and then decreased to intermediate values in adulthood.

exists early in life. Instead there appears to be a nearly equal complement of synaptic contacts per cell on day 10–14 and in adulthood.

These results have led to an alternative explanation of how network excitability may arise on postnatal days 10–14. This explanation is based on the dramatic decrease in axon *branching* that takes place between days 10–14 and adulthood. There appears to be a major decrease in axon arbor complexity with maturation. But why should such a major loss in axon branches not be accompanied by a complementary decrease in axon length and varicosity number? This apparent discrepancy is explained by the fact that a network of mature hippocampal neurons occupies a considerably larger volume than a network of the same number of immature neurons. That is, as the hippocampus expands in volume and neurons grow and move away from each other, axons from any given neuron will have to lengthen in order to remain in synaptic contact with the cells it contacted earlier in life. Thus during maturation, long but simple axon arbors replace short, complex arbors of immature hippocampus. These results of age-dependent remodeling of hippocampal recurrent collaterals are consistent with comparable findings in other areas of the CNS.

Synthesis and Speculation

In summary, our results suggest that age-dependent recurrent collateral and excitatory synapse remodeling takes place. Many early-formed recurrent collaterals and excitatory synapses appear to be eliminated as the hippocampus matures only to be replaced by a different complement of synapses in adulthood. Concurrent with this remodeling, hippocampal seizure susceptibility decreases. Early-life seizure susceptibility does not appear to be produced by an excess in recurrent excitatory contacts per cell. Instead, it seems possible that age-dependent differences in the biophysical properties of early-formed synapses (such as those reviewed earlier in this chapter) contribute to seizure generation in the developing hippocampus.

These recent anatomical findings suggest that CA_3 recurrent excitatory axon collaterals are remodeled in early postnatal life. Earlier in this chapter results showing that excitation spreads very easily through networks of immature hippocampal neurons were discussed. Thus it seems plausible that early-formed synaptic contacts may result in EPSPs which more easily evoke action potentials in postsynaptic cells and thus promote the spread of excitation through immature neuronal networks.

As reviewed in this chapter, a substantial number of studies have shown that cortical and hippocampal networks have a pronounced capacity to generate electrographic seizures during a critical period in postnatal life. Local recurrent excitatory networks using an excitatory amino acid neurotransmitter appear to play a critical role in these seizures. Anatomical studies suggest that local circuits in neocortex and hippocampus remodel during postnatal life and substantial numbers of axon collaterals are lost only to be replaced by a new set of connections as the brain matures. At least in neocortex this remodeling has been shown to be dependent on neuronal activity.

In some instances synchronized discharging of neuronal populations has been demonstrated to alter or prevent axon remodeling. Thus one must wonder if the synchronized discharging that underlies seizures in developing cortical networks might alter the remodeling of axon arbors that normally takes place within these networks. The maintenance of diffuse patterns of early-life connections could conceivably contribute to the formation of epileptogenic circuits and possibly the development of chronic and intractable seizure disorders.

To examine this possibility, new animal models are needed in which focal neocortical or hippocampal seizures are experimentally induced during a critical period of pronounced seizure susceptibility. Seizures should occur frequently throughout the critical period when network remodeling is thought to take place. If a pharmacologic agent is used to induce seizures, its effects should persist for 5 to 10 days. But thereafter its efficacy should be greatly reduced or eliminated so that the consequences of the seizures can be assessed in the absence of the convulsant agent. Only with the availability of such models will we be able to determine if seizures alter network remodeling that takes place in early life and whether these alterations contribute in any way to the persistence of epileptiform activity in adulthood.

Conclusion

During periods in early postnatal life, local circuits in hippocampus and neocortex demonstrate an unusual propensity to produce electrographic seizures. In some instances the late appearance of functional inhibitory synapses may contribute to seizure generation. However, often during neonatal life, when synaptic inhibition is poorly developed, synaptic excitation appears to be equally immature. At this time epileptic discharging is usually absent or largely asynchronous in nature. However, in rodents, the second postnatal week marks a time of major transition in seizure susceptibility. Large prolonged ictallike discharges are produced in both hippocampus and neocortex. Recurrent IPSPs are easily elicited at this time and the application of $GABA_A$ receptor antagonists produces 30- to 60-second synchronized discharges. In adults, the same treatment results in only brief (100 msec) interictal events. Results from numerous laboratories have shown that the epileptiform discharges in both immature and mature cortical circuits are blocked by excitatory amino acid receptor antagonists. Thus attention has turned to a study of the ontogeny of recurrent excitatory networks in brain.

In general, there are two major phases in the formation of synaptic connections in the central nervous system. The first phase is pathway and target selection. During this time, axons grow long distances over what appear to be preordained pathways. Local molecular cues as well as gradients of chemotaxic agents appear to guide axons and their leading growth cones to their target. At these sites, an early complement of anatomically dispersed axon arbors and synapses is usually formed. As the brain matures, the second phase of network formation takes place. The early plexus of dispersed axons and synapses is remodeled. Many of the wide-ranging branches are pruned, remaining axons grow within a more restricted field, and an adult complement of more highly targeted synaptic connections gradually evolves.

It is perhaps not surprising that during both phases of synaptogenesis molecular markers for excitatory and inhibitory synapses undergo dramatic changes. Reported changes in neurochemical markers and pharmacologic sensitivity of amino acid neurotransmitter receptors will likely be explained by complementary changes in the expression of newly identified molecular subunits for these receptors. These changes appear to be reflected in dramatic age-dependent alterations in the physiology of synapses in both hippocampus and neocortex. For instance, in early life EPSPs are unusually prolonged and NMDA receptors make a large contribution to EPSP amplitude and time course. So-called neonatal forms of these receptors appear to have unusual biophysical properties that are different from their adult counterparts.

The remodeling of neuronal connections that takes place in postnatal life is largely dependent on patterned neuronal activity, not only for long afferent projections (e.g., to visual cortex) but also for some local circuit connections. When discharging of neurons is synchronized by artificial means the neuronal remodeling of axons fails to occur. Recent studies in hippocampus demonstrate that remodeling of recurrent excitatory collaterals parallels changes in seizure susceptibility. One challenge for the future is to determine whether synchronized discharging that occurs during seizures prevents the remodeling of connections that normally takes place within hippocampal and neocortical local circuits. It seems plausible that such alterations in the normal course of neural network maturation could result in hyperexcitable neural networks and the establishment of an epileptic focus that could underlie chronic and intractable forms of epilepsy throughout life.

Acknowledgments

I would like to thank Dr. Martha Pierson, Dr. Robert Brady, Karen Smith, Dr. Caroline Gomez-Di Cesare, and Dr. Chong Lee for their thoughtful discussions and contributions to ideas presented in this chapter. The work of my laboratory was supported by NIH grant NS-18309.

References

Alger, B. E., and Nicoll, R. A. (1982a) Feed-forward dendritic inhibition in rat hippocampal pyramidal cells studied *in vitro. J. Physiol. 328:*105–123.

Alger, B. E., and Nicoll, R. A. (1982b) Pharmacological evidence for two kinds of GABA receptor on rat hippocampal pyramidal cells studies *in vitro. J. Physiol. 328:*125–141.

Amaral, D. G., and Kurz, J. (1985) The time of origin of cells demonstrating glutamic acid decarboxylase-like immunoreactivity in the hippocampal formation of the rat. *Neurosci. Lett. 59:*33–39.

Angelotti, T. P., and Macdonald, R. L. (1993) Assembly of $GABA_A$ receptor subunits: $\alpha_1\beta_1$ and $\alpha_1\beta_{12S}$ subunits produce unique ion channels with dissimilar single-channel properties. *J. Neurosci. 13:*1429–1440.

Balice-Gordon, R. J., and Lichtman, J. W. (1993) *In vivo* observations of pre- and postsynaptic changes during the transition from multiple to single innervation at developing neuromuscular junctions. *J. Neurosci. 13:*834–855.

Bear, M. F., Kleinschmidt, A., Gu, Q., and Singer, W. (1990) Disruption of experience-dependent synaptic modifications in striate cortex by infusion of an NMDA receptor antagonist. *J. Neurosci. 10:*909–925.

Ben-Ari, Y., Cherubini, E., and Krnjevic, K. (1988) Changes in voltage dependence of NMDA currents during development. *Neurosci. Lett. 94:*88–92.

Bergmann, I., Nitsch, R., and Frotscher, M. (1991) Area-specific morphological and neurochemical maturation of non-pyramidal neurons in the rat hippocampus as revealed by parvalbumin immunocytochemistry. *Anat. Embryol. (Berlin) 184:*403–409.

Blanton, M. G., Lo Turco, J. J., and Kriegstein, A. R. (1990) Endogenous neurotransmitter activates N-methyl-D-aspartate receptors on differentiating neurons in embryonic cortex. *Proc. Natl. Acad. Sci. 87:*8027–8030.

Bovolin, P., Santi, M.-R., Memo, M., Costa, E., and Grayson, D. R. (1992) Distinct developmental patterns of expression of rat α_1, α_5, γ_{2S}, and gamma$_{2L}$ gamma-aminobutyric acid$_A$ receptor subunit mRNAs *in vivo* and *in vitro*. *J. Neurochem. 59:*62–72.

Bowe, M. A., and Nadler, J. V. (1990) Developmental increase in the sensitivity to magnesium of NMDA receptors on CA$_1$ hippocampal pyramidal cells. *Dev. Brain Res. 56:*55–61.

Brady, R. J., Smith, K. L., and Swann, J. W. (1991) Calcium modulation of the NMDA response and electrographic seizures in immature hippocampus. *Neurosci. Lett. 124:*92–96.

Brady, R. J., and Swann, J. W. (1984) Postsynaptic actions of baclofen associated with its antagonism of bicuculline-induced epileptogenesis in hippocampus. *Cell. Mol. Neurobiol. 4:*403–408.

Brady, R. J., and Swann, J. W. (1986) Ketamine selectively suppresses synchronized afterdischarges in immature hippocampus. *Neurosci. Lett. 69:*143–149.

Brady, R. J., and Swann, J. W. (1988) Suppression of ictal-like activity by kynurenic acid does not correlate with its efficacy as an NMDA receptor antagonist. *Epilepsy Res. 2:*232–238.

Burgard, E. C., and Hablitz, J. J. (1993) Developmental changes in NMDA and non-NMDA receptor-mediated synaptic potentials in rat neocortex. *J. Neurophysiol. 69:*230–240.

Burkhalter, A., Bernado, K. L., and Charles, V. (1993) Development of local circuits in human visual cortex. *J. Neurosci. 13:*1916–1931.

Callaway, E. M., and Katz, L. C. (1990) Emergence and refinement of clustered horizontal connections in cat striate cortex. *J. Neurosci. 10:*1134–1153.

Callaway, E. M., and Katz, L. C. (1991) Effects of binocular deprivation on the development of clustered horizontal connections in cat striate cortex. *Proc. Natl. Acad. Sci. 88:*745–749.

Callaway, E. M., and Katz, L. C. (1992) Development of axonal arbors of layer 4 spiny neurons in cat striate cortex. *J. Neurosci. 12:*570–582.

Carmignoto, G., and Vicini, S. (1992) Activity-dependent decrease in NMDA receptor responses during development of the visual cortex. *Science 258:*1007–1011.

Chen, C. S., and Aberdeen, G. C. (1981) The sensitive period for induction of susceptibility to audiogenic seizures by kanamycin in mice. *Arch. Otorhinolaryngol. 232:*215–220.

Chen, C. S., Gates, G. R., and Bock, G. R. (1973) Effect of priming and tympanic membrane destruction on development of GAS susceptibility in BALB/c mice. *Exp. Neurol. 39:*277–284.

Cherubini, E., Ben-Ari, Y., Ito, S., and Krnjevic, K. (1991) Persistent pulsatile release of glutamate induced by N-methyl-D-aspartate in neonatal rat hippocampal neurones. *J. Physiol. (London) 436:*531–547.

Cherubini, E., Gaiarsa, J. L., and Ben-Ari, Y. (1991) GABA: An excitatory transmitter in early postnatal life. *Trends Neurosci. 14:*515–519.

Chisholm, J., Kellogg, C., and Lippa, A. (1983) Development of benzodiazepine binding subtypes in three regions of rat brain. *Brain Res. 267:*388–391.

Cline, H. T., Debski, E. A., and Constantine-Paton, M. (1987) N-methyl-D-aspartate receptor antagonist desegregates eye-specific stripes. *Proc. Natl. Acad. Sci. 84:*4342–4345.

Colley, P. A., and Routtenberg, A. (1993) Long-term potentiation as synaptic dialogue. *Brain Res. Rev. 18:*115–122.

Colman, H., and Lichtman, J. W. (1993) Interactions between nerve and muscle: Synapse elimination at the developing neuromuscular junction. *Dev. Biol. 156:*1–10.

Connors, B. W. (1984) Initiation of synchronized neuronal bursting in neocortex. *Nature 310:*685–687.

Connors, B. W., Benardo, L. S., and Prince, D. A. (1983) Coupling between neurons of the developing rat neocortex. *J. Neurosci. 3:*773–782.

Connors, B. W., Malenka, R. C., and Silva, L. R. (1988) Two inhibitory postsynaptic potentials, and GABA$_A$ and GABA$_B$ receptor-mediated responses in neocortex of rat and cat. *J. Physiol. 406:*443–468.

Constantine-Paton, M., Cline, H. T., and Debski, E. (1990) Patterned activity, synaptic convergence, and the NMDA receptor in developing visual pathways. *Ann. Rev. Neurosci. 13:*129–154.

Coyle, J. T., and Enna, S. J. (1976) Neurochemical aspects of the ontogenesis of GABAergic neurons in the rat brain. *Brain Res. 111:*119–133.

Crabtree, J. W., Chow, K. L., Ostrach, L. H., and Baumbach, H. D. (1981) Development of receptive field properties in the visual cortex of rabbits subjected to early epileptiform cortical discharges. *Dev. Brain Res. 1:*269–281.

Dan, Y., and Poo, M.-M. (1992) Hebbian depression of isolated neuromuscular synapses *in vitro*. *Science 256:*1570–1573.

Deitch, J. S., Smith, K. L., Swann, J. W., and Turner, J. N. (1991) Ultrastructural investigation of neurons identified and localized using the confocal scanning laser microscope. *J. Electron Microsc. Tech. 18:*82–90.

Dunwiddie, T. V. (1981) Age-related differences in the *in vitro* rat hippocampus: Development of inhibition and the effects of hypoxia. *Dev. Neurosci. 4:*165–175.

Evers, J., Laser, M., Sun, Y.-A., Xie, Z.-P., and Poo, M.-M. (1989) Studies of nerve–muscle interactions in *Xenopus* cell culture: Analysis of early synaptic currents. *J. Neurosci. 9:*1523–1539.

Fox, K., and Daw, N. W. (1993) Do NMDA receptors have a critical function in visual cortical plasticity? *Trends Neurosci. 16:*116–122.

Furshpan, E. J., and Potter, D. D. (1989) Seizure-like activity and cellular damage in rat hippocampal neurons in cell culture. *Neuron 3:*199–207.

Goodman, C. S., and Shatz, C. J. (1993) Developmental mechanisms that generate precise patterns of neuronal activity. *Cell 10:*77–98.

Goodman, C. S., and Spitzer, N. C. (1979) Embryonic development of identified neurones: Differentiation from neuroblast to neurone. *Nature 280:*208–214.

Goodman, C. S., and Spitzer, N. C. (1981) The development of electrical properties of identified neurons in grasshopper embryos. *J. Physiol. 313:*385–413.

Grover, L. M., Lambert, N. A., Schwartzkroin, P. A., and Teyler, T. J. (1993) Role of HCO$_3^-$ ions in depolarizing GABA$_A$ receptor-mediated responses in pyramidal cells of rat hippocampus. *J. Neurophysiol. 69:*1541–1555.

Hablitz, J. J. (1987) Spontaneous ictal-like discharges and sustained depolarization shifts in the developing rat neocortex. *Neurophysiol. 58:*1052–1065.

Hablitz, J. J., and Heinemann, U. (1987) Extracellular K$^+$ and Ca^{2+} changes during epileptiform discharges in the immature rat neocortex. *Dev. Brain Res. 36:*299–303.

Harish, O. E., and Poo, M. (1992) Retrograde modulation at developing neuromuscular synapses: Involvement of G protein and arachidonic acid cascade. *Neuron 9:*1201–1209.

Harris, K. M., and Teyler, T. J. (1983) Evidence for late development of inhibition in area CA₁ of the rat hippocampus. *Brain Res. 268:*339–343.

Haydon, P. G., and Zoran, M. J. (1989) Formation and modulation of chemical connections: Evoked acetylcholine release from growth cones and neurites of specific identified neurons. *Neuron 2:*1483–1490.

Henry, K. R. (1967) Audiogenic seizure susceptibility induced in C57B1/6J mice by prior auditory exposure. *Science 158:*938–940.

Hestrin, S. (1992) Developmental regulation of NMDA receptor-mediated synaptic currents at a central synapse. *Nature 357:*686–689.

Hollmann, M., Boulter, J., Maron, C., Beasley, L., Sullivan, J., Pecht, G., and Heinemann, S. (1993) Zinc potentiates agonist-induced currents at certain splice variants of the NMDA receptor. *Neuron 10:*943–954.

Hubel, D. H., and Wiesel, T. N. (1970) The period of susceptibility to the physiological effects of unilateral eye closure in kittens. *J. Physiol. 206:*419–436.

Ishizuka, N., Weber, J., and Amaral, D. G. (1990) Organization of intrahippocampal projections originating from CA₃ pyramidal cells in the rats. *J. Comp. Neurol. 295:*580–623.

Iturrian, W. B., and Fink, G. B. (1969) Influence of age and brief auditory conditioning upon experimental seizures in mice. *Dev. Psychobiol. 2:*10–18.

Janigro, D., and Schwartzkroin, P. A. (1988a) Effects of GABA and CA₃ pyramidal cell dendrites in rabbit hippocampal slices. *Brain Res. 453:*265–274.

Janigro, D., and Schwartzkroin, P. A. (1988b) Effects of GABA and baclofen on pyramidal cells in the developing rabbit hippocampus: An "in vitro" study. *Dev. Brain Res. 41:*171–184.

Katz, L. C. (1991) Specificity in the development of vertical connections in cat striate cortex. *J. Neurosci. 3:*1–9.

Katz, L. C., and Callaway, E. M. (1992) Development of local circuits in mammalian visual cortex. *Ann. Rev. Neurosci. 15:*31–56.

Kleckner, N. W., and Dingledine, R. (1991) Regulation of hippocampal NMDA receptors by magnesium and glycine during development. *Mol. Brain Res. 11:*151–159.

Kleinschmidt, A., Bears, M. F., and Singer, W. (1987) Blockade of "NMDA" receptors disrupts experience-dependent plasticity of kitten striate cortex. *Science 238:*355–358.

Kriegstein, A. R., Suppes, T., and Prince, D. A. (1987) Cellular and synaptic physiology and epileptogenesis of developing rat neocortical neurons *in vitro*. *Dev. Brain Res. 34:*161–171.

Kunkel, D. D., Hendrickson, A. E., Wu, J.-Y., and Schwartzkroin, P. A. (1986) Glutamic acid decarboxylase (GAD) immunocytochemistry of developing rabbit hippocampus. *J. Neurosci. 6:*541–552.

LaMantia, A.-S., and Rakic, P. (1990) Axon overproduction and elimination in the corpus callosum of the developing Rhesus monkey. *J. Neurosci. 10:*2156–2175.

Lang, U., and Frotscher, M. (1990) Postnatal development of nonpyramidal neurons in the rat hippocampus (areas CA₁ and CA₃): A combined Golgi/electron microscope study. *Anat. Embryol. 181:*533–545.

Laurie, D. J., Wisden, W., and Seeburg, P. H. (1992) The distribution of thirteen GABA_A receptor subunit mRNAs in the rat brain: III. Embryonic and postnatal development. *J. Neurosci. 12:*4151–4172.

Lee, C. L., Hrachovy, R. A., Smith, K. L., Frost, J. D. J., and Swann, J. W. (1993) Seizures produced in neonatal rats by stereotaxis injections of tetanus toxin

(TT): *In vivo* and *in vitro* models of seizures in early infancy. *Neurosci. Abstr.* *19:*1870.

Lee, W.-L., and Hablitz, J. J. (1991) Excitatory synaptic involvement in epileptiform bursting in the immature rat neocortex. *J. Neurophysiol. 66:*1894–1901.

LeVay, S., Stryker, M. P., and Shatz, C. J. (1978) Ocular dominance columns and their development in layer IV of the cat's visual cortex. *J. Comp. Neurol. 179:*223–244.

LeVay, S., Wiesel, T. N., and Hubel, D. H. (1980) The development of ocular dominance columns in normal and visually deprived monkeys. *J. Comp. Neurol. 191:*1–51.

Lo, Y.-J., and Poo, M. (1991) Activity-dependent synaptic competition in vitro: Heterosynaptic suppression of developing synapses. *Science 254:*1019–1022.

Lo Turco, J. J., Blanton, M. G., and Kriegstein, A. R. (1991) Initial expression and endogenous activation of NMDA channels in early neocortical development. *J. Neurosci. 11:*792–799.

Lomeli, H., Sprengel, R., Laurie, D. J., Köhr, G., Herb, A., Seeburg, P. H., and Wisden, W. (1993) The rat delta-1 and delta-2 subunits extend the excitatory amino acid receptor family. *FEBS Lett. 315:*318–322.

Lowel, S. and Singer, W. (1992) Selection of intrinsic horizontal connections in the visual cortex by correlated neuronal activity. *Science 255:*209–212.

Luhmann, H. J., and Prince, D. A. (1990) Control of NMDA receptor-mediated activity by GABAergic mechanisms in mature and developing rat neocortex. *Dev. Brain. Res. 54:*287–290.

Luhmann, H. J., and Prince, D. A. (1991) Postnatal maturation of the GABAergic system in rat neocortex. *J. Neurophysiol. 65:*247–263.

MacLennan, A. J., Brecha, N., Khrestchatisky, M., Sternini, C., Tillakaratne, N. J. K., Chiang, M.-Y., Anderson, K., Lai, M., and Tobin, A. J. (1991) Independent cellular and ontogenetic expression of mRNAs encoding three α polypeptides of the rat $GABA_A$ receptor. *Neuroscience 43:*369–380.

Malenka, R. C., and Nicoll, R. A. (1993) NMDA-receptor-dependent synaptic plasticity: Multiple forms and mechanisms. *TINS 16:*521–527.

McBain, C., and Dingledine, R. (1992) Dual-component miniature excitatory synaptic currents in rat hippocampal CA_3 pyramidal neurons. *J. Neurophysiol. 68:*16–27.

McDonald, J. W., and Johnston, M. V. (1990) Physiological and pathophysiological roles of excitatory amino acids during central nervous system development. *Brain Res. Rev. 15:*41–70.

McGinn, M. D., Willot, J. F., and Henry, K. R. (1973) Effects of conductive hearing loss on auditory evoked potentials and audiogenic seizures in mice. *Nature 244:*255–256.

McNaughton, B. L. (1993) The mechanism of expression of long-term enhancement of hippocampal synapses: Current issues and theoretical implications. *Annu. Rev. Physiol. 55:*375–396.

Meister, M., Wong, R. O. L., Baylor, D. A., and Shatz, C. J. (1991) Synchronous bursts of action potentials in ganglion cells of the developing hippocampus mammalian retina. *Science 252:*939–943.

Michelson, H. B., and Wong, R. K. S. (1991) Excitatory synaptic reponses mediated by $GABA_A$ receptors in the hippocampus. *Science 253:*1420–1423.

Miles, R. (1990) Synaptic excitation of inhibitory cells by single CA_3 hippocampal pyramidal cells of the guinea-pig *in vitro*. *J. Physiol. (London) 428:* 61–77.

Miles, R., and Wong, R. K. S. (1983) Single neurons can initiate synchronized population discharge in the hippocampus. *Nature 306:*371–373.

Miles, R., and Wong, R. K. S. (1984) Unitary inhibitory synaptic potentials in the guinea-pig hippocampus *in vitro. J. Physiol. (London) 356:*97–113.

Miles, R., and Wong, R. K. S. (1986) Excitatory synaptic interactions between CA3 neurones in the guinea-pig hippocampus. *J. Physiol. (London) 373:*397–418.

Miles, R., and Wong, R. K. S. (1987) Inhibitory control of local excitatory circuits in the guinea-pig hippocampus. *J. Physiol. (London) 388:*611–629.

Misgeld, U., Deisz, R. A., Dodt, H. U., and Lux, H. D. (1986) The role of chloride transport in postsynaptic inhibition of hippocampal neurons. *Science 232:*1413–1415.

Monyer, H., Seeburg, P. H., and Wisden, W. (1991) Glutamate-operated channels: Developmentally early and mature forms arise by alternative splicing. *Neuron 6:*799–810.

Mueller, A. L., Chesnut, R. M., and Schwartzkroin, P. A. (1983) Actions of GABA in developing rabbit hippocampus: An in vitro study. *Neurosci. Lett. 39:*193–195.

Nelson, S. B., and Sur, M. (1992) NMDA receptors in sensory information processing. *Curr. Opin. Neurobiol. 2:*484–488.

Newberry, N. R., and Nicoll, R. A. (1985) Comparison of the action of baclofen with gamma-aminobutyric acid on rat hippocampal pyramidal cells *in vitro. J. Physiol. 360:*161–185.

Norris, C. H., Cawthorn, T. H., and Carroll, R. C. (1977) Kanamycin priming for audiogenic seizures in mice. *Neuropharmacology 16:*375–380.

O'Dell, T. J., Hawkins, R. D., Kandel, E. R., and Arancio, O. (1991) Tests of the roles of two diffusible substances in long-term potentiation: Evidence for nitric oxide as a possible early retrograde messenger. *Proc. Natl. Acad. Sci. 88:*11285–11289.

O'Leary, D. D. M., Heffner, C. D., Kutka, L., Lopez-Mascaraque, L., Missias, A., and Reinoso, B. S. (1991) A target-derived chemoattractant controls the development of the corticopontine projection by a novel mechanism of axon targeting. *Development 2* (Suppl.):123–130.

O'Leary, D. D. M., and Koester, S. E. (1993) Development of projection neuron types, axon pathways, and patterned connections of the mammalian cortex. *Neuron 10:*991–1006.

Peinado, A., Yuste, R., and Katz, L. C. (1993) Extensive dye coupling between rat neocortical neurons during the period of circuit formation. *Neuron 10:*103–114.

Pellegrini-Giampietro, D. E., Bennett, M. V. L., and Zukin, R. S. (1991) Differential expression of three glutamate receptor genes in developing rat brain: An in situ hybridization study. *Proc. Natl. Acad. Sci. 88:*4157–4161.

Persohn, E., Malherbe, P., and Richards, J. G. (1992) Comparative molecular neuroanatomy of cloned GABA$_A$ receptor subunits in the rat CNS. *J. Comp. Neurol. 326:*193–216.

Pierson, M., and Snyder-Keller, A. (1994) Development of frequency-selective domains in inferior colliculus of normal and neonatally noise-exposed rats. *Brain Res. 636:*55–67.

Pierson, M. G., and Swann, J. W. (1988) The sensitive period and optimum dosage for induction of audiogenic seizure susceptibility by kanamycin in the Wistar rat. *Hear. Res. 32:*1–10.

Pierson, M. G., and Swann, J. W. (1991) Ontogenetic features of audiogenic seizure susceptibility induced in immature rats by noise. *Epilepsia 32*:1–9.

Pritchett, D. B., Luddens, H., and Seeburg, P. H. (1989) Type I and type II GABA_A–benzodiazepine receptors produced in transfected cells. *Science 245*:1389–1392.

Pritchett, D. B., Sontheimer, H., Shivers, B. D., Ymer, S., Kettenmann, H., Schofield, P. R., and Seeburg, P. H. (1989) Importance of a novel GABA_A receptor subunit for benzodiazepine pharmacology. *Nature 338*:582–585.

Purpura, D. P. (1969) Stability and seizure susceptibility of immature brain. In H. H. Jaspar, A. A. Ward, and A. Pope (eds.), *Basic Mechanisms of the Epilepsies*. Boston: Little, Brown, pp. 481–505.

Purpura, D. P., Prelevic, S., and Santini, M. (1968) Postsynaptic potentials and spike variations in the feline hippocampus during postnatal ontogenesis. *Exp. Neurol. 22*:408–422.

Purpura, D. P., Shofer, R. J., and Scarff, T. (1965) Properties of synaptic activities and spike potentials of neurons in immature neocortex. *J. Neurophysiol. 28*:925–942.

Rauschecker, J., and Hahn, S. (1987) Ketamine-xylazine anaesthesia blocks consolidation of ocular dominance changes in kitten visual cortex. *Nature 326*:183–185.

Reichelt, R., Hofmann, D., Fodisch, H.-J., Mohler, H., Knapp, M., and Hebebrand, J. (1991) Ontogeny of the benzodiazepine receptor in human brain: Fluorographic, immunochemical and reversible binding studies. *J. Neurochem. 57*:1128–1135.

Sanes, J. R. (1993) Topographic maps and molecular gradients. *Curr. Opin. Neurobiol. 3*:67–74.

Scherer, W. S., and Udin, S. B. (1989) N-methyl-D-aspartate antagonists prevent interaction of binocular maps in *Xenopus* tectum. *J. Neurosci. 9*:3837–3843.

Schmidt, J. T., and Eisele, L. E. (1985) Stroboscopic illumination and dark rearing block the sharpening of the regenerated retinotectal map in goldfish. *Neuroscience 14*:535–546.

Schoepp, D. D., and Conn, P. J. (1993) Metabotropic glutamate receptors in brain function and pathology. *TIPS 14*:13–20.

Schofield, P. R., Darlison, M. G., Fujita, N., Burt, D. R., Stephenson, F. A., Rodriguez, H., Rhee, L. M., Ramachandran, J., Reale, V., Glencorse, T. A., Seeburg, P. H., and Barnard, E. A. (1987) Sequence and functional expression of the GABA_A receptor shows a ligand-gated receptor super-family. *Nature 328*:221–227.

Schwartzkroin, P. A. (1982) Development of rabbit hippocampus: Physiology. *Dev. Brain Res. 2*:469–486.

Schwartzkroin, P. A., and Altschuler, R. J. (1977) Development of kitten hippocampal neurons. *Brain Res. 134*:429–444.

Seeburg, P. H. (1993) The TINS/TIPS lecture: The molecular biology of mammalian glutamate receptor channels. *TINS 16*:359–365.

Segal, M. M. (1991) Epileptiform activity in microcultures containing one excitatory hippocampal neuron. *J. Neurophysiol. 65*:761–770.

Segal, M. M., and Furshpan, E. J. (1990) Epileptiform activity in microcultures containing small numbers of hippocampal neurons. *J. Neurophysiol. 64*:1390–1398.

Seress, L., Frotscher, M., and Ribak, C. E. (1989) Local circuit neurons in both the

dentate gyrus and Ammon's horn establish synaptic connections with principal neurons in five-day-old rats: A morphological basis for inhibition in early
development. *Exp. Brain Res.* 78:1–9.

Seress, L., and Ribak, C. E. (1988) The development of GABAergic neurons in the
rat hippocampal formation: An immunocytochemical study. *Dev. Brain Res.*
44:197–209.

Shatz, C. J. (1990) Impulse activity and the patterning of connections during CNS
development. *Neuron* 5:745–756.

Skerritt, J. H., and Johnston, A. R. (1982) Postnatal development of GABA binding
sites and their endogenous inhibitors in rat brain. *Dev. Neurosci.* 5:189–197.

Smith, K. L., and Swann, J. W. (1993) The formation of hippocampal CA₃ networks
in explant cultures of neonatal rat. *Neurosci. Abstr.* 19:1292.

Sperry, R. W. (1963) Chemoaffinity in the orderly growth of nerve fiber patterns and
connections. *Proc. Natl. Acad. Sci.* 50:703–710.

Stryker, M. P., and Harris, W. A. (1986) Binocular impulse blockade prevents the
formation of ocular dominance columns in cat visual cortex. *J. Neurosci.*
6:2117–2133.

Stryker, M. P., and Strickland, S. L. (1984) Physiological segregation of ocular dominance columns depends on the pattern of afferent electrical activity. *Invest.
Ophthalmol. Vis. Sci.* 25 (Suppl.):278.

Sugihara, H., Moriyoshi, K., Ishii, T., Masu, M., and Nakanishi, S. (1992) Structures and properties of seven isoforms of the NMDA receptor generated by
alternative splicing. *Biochem. Biophys. Res. Commun.* 185:826–832.

Swann, J. W., and Brady, R. J. (1984) Penicillin-induced epileptogenesis in immature
rat CA₃ hippocampal pyramidal cells. *Dev. Brain Res.* 12:243–254.

Swann, J. W., and Gomez-Di Cesare, C. M. (1994) Developmental plasticity and
hippocampal epileptogenesis. *Hippocampus,* 4:266–269.

Swann, J. W., Brady, R. J., and Martin, D. (1989) Postnatal development of GABA-
mediated synaptic inhibition in rat hippocampus. *Neuroscience* 28:551–561.

Swann, J. W., Smith, K. L., and Brady R. J. (1986) Extracellular K⁺ accumulation
during penicillin-induced epileptogenesis in the CA3 region of immature rat
hippocampus. *Dev. Brain Res.* 30:243–255.

Swann, J. W., Smith, K. L., and Brady, R. J. (1993) Localized excitatory synaptic
interactions mediate the sustained depolarization of electrographic seizures in
developing hippocampus. *J. Neurosci.* 13:4680–4689.

Swann, J. W., Smith, K. L., Brady, R. J., and Pierson, M. G. (1993) Neurophysiological studies of alterations in seizure susceptibility during brain development. In: P. Schwartzkroin (ed.), *Concepts and Models in Epilepsy Research.*
New York: Cambridge University Press, pp. 209–243.

Tanabe, Y., Masu, M., Ishii, T., Shigemoto, R., and Nakanishi, S. (1992) A family
of metabotropic glutamate receptors. *Neuron* 8:169–179.

Tepper, J. M., and Schlesinger, J. (1980) Acoustic priming and kanamycin-induced
cochlear damage. *Brain Res.* 187:81–95.

Tessier-Lavigne, M. (1992) Axon guidance by molecular gradients. *Curr. Opin. Neurobiol.* 2:60–65.

Thompson, W. J., Kuttler, D. P., and Jansen, J. K. S. (1979) The effects of prolonged, reversible block of nerve impulses on the elimination of polyneuronal
innervation of new-born rat skeletal muscle fibers. *Neuroscience* 4:271–281.

Werner, P., Voigt, M., Keinänen, K., Wisden, W., and Seeburg, P. H. (1991) Cloning of a putative high-affinity kainate receptor expressed predominantly in hippocampal CA₃ cells. *Nature 351:*742–744.

Wigstrom, D. J., and Gustafsson, B. (1985) On long-lasting potentiation in the hippocampus: A proposed mechanism for its dependence on coincident pre- and post-synaptic activity. *Acta Physiol. Scand. 123:*519–522.

Williams, K., Russell, S. L., Shen, Y. M., and Molinoff, P. B. (1993) Developmental switch in the expression of NMDA receptors occurs *in vivo* and *in vitro*. *Neuron 10:*267–278.

Wisden, W., Laurie, D. J., Monyer, H., and Seeburg, P. H. (1992) The distribution of 13 GABA_A receptor subunit mRNAs in the rat brain: I. Telencephalon, diencephalon, mesencephalon. *J. Neurosci. 12:*1040–1062.

Wisden, W., and Seeburg, P. H. (1992) GABA_A receptor channels: From subunits to functional entities. *Curr. Opin. Neurobiol. 2:*263–269.

Xie, Z.-P., and Poo, M.-M. (1986) Initial events in the formation of neuromuscular synapse: Rapid induction of acetylcholine release. *Proc. Natl. Acad. Sci. 83:*7069–7073.

Yuste, R., Peinado, A., and Katz, L. C. (1992) Neuronal domains in developing neocortex. *Science 257:*665–669.

Zhang, L., Spigelman, I., and Carlen, P. L. (1990) Whole-cell patch study of GABAergic inhibition in CA₁ neurons of immature rat hippocampal slices. *Dev. Brain Res. 56:*127–130.

Zhang, L., Spigelman, I., and Carlen, P. L. (1991) Development of GABA-mediated, chloride-dependent inhibition in CA₁ pyramidal neurones of immature rat hippocampal slices. *J. Physiol. (London) 444:*25–49.

9

Plasticity and Repair in the Immature Central Nervous System

PHILIP A. SCHWARTZKROIN

Investigators have long believed that the immature central nervous system (CNS) is far more flexible—"plastic"—than the adult brain. Clinical observations have led investigators to the conclusion that nervous system injury is often less likely to have irreparable consequence if it occurs in the young, developing nervous system than if the injury is to the mature and stable CNS. For example, the immature brain is more likely to compensate for trauma or surgically-induced tissue loss in language areas or in critical motor regions (Kennard, 1942; Milner, 1974). Various hypotheses have been offered to account for this striking plasticity in the young CNS and its decay as the animal matures. Complementing the investigations of immature mammalian CNS are both studies of nonmammalian nervous system (where injury and lesions are often not "permanent"; (Borgens et al., 1981; Jacobson and Baker, 1969; Yoon, 1973) and observations of cells grown in controlled culture environments. These studies have led to a number of insights into key properties of immature CNS plasticity, such as the importance of (1) timing of cell "commitment" to a given fate or function (Walsh and Cepko, 1992; see also Walsh, Chapter 5); (2) location- and time-specific expression of neurotrophic factors in young animals (Enfors et al., 1993; Maisonpierre et al., 1990); (3) developmentally timed expression of guidance cues—for example, extracellular matrix molecules (Reichardt and Tomaselli, 1991), cell adhesion molecules (Rutishauser and Jessell, 1988), and inhibitory molecules (Patterson, 1988)—that favor neurite outgrowth in immature brain; (4) development of physical barriers (e.g., glial cells) as the CNS matures (Schwab and Caroni, 1988); and (5) differential effects of neurotransmitter release with age (Lipton and Kater, 1989).

Given a general consensus that the immature CNS does indeed exhibit far more plasticity than the mature system (Finger and Stein, 1982), why should we be particularly concerned about the ill effects of seizure activity (or of the abnormalities that lead to seizures) in the developing nervous system?

One answer is that many of the issues that we are concerned about—or at least think we should be concerned about—do not focus on a young nervous system which has already taken its final form, but rather involve a developing system in which the determination of cell identities, migration targets, contact sites, and so on, are yet to be established. Disruption of the normal patterns of development might lead to serious and irreversible consequences. These consequences occur in spite of the fact that the immature nervous system may still exhibit the capability for change, since "plasticity" serves little function in the absence of an appropriate structural framework. For example, axon sprouting is of no benefit if that growth occurs in the "wrong" brain region or at a time when "correct" targets are not available. Indeed, the ability of the young neurons to continue to grow and make contacts may aggravate a pathological situation, as the system may make aberrant connections or respond inappropriately to stimuli. It is, in fact, precisely this enhanced plasticity that may lead to the abnormalities that express themselves as seizure activity. This consequence may not be seen immediately (in the immature nervous system) but may manifest finally in the adult.

This chapter will focus on a number of issues that are related to the cellular and molecular "plasticities" that are characteristic of the immature nervous system. Its goal is to provide a view of the forms of plasticity that occur during development and to discuss how they are related to mature forms of plasticity (e.g., involvement in learning or repair from injury) and how these mechanisms might lead to expression of CNS abnormalities (Table 9-1). Examples of developmental plasticities, studied in a variety of systems, will be used to suggest how they may contribute to abnormal electrical activities in the immature mammalian CNS; how they may, over time, lead to seizures in the adult brain; and how they may also provide us with a window of opportunity for therapy. In the model systems examined here, it is clear that manipulations of the environment, direct injuries to the nervous system, or alterations in the electrophysiologic status of the brain can all lead to changes that leave a permanent mark on the CNS; the particular effects of these manipulations are peculiar to the developing nervous system inasmuch as similar perturbations or injuries in the mature brain lead to quite difference consequences.

Activity-Dependence and Mammalian CNS Plasticity

A number of mechanisms (reviewed in Chapters 4–7) provide guidance cues independent of neural activity (e.g., genetic makeup and environmental determinants, contact guidance cues). In general, such signals enable devel-

TABLE 9-1. Parallel and Related "Plastic" Processes in Developing, Mature, and Pathologic CNS Tissue

Developing (immature) Cortices	Mature Plasticity	Pathological (epileptic) Tissue
Synaptic excitation Changing pattern of expression of glutamate receptor subunits High levels of NMDA receptor function Lesser voltage (Mg^{2+})-dependency of NMDA receptors Non-NMDA receptor-gated channels admit Ca^{2+} Peak long-term potentiation	Synaptic excitation Long-term potentiation and depression mediated primarily via NMDA receptor activation LTP and LTD can be "associative" processes Potentiation (or depression) mediated by rise of intracellular Ca^{2+} concentration Potentiation (or depression) increases with repetitive stimulation	Synaptic excitation Excitation enhanced relative to inhibition Major role for NMDA-mediated processes (NMDA blockers reduce pathology, are anticonvulsant) Large changes in ion flux, including Ca^{2+} influx during epileptiform events Activity-dependent changes in glutamate receptor subunits
Synaptic inhibition Changing pattern of expression of GABA receptor subunits Late deveopment of hyperpolarizing inhibition GABA induces depolarizing response Labile IPSP	Synaptic inhibition Mediated via hyperpolarizing (and conductance increase) mechanism Hyperpolarizing IPSP decreases with repetitive stimulation Depolarizing GABA-mediated synaptic process (in dendrites) is facilitated by repetitive stimulation Loss (or blockade) of hyperpolarizing IPSP important for LTP	Synaptic inhibition Functional inhibition often decreased GABA-enhancing drugs effective against some forms of epilepsy Synchronization and rhythmic activity sometimes associated with depolarizing GABA effect
Morphologic plasticity Changes in dendritic and axonic patterns (length, branching) Establishment of specific synaptic contacts—associative process-dependent on NMDA activation and/or afferent activity Cell growth and guidance enhanced by neurotrophic factors, etc.	Morphologic plasticity Stimulation/experience can modify dendritic branching Change in spines and synaptic contacts accompanies LTP-like stimulation LTP associated with changes in neurotrophin expression	Morphologic plasticity Spine loss Sprouting of axon collaterals Large changes in immediate early gene expression, neurotrophin mRNAs, etc.

oping neurons to differentiate, migrate, and project processes toward their appropriate targets. However, investigators have also shown that normal activity—both spontaneous and sensory-mediated—is critical for the refinement of synaptic connections and consequent development of normal physiologic function (Goodman and Shatz, 1993).

As is the case for many of the following examples of developmental plasticity, the functional result of these activity-dependent processes has been most extensively examined in the developing visual system. In the immature animal (or, indeed, in the human patient), loss of normal visual input—even transiently—may leave the individual visually impaired, although a neural response to sensory input may still be transmitted from the retina to the cortex. To have a long-lasting and significant effect on behavior, the visual deprivation experience must occur during the "critical" period for development of cortical connections. Following childhood periods of such sensory disruption, the adult nervous system is permanently changed; while some individuals have been able to "relearn" how to see, processes such as visual acuity often remain impaired.

Visual deficits (e.g., the displaced images in strabismus) which result in imbalanced visual input also lead to abnormal visual system development. In their influential studies, Hubel and Wiesel (1970) showed that when visual input is mediated primarily through one eye, that eye quickly dominates the animal's visually guided behavior and also "controls" the electrophysiologic properties of individual cells in visual cortex. More recently, Shatz and Stryker (1988) showed that blockade of activity in visual pathways (via injections of tetrodotoxin) at a critical period of development disrupts the formation of eye-specific layers in the lateral geniculate nucleus (Fig. 9-1A; see also Sretavan et al., 1988); Stryker and Harris (1986) found that such treatment also disrupted the normal morphology of the ocular dominance pattern in visual cortex. The result of this treatment is a loss of function that lasts well beyond the time attributable directly to the toxin. Perhaps even more dramatic examples are reported in studies in which young animals were exposed selectively to restricted visual patterns—for example, horizontal or vertical lines—during the critical period of visual development. In the majority of these studies investigators reported that the receptive fields of cortical neurons in these animals were responsive primarily to orientation of visual patterns that corresponded to the patterns to which the animal had been exposed (Blakemore and Cooper, 1970; Stryker and Sherk, 1975). Animals also exhibited some deficits in visually guided behavior, although interpretation of the behavioral data is confounded by the unusual nature of the visual exposure.

The effects of manipulating sensory input are reflected in alterations in the structure of cortical organization. In the studies just described, loss of input to one eye results in a shrinkage of the ocular dominance column normally controlled by that eye. Similarly, in the rat somatosensory cortex, activity appears to play a role in the developmental plasticity of whisker barrel-field representation. Although barrel-field development apparently

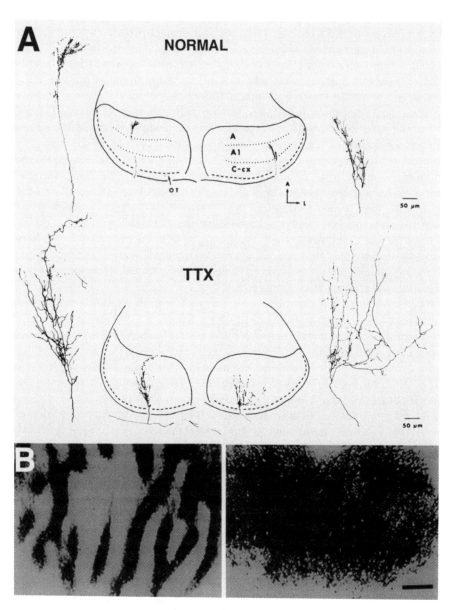

Figure 9-1. (A) Effects of tetrodotoxin (TTX) blockade of neuronal activity on retino-geniculate axon arborization. TTX was administered between embryonic day 42 and embryonic day 56 to the optic chiasm (minipumps implanted in utero). Intracellular horseradish peroxidase (HRP) labeling of individual axons showed that at day 58 in normal cats, the terminal arborizations from contralateral (left) and ipsilateral (right) eyes are restricted to appropriate layers of lateral geniculate nucleus (LGN). With tetrodotoxin treatment, the axon terminal arborization is much more extensive, branching indiscriminately, without regard to the lamina associated with each eye. (Reproduced with permission from Sretavan et al., 1988.)

does not depend on activity in the afferent nerves from vibrissae (Henderson et al., 1992), anatomical changes that occur in response to damage (e.g., whisker removal) *are* dependent on remaining activity (Schlaggar et al., 1993). Transient changes have been reported in other systems when afferent input is removed during critical periods of development. For example, in the chick auditory pathway, blockade of activity from the auditory nerve of one ear to the relay nuclei in the brainstem results in a selective shrinkage of that part of the dendritic tree to which the blocked nerve normally projects. This effect is accompanied by glial proliferation as well as decreased protein formation in the brainstem nucleus (Rubel and Hyson, 1992). Complex environmental stimulation has long been known to affect the gross morphology of neocortex. For example, comparing rats raised in an "enriched" environment with those raised in a sensory-"deprived" environment, investigators found that the thickness of the neocortex is clearly greater for the enriched population, and that the enriched-environment animals perform better on a variety of behavioral tasks (Diamond, 1967; Greenough, 1976). These effects on cortical structure—primarily a reflection of the complexity of dendritic arborization—can be demonstrated in the adult, but they appear to be much more dramatic in young animals.

Although the cellular basis for this activity-dependency is still poorly understood, a number of in vitro studies are beginning to provide interesting clues. Cell culture studies (Bergey et al., 1981; Lo and Poo, 1991; Nelson et al., 1989) have shown that strength of connectivity among neurons depends on baseline level of spontaneous discharge; further, if the cells are silenced (e.g., with tetrodotoxin) during initial periods of synapse formation, the viability of the culture may be impaired. Cellular activity and the consequent release of neurotransmitter from terminals have also been postulated to have trophic influences which help determine the growth of dendrites and spines as well as modulate "consolidation" of synaptic contacts (i.e., establishment of stable connections). For example, cell culture studies have shown that cell exposure to a variety of neurotransmitters can influence the growth of dendrites and spines, exerting effects over a remarkably short time frame (Lipton and Kater, 1989; Mattson and Kater, 1989; Patterson, 1988). Gluta-

---

(B) Effect of NMDA, and the NMDA blocker MK801, on retinotectal arborization in the three-eyed tadpole model. MK801 and NMDA were slowly released from Elvax plastic polymer implanted over the optic tectum of tadpoles for 14 weeks, and ocular dominance stripes were assessed in tectum by labeling the supernumerary retinal projection with HRP. In the normal, untreated tectum, clear eye-specific stripes are visible (left). However, when the tectum was treated with MK801 and NMDA (NMDA was found to be a necessary cotreatment, presumably because MK801 blockade is "use-dependent" at the NMDA receptor), growing retinal afferents arborize in an apparently indiscriminate manner; no eye-specific stripes are seen. Scale bar = 200 µM. (Reproduced with permission from Cline and Constantine-Paton, 1990.)

mate effects have been shown to be age- and concentration-dependent. The primary effect of glutamate release in hippocampal cultural systems appears to be inhibition of dendritic outgrowth; blockade of glutamate receptors, or of presynaptic electrical activity which normally releases transmitter, gives rise to increased dendritic growth and reduction of presumed synapses (Mattson et al., 1988). Further, the release of transmitter can have significant effects on the surrounding glia (Cornell-Bell et al., 1990).

In more complex preparations, a variety of observations are consistent with these culture system results. Recent reports suggest that there is a reversible loss of dendritic spines in organotypic hippocampal slice cultures made epileptogenic—a condition under which large amounts of transmitter are likely to be released (Müller et al., 1993). In in vitro hippocampal slice preparations from immature rat, activity-dependent release of zinc from mossy fiber terminals has been hypothesized to interact with spontaneously occurring giant depolarizing potentials to affect synapse formation of mossy fibers on CA_3 pyramidal cells (Xie and Smart, 1991). In entorhinal-hippocampal cultures, glutamate has been shown to have an important effect on determining the appropriate formation of perforant path–to–hippocampus synapses (Mattson et al., 1988). In all these cases, the critical variable associated with this activity-dependent establishment of synaptic contacts appears to be the release of transmitter (or an associated molecule).

The underlying bases of these plasticities are still to be elucidated. These activity-dependent processes are often modulated by the same traditional neurotransmitters which are functional in the adult animal. How, then, can we account for these age-specific processes in the immature CNS? Perhaps at critical times during development specific responsive elements or cell properties are expressed in parallel with an appropriate "activating" stimulus (i.e., a stimulus to which the response element is sensitive). Such critical periods are characteristic of the entire developmental process, from the time of cell migration and differentiation to the establishment of appropriate synaptic contacts.

Neurotransmitter- and Modulator-Induced Plasticity

A variety of experimental systems have been exploited to examine the role of neurotransmitter systems in the determination of synaptic connectivity and function in CNS structures. Among the most elegant of these models is the ectopic eye model developed by Constantine-Paton and collaborators (Constantine-Paton et al., 1990; Simon et al., 1993). They have shown that in the growth of visual afferents from the eye to the tectum of frog, competition among afferent inputs results in the "sorting" of connections. This process, which establishes functional receptive fields and ocular dominance columns, is very much dependent on the activation of the NMDA receptor (Fig. 9-1B). As described by Swann (Chapter 8), this sorting process involves more than simply an initial exuberance of afferent fibers and subsequent "programmed cell death" (see also Murakami et al., 1992). Only associated activity in neighboring inputs at an NMDA receptor provides sufficient depolarization to activate the NMDA receptor; this "activation" then triggers secondary processes required to consolidate those inputs at that postsynaptic site. Thus the concomitant pattern of activities in functionally related fibers—fibers with related retinal fields—appears to play a key role in determining connections at CNS targets.

In an early chemoaffinity hypothesis, Sperry and colleagues showed that a variety of tropic cues apparently provided the signal necessary to guide visual afferents to their appropriate targets in frog tectum (Attardi and Sperry, 1963; Sperry, 1963; see also Purves and Lichtman, 1985). The relative organization of these afferents was maintained despite manipulations of both the sensory surface (e.g., rotating the eyeball) and the receptive neural surface (e.g., rotating the tectum). Diffusion of chemical cues may indeed be responsible for a general pattern of receptive field relationships in this system, but this mechanism cannot adequately specify the precision that is typical of retinotectal input. Nor do such signals explain why only some afferents establish viable and lasting contacts—as is typical of competitive "consolidation" of inputs in the developing CNS. The work of the Constantine-Paton group on "Hebbian" synaptic stabilization provides us with an insight into at least one of the cues responsible for providing a precise level of organization, even in the face of abnormal manipulation of the system. Interestingly, the dependence of this organization on the NMDA receptor, and on associative activities of related (and/or neighboring) afferents, is reminiscent of the associative potentiation phenomena thought by many investigators to underlie learning-related behaviors (see "Long-Term Potentiation," below).

"Associative" activity processing seems to be characteristic of developmental organization at many levels. Even earlier than the cortical "critical periods" already described, organization within the retina appears to arise, at least in part, from coincident or near-coincident retinal (receptor) activity (Meister et al., 1991). In the immature retina of cat and ferret, even before connections are made in central nervous system structures such as tectum or cortex, retinal organization appears to be determined and maintained by spontaneous activity in the ganglion cells. Although the retinal ganglion cells are not synaptically connected, some interactive signaling process supports a synchronized discharge pattern within neighboring neurons; thus groups of cells within a given retinal region tend to fire "spontaneously" at the same time. As a reflection of this regional synchrony, a "wave" of activity sweeps across the retina. These observations suggest that correlated activity in neighboring elements, even before synaptic contacts are made, appears to be a major organizing principle in the visual system. The relatively greater occurrence of electrical coupling and gap junctions in immature mammalian neocortex, but not mature cortex (Connors et al., 1983; Lo Turco and Kriegstein, 1991; Peinado et al., 1993), may be a mechanism for providing such correlated activity among neighboring neurons, at a time that precedes effective chemical synaptic coupling—and might indeed guide this later development.

As suggested, activation of NMDA receptors via associative inputs and the subsequent triggering of intracellular messenger systems appear to be an important means for shaping CNS organization. Thus it is perhaps not surprising that the NMDA contribution to excitatory postsynaptic potentials (EPSPs) in immature cortex appears to be much larger than in mature animals (Fig. 9-2; Burgard and Hablitz, 1993; Tremblay et al., 1988). The NMDA receptor has also been found to change in its characteristics during development, showing different kinetics (Fig. 9-2; Hestrin, 1992) and/or Mg^{2+} voltage-dependency (Ben-Ari et al., 1988) in the immature brain. Given the hypothesis that the critical role of these NMDA channels is to mediate calcium flux across the cell membrane, it seems likely that non-NMDA glutamate receptors, which may also admit calcium, play a similar role at some synapses. Recent studies have shown that AMPA/kainate receptors may modulate calcium flux, depending on the receptor's subunit composition; posttranslational modifications of the protein subunits that make up these channels are critical in determining this calcium permeability (Dingledine et al., 1992; Köhler et al., 1993; Seeburg, 1993). Further, the subunit composition of these receptors is known to change during development (Pellegrini-Giampietro et al., 1991), with the calcium-permeant forms more prevalent in immature CNS (Monyer et al., 1991; Williams et al., 1993). Finally, the subunit composition of glutamate receptors has been shown to be sensitive to levels of activity, such as kindling-evoked seizurelike discharge (Kamphuis et al., 1992).

Other receptors and modulators, of course, may also play a role in shaping this neuronal development and organization. For example, activity-dependent release of factors from target neurons—in order to stabilize synaptic connections—has long been hypothesized (Goodman and Shatz, 1993; O'Leary and Koester, 1993). It is now clear that in addition to nerve growth factor (NGF), which is found to support a rather limited set of neurons in the CNS, primarily cholinergic cells in the basal forebrain, there are a number of related substances whose functions we have yet to clarify (e.g., extracellular matrix proteins [Dodd and Jessell, 1988; Taira et al., 1993], cell adhesion molecules [Jessell, 1988], and nonneural growth factors such as fibroblast growth factor [Mattson et al., 1989]). Recent experiments suggest that these substances may play a role in such activity-related functions as synaptic plasticity and synaptic stabilization. For example, neurotrophic factors are significantly upregulated in conjunction with seizure activity (Fig. 9-3A; Dugich-Djordjevic et al., 1992; Gall and Lauterborn, 1992) and can also be shown to increase during more "normal" physiological activity such as stimulation to induce long-term potentiation (Figure 9-3B; Patterson et al., 1992). A recent report has shown that the function of developing synapses (neuromuscular junction contacts) may be potentiated by neurotrophins (Lohof et al., 1993). While most available results are primarily correlative—they establish only a correlation between neurotrophin expression and changes in synaptic efficacy—the suggestion of neurotrophin involvement in synaptic plasticity is intriguing. It may be particularly relevant for the developing CNS, where changing patterns of trophic factor expression indicate specific roles for each factor at different stages of development (Fig. 9-3C; Enfors et al., 1993; Maisonpierre et al., 1990; Rocamora et al., 1993).

CNS plasticity has also been shown to have significant dependence on inhibitory neurotransmitters, and particularly on GABA. Again, using the visual system as an accessible model, investigators have found that acute systemic injections of GABA antagonists can have significant effects on receptive field organization in the adult animal. In particular, complex cortical receptor fields lose considerable specificity in the presence of GABA blockade, with cells firing in response to much more diffuse inputs (Sillito, 1975). The critical role of GABA in sharpening receptive fields during development was shown in experiments in which GABA blockers were topically applied, repetitively, throughout the "critical period" for development of rabbit visual cortical receptive fields (Baumbach and Chow, 1981; Crabtree et al., 1983). Such penicillin treatment not only changed receptive fields acutely, but yielded a mature cortex in which receptive fields were dramatically different from those of the normal adult. A number of investigations have shown that the conventional inhibitory GABA effect is late-developing in many cortical tissues (Kriegstein et al., 1987; Schwartzkroin, 1982)—perhaps due to a developmental alteration in the nature of the $GABA_A$ subunit composition (Killisch et al., 1991; Laurie et al., 1992; Zhang et al., 1993). A depolarizing effect of GABA has been seen in many immature cell types (Cherubini et al., 1991; Luhmann and Prince, 1991; Mueller et al., 1984; see Fig. 9-2). Developmental changes in benzodiazepine binding (Rovira and Ben-Ari, 1991), zinc sensitivity (Xie and Smart, 1991), and calcium permeability (Connor et al., 1987; Yuste and Katz, 1991) have been associated with changes in the subunit composition of these receptors and channels. These developmental changes may determine the appropriate involvement of the inhibitory transmitter during critical periods, which in turn may be key to maturation of normal and highly specific synaptic responsivity, such as responsivity to sensory stimuli.

Other neuroactive substances play somewhat less specific, more "modulatory" roles in development and maintenance of cell properties and connectivities and in the plasticity of CNS structures. In the visual system, both acetylcholine and norepinephrine appear to have significant modulatory action during critical periods of development (Bear and Singer, 1986). In the absence of norepinephrine (e.g., with 6-OH-dopamine lesions), the expected shifts in ocular dominance of neocortex neurons do not occur when the animal is subjected to short periods of monocular deprivation (Kasamatsu and Pettigrew, 1979); exogenous application of norepinephrine (NE) reverses this loss of plasticity (Kasamatsu et al., 1979). The second-messenger systems that might be responsible for this effect of norepinephrine have yet to

A

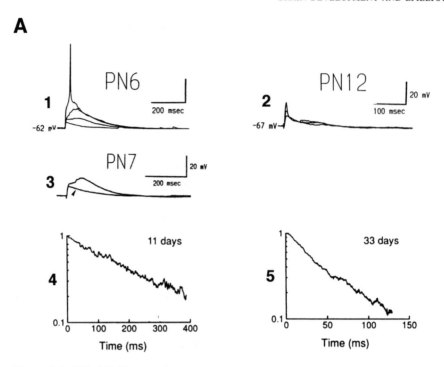

Figure 9-2. (A1–A3) Changes in the NMDA component of the EPSP in rat neocortex during development. A comparison of the traces in 1 and 2 show that a large, slow EPSP component is present at postnatal day 6 (PN6) but not at PN12. Traces in 3 show that this large, slow component is due, in large part, to NMDA channel activation; NMDA antagonism with APV (lower trace, arrowhead) blocks this component of the EPSP. (Reproduced with permission from Burgard and Hablitz, 1993.)

(A4–A5) The kinetics of the NMDA response also changes during development, as shown in these plots of EPSC decay in rat superior colliculus. The response becomes much faster as the animal matures (note the difference in abscissa calibrations for the 11- and 33-day-old tissue), but it remains voltage-dependent. (Reproduced with permission from Hestrin, 1992.)

(B1–B2) Depolarizing response to a brief somatic GABA application, as seen in a hippocampal CA_1 neuron from an 8-day-old rabbit. The reversal potential for this GABA response was near −40mV, much more positive than the reversal potential reported for mature tissue. (Reproduced with permission from Janigro and Schwartzkroin, 1988.)

(B3–B4) Giant depolarizing responses (GDRs) are produced spontaneously in immature (4-day-old) rat hippocampal tissue. The burst discharge can be blocked with bicuculline, suggesting that the response is mediated by a $GABA_A$ mechanism. (Reproduced with permission from Ben-Ari et al., 1989.)

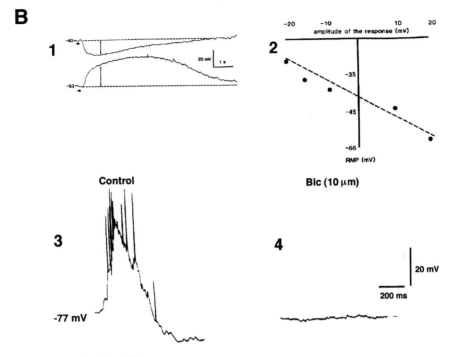

Figure 9-2. (Continued)

be identified, but it is striking that a similar NE modulatory effect has been shown in studies of long-term potentiation in at least some regions of adult hippocampus and neocortex (Bröcher et al., 1992a; Hopkins and Johnston, 1984). Indeed, NE itself can produce long-lasting synaptic potentiation in the dentate granule cells (Sarvey, 1988).

Neuromodulatory effects are exerted by circulating steroids, including gonadal and adrenal hormones. Studies of cortical and hippocampal architecture have shown that exposure to thyroid hormone at critical periods of development is absolutely necessary for the development of normal dendritic trees; abnormal exposures give rise to altered neuronal structure (Fig. 9-4; Gould et al., 1991; Rami et al., 1986). Similarly, glucocorticoids and mineralocorticoids have profound effects on various hippocampal neurons, maintaining (or reducing) their viability (McEwen, Angulo et al., 1991) and dramatically affecting the extent of their dendritic trees and spines (see Chapters 1 and 11 for discussion of steroid-related treatment and infantile spasms). In the female, estradiol and progesterone also have significant effects on spine and synaptic density, effects that occur on a relatively short time scale and are reversible with changes in hormone level (Woolley and McEwen, 1992). Some of these changes in dendritic profiles are strikingly reminiscent of changes associated with seizure activity in organotypic hippocampal cultures (Müller et al., 1993).

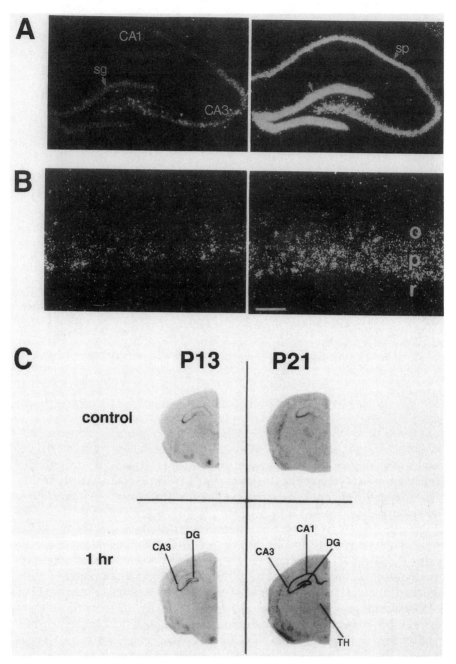

Figure 9-3. (A) Upregulation of mRNA for brain-derived neurotrophic factor (BDNF) in hippocampus of adult rat 6 hours following experimentally induced seizure activity. Note the strong activation of BDNF expression in pyramidal and dentate granule cell regions. (Reproduced with permission from Gall and Lauterborn, 1992.)

(B) Upregulation of mRNA for BDNF in the CA$_1$ region of hippocampal slices following LTP-inducing stimulation in stratum radiatum. (Reproduced with permission from Patterson et al., 1992.)

Long-Term Potentiation and Depression during Development and Their Potential Role in Kindling Epileptogenesis

Perhaps more than any other "plastic" phenomenon, long-term potentiation (LTP) has captured the imagination of neuroscience researchers. Because of its "associative" nature (note the analogy to associative processes underlying consolidation of synaptic contacts, as discussed previously), LTP has been viewed as a major candidate for the cellular basis of learning and memory. Many researchers have sought to identify the underlying mechanisms responsible for activity-dependent changes in synaptic strength associated with LTP. Long-term potentiation has been studied intensively (but not exclusively) in hippocampus; the term LTP refers to the phenomenon of enhanced synaptic efficacy which endures for long periods and is brought about by relatively moderate levels of brief, repetitive stimulation (Bliss and Lømo, 1973; Madison et al., 1991). Investigators have shown that most forms of LTP are mediated by an NMDA receptor linked process (Artola and Singer, 1987; Collingridge et al., 1983). However, in some cells LTP apparently can occur without NMDA receptor activation (Grover and Teyler, 1992). What appears critical in virtually all forms is a rise in intracellular calcium that is produced by membrane depolarization (to open voltage-dependent calcium channels and/or to relieve the magnesium blockade of the NMDA receptor). The critical role of calcium in this plastic process reinforces the focus on calcium influx (discussed by Spitzer, Chapter 6) as a major contributor to a number of developmental processes. LTP has been induced in hippocampal neurons as young as 5 days postnatal, but the most vigorous response is not reached until somewhat later (Fig. 9-5; Harris and Teyler, 1984)—2–3 weeks postnatal in hippocampus and somewhat later in neocortex (Perkins and Teyler, 1988). The NMDA contribution to LTP in the immature animal is not entirely clear. Given that at least in hippocampal neurons the NMDA receptor does not experience as significant a voltage-dependent magnesium block as in the adult (Ben-Ari et al., 1988; Bowe and Nadler, 1990), one might expect that NMDA-dependent processes would occur more readily. Certainly, extremely large depolarizing NMDA-mediated synaptic potentials can be induced in immature hippocampal cells (Ben-Ari et al., 1989). Recent studies have shown, further, that the susceptibility to LTP in relatively immature rat visual cortex appears to be correlated with the extent of NMDA contribution to the EPSP (Kato et al., 1991). As indicated earlier, AMPA/kainate receptor subunits in immature brain appear to be of a type that mediate high calcium permeability, and thus could

(C) Differential sensitivity of BDNF/mRNA expression to seizure-inducing activation at different stages of development. In rat hippocampus (and elsewhere, such as in piriform cortex), seizures induce little change of BDNF/mRNA in animals at 13 days postnatal, but a large change at 21 days. (Reproduced with permission from Dugich-Djordjevic et al., 1992.)

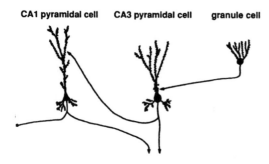

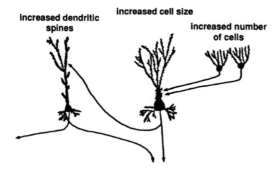

Figure 9-4. Schematic diagram of changes in hippocampal cell morphology when immature rats are treated with thyroid hormone during development. Excess thyroid hormone could result in increased spine density in CA_1 pyramidal cells, increased cell size in CA_3, and increased numbers of granule cells. (Reproduced with permission from Gould et al., 1991.)

also, theoretically, support LTP initiation. The ratio of calcium-permeable to calcium-impermeable AMPA/kainate receptors is particularly high in rat hippocampus between postnatal days 7 and 21 (Pellegrini-Giampietro et al., 1992)—just at the time that LTP peaks in this structure (See Figure 9-5). Finally, there has been much interest in metabotropic glutamate receptors, subtypes of which trigger calcium release from intracellular stores (Shoepp and Conn, 1993). These metabotropic receptors, which also show a developmentally specific profile (Minakami et al., 1992), have been implicated in LTP in adult CNS (Bashir et al., 1993; Zheng and Gallagher, 1992). Their role in immature neurons remains to be determined.

The same general stimulation protocols that induce long-term potentiation, when slightly modified, induce synaptic depression at many CNS synapses (Bröcher et al., 1992b; Mulkey and Malenka, 1992; Tsumoto, 1993). Investigators have hypothesized that the level of intracellular calcium

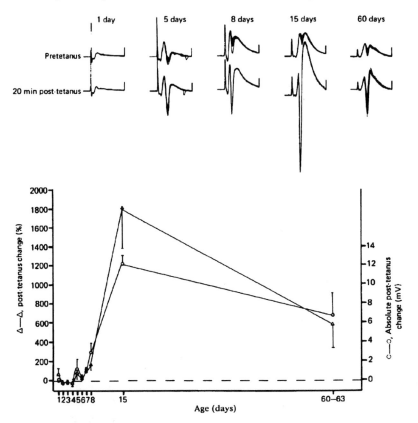

Figure 9-5. Developmental time course of long-term potentiation (LTP) in the CA₁ region of rat hippocampus. Top traces illustrate the changes in response to tetanic stimulation at different postnatal ages. These changes are graphed below, showing a peak expression at 15 days. (Reproduced with permission from Harris and Teyler, 1984.)

evoked by the stimulation determines whether potentiation or depression occurs, with higher levels of calcium required for potentiation (Artola et al., 1990; Dudek and Bear, 1992). Long-term synaptic depression can also be induced in relatively immature (i.e., about 2 weeks postnatal) rats and is at least partially NMDA receptor-dependent (as in adult animals), but it shows less NMDA dependency in the immature hippocampus (Velísek et al., 1993). Still, regulation of intracellular calcium appears to be the critical factor in induction of such synaptic plasticities. Developmental differences in regulation of intracellular calcium levels (e.g., via calcium exchange mechanisms) or in the calcium sensitivities of intracellular mechanisms (e.g., via kinase activation) may determine the nature and/or degree of such plasticities in immature neurons.

If one thinks of the rise in calcium as a critical intracellular process that mediates potentiation (or depression), then many transmitter and modulatory factors should be able to influence these mechanisms. With respect to LTP, the initiating role of glutamate action at NMDA receptors, the modulatory role of GABA (GABA$_A$ inhibition is an important modulatory factor in the initiation of associative LTP; Wigstrom and Gustafsson, 1985), and even the potentiation-inducing effects of norepinephrine (for some forms of LTP in the hippocampal CA$_3$ region and as an inducer of potentiation in the dentate; Hopkins and Johnston, 1984; Sarvey, 1988) are noteworthy; these effects show striking parallels to normal developmental processes. Many of the cellular mechanisms underlying transmitter-induced actions (e.g., modulation by calcium-dependent kinases) may be common to diverse forms of plasticity—from development of afferent synapses to induction of epileptogenic activities.

From the point of view of the developmental epileptologist, the synaptic potentiation phenomenon is particularly interesting as a potential contributor to seizure generation. In particular, the kindling model of temporal lobe epilepsy employs stimulation paradigms for generating a seizure state which are similar to those used for inducing long-term potentiation. The peculiarities of kindling in the immature animal are described in Chapter 2. However, it is worthwhile considering here what the relationship between synaptic potentiation and kindling might really be (Cain, 1989), and whether the association is likely to be of importance in the developing animal. There has been considerable controversy about whether kindling is simply an extension of long-term potentiation, is completely independent of it, or is based on some (but not all) of the LTP mechanisms. Investigators have found that animals that are initially subjected to LTP stimulation protocols (and display long-term potentiation of their synaptic activities) can be kindled more easily than unpotentiated controls (Sutula and Steward, 1986, 1987). It has also been noted, however, that animals could be subjected to many periods of potentiating stimulation without seizure induction. The critical difference between LTP and kindling—indeed, the key to successful kindling—appears to be the triggering of afterdischarge (AD) activity. Afterdischarge typically does not occur in response to LTP-inducing stimulation. In fact, some studies have suggested that afterdischarge can "depotentiate" synaptic responses and/or lead to synaptic depression (Hesse and Teyler, 1976; Moore et al., 1993). Thus it is likely that although kindling may initially involve some form of the LTP mechanism, it also requires additional and/or novel processes. Just as in LTP, however, kindling apparently establishes increased synaptic efficacy in affected regions; stimulus intensities subthreshold for triggering AD can be shown to evoke enhanced synaptic responses. Pathways for propagation of electrical signaling appear to be strengthened and provide for relatively stereotyped spread of activity. Thus as a model of enhanced synaptic activity, and as a means of obtaining access to neuronal pathways through sensitive brain regions, LTP seems to be an important substrate for kindling—or, for that matter, for any epileptogenic mechanism.

Of particular interest in this regard are a pair of recent findings that bear upon potentiationlike effects that can be induced by experiences not uncommon for the immature CNS. Crepel et al. (1993), studying LTP in adult animals, found that brief periods of anoxia produce an LTP of NMDA responses in slice tissue. Jensen et al. (1991) found that immature animals which have been subjected to brief hypoxic episodes are more seizure-prone as they mature (Jensen et al., 1993). Taken together, these data suggest that trauma in the immature CNS, under certain conditions, can lead to a significant upregulation of excitatory synaptic interactions, which in turn could provide a basis for later seizure susceptibility.

Seizure-Induced Plastic Changes

Why should we, as developmental neurobiologists and pediatric epileptologists, be interested in such phenomena as LTP and kindling? Certainly they represent a form of plasticity, but the processes are as apparent in the adult CNS as in the immature brain. True, they appear to depend on a number of transmitter and neuromodulatory factors that are involved in developmental plasticity—but these factors are also involved in normal, mature CNS function (Table 9-1). One significant reason for interest in these processes in the immature CNS revolves around the issue of whether and/or how seizures themselves induce plastic changes in the brain. This issue becomes particularly important given the high degree of plasticity of the developing central nervous system. The concern is that aberrant long-term changes in CNS function may result from *apparently* benign—but abnormal—early experiences. Therefore, an important question is whether seizures can induce alterations in normal neuronal structure and function. A related question is whether epilepsy and epilepsy-related brain damage are "progressive" processes that can arise from relatively subtle plastic changes in of the immature nervous system. Do repeated seizures arising from a particular focus in the brain lead to development of additional seizure foci (secondary epileptogenesis) or generalization of seizure activity (secondary generalization)? Although some clinical observations argue against such dangers (see Chapter 1), there remains unsettling doubt.

Seizure generalization is a common occurrence; in a large percentage of clinical cases a focal epileptic lesion triggers generalized seizure activity that engulfs the entire brain (see Chapters 1 and 2). It is unclear, however, if generalization depends on pathological changes over widespread regions of the brain (perhaps as a result of a "kindling"-like process), or whether secondary generalization reflects normal CNS properties. This issue is of considerable importance, especially in trying to analyze seizure types that characterize the immature brain—some of which initially appear to be focal, but which can become more generalized as the brain matures. Does such generalized activity require an initiation point, some abnormal but heretofore hidden "lesion," which provides the initial drive for the seizure? A number of experimental approaches have been used to investigate the ideas of secondary epileptogenesis and secondary "sensitivity" to seizures. In early experiments, Morrell et al. (1975) reported the development of secondary (and even tertiary) seizure foci, presumably as a result of bombardment of normal tissue by discharge from the primary focus. However, in the monkey alumina cream model, contralateral "foci" were shown to disappear when the primary epileptogenic zone was removed, thus failing to support the notion that *independent* foci were established as a result of a chronically discharging cortex (Harris and Lockard, 1981). Such studies leave it unclear whether abnormal projections to a relatively normal brain region can ultimately result in pathology (Morrell, 1985). This issue is especially important in thinking about tissue in which synaptic contact number, pattern, and strength appear so dependent on activity and transmitter release (see above).

This phenomenon of secondary epileptogenesis is seen in the kindling model, where electrical activity induces an afterdischarge from a primary site (e.g., the amygdala). Repeated afterdischarges in this primary site lead, in turn, to propagated seizure activity into connected regions (e.g., the hippocampus). Cellular and synaptic alterations in the "secondary" sites have been demonstrated, suggesting that the secondary sites might play critical roles in supporting the induced epilepsy. Changes in synaptic inhibition (Oliver and Miller, 1985), in the NMDA component in the excitatory synaptic potential (Fig. 9-6A; Mody et al., 1988), in the flux of calcium across affected cell membranes (Fig. 9-6B; Mody et al., 1990), and in cell sensitivity to exogenously applied potassium (King et al., 1985) have all been reported in the hippocampus of kindled animals. One might argue that the hippocampus in these experiments does not really assume the role of a "secondary focus," since it does not discharge independently in this kindling model. It is worth noting, however, that kindling susceptibility can be conferred upon (or discouraged in) structures that were not the primary site of the initial kindling procedures. The "transference" of susceptibility leads to increased sensitivity in distant regions (Racine, 1978), such that the animal can be kindled from these sites much more quickly than from the same regions in animals that had not previously received kindling stimulations.

The evidence that an initially restricted discharging "focus" can give rise to additional areas of hyperexcitability is somewhat alarming, especially given that "benign" epilepsy syndromes are relatively common in young children (see Chapters 1 and 10). Do such seizures have significant long-term consequences? Can surrounding regions of the immature human brain be "kindled" as in experimental animal models? Evidence that kindling occurs in humans is controversial, and kindling clearly becomes more difficult to demonstrate as one looks higher on the phylogenetic tree (Moshé and Ludvig, 1988). However, ease of kindling (similar to likelihood of seizures) is significantly greater in immature than in mature rat brain (Moshé et al., 1991; Moshé, Shinnar, and Swann, Chapter 2). Thus the increased possibility of secondary epileptogenesis in the developing nervous system cannot be ignored (Moshé and Shinnar, 1993). One can argue regarding this potential danger. On the one hand, there appears to be enhanced plasticity in the immature brain, and (at least in some regions) an exuberant profusion of

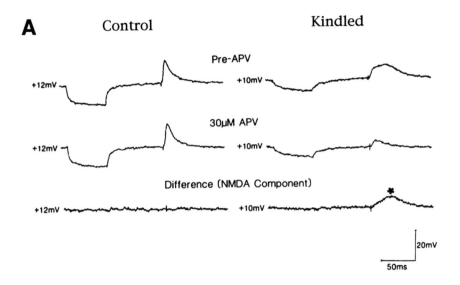

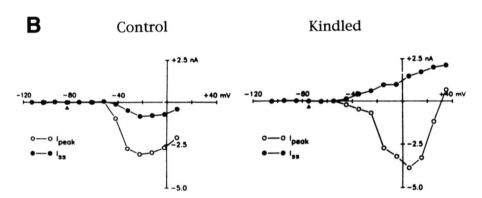

Figure 9-6. (A) Effects of kindling on NMDA contribution to the EPSP in the perforant path-to-granule cell synapse of adult rat. In the control animal, the APV-sensitive component of the EPSP (i.e., the component mediated by the NMDA receptor) is not evident (as shown in the result of subtraction of the two upper traces). Following kindling, there is a signficant increase in the APV-sensitive component of the EPSP (asterisk in the difference trace). (Reproduced with permission from Mody et al., 1988.)

(B) In parallel to this change in NMDA contribution to the EPSP, there is a kindling-induced change in the inward voltage-dependent calcium current seen in hippocampal granule cells. Voltage-clamp studies show a larger peak (transient) inward current, and the absence of a steady state (ss) inward current (actually, a net outward current) following kindling; these changes are not seen when the cell is injected with a calcium chelator. (Reproduced with permission from Mody et al., 1990.)

connections that would encourage spread of activity (see Chapter 8). Further, as indicated previously, inhibitory synaptic mechanisms appear relatively late in development, and LTP-like phenomena are known to be facilitated by the reduction of $GABA_A$-mediated inhibition. Thus a number of factors coalesce in the immature brain to encourage secondary epileptogenic processes. On the other hand, the capacity of individual neurons to discharge (particularly to generate repetitive activities) and fidelity of fiber connections (including speed of discharge and synchrony of output) are reduced in the immature brain compared to the adult (Gutnick et al., 1982; Schwartz-kroin, 1982); thus the repetitive nature of the "input" and the synchrony of associated afferents may be insufficient to support LTP-like plasticity in the immature CNS.

Postseizure Damage and Repair

There has been relatively little experimental work done on the effects of seizures on the immature brain and the capacity of the immature CNS to compensate for and/or repair damage induced by seizures. We know that in the adult CNS high levels of electrical activity such as seizures can induce a variety of changes, including cell damage and death, receptor modifications, induction of mRNA expression for neurotrophic factors, sprouting of axonal collaterals and establishment of new receptors, and development of new cell-to-cell connections. On the basis of the adult literature, it would appear that seizures can damage—or at least alter—the brain. Interestingly, there is evidence that pathologies produced by seizure activity in the adult do not occur (or are much milder) in the immature CNS (see Chapter 10). Experimentally induced seizure damage and reorganization—for example, as produced in the kainate model, where the drug selectively destroys hippocampal CA_3 and hilar cells and induces mossy fiber sprouting—is not easily produced in the immature animal (Sperber et al., 1991), although this treatment does cause seizures in rats as young as 1 day postnatal. Similarly, in a genetic model of generalized seizures, Qiao and Noebels (1993) found that seizure activity precedes mossy fiber sprouting during development. Other experimental models of seizures in the immature rat have also been relatively benign, at least in terms of the associated structural damage and long-term consequences for increased seizure susceptibility (Holmes and Thompson, 1988; Okada et al., 1984; Stafstrom et al., 1992).

Despite these data, the prospect of seizure-induced damage in the immature brain—or damage produced by other means which can then lead to seizure activity—remains a concern. Recent studies of kainate-induced seizure activity in young rats suggest that mossy fiber sprouting—a dramatic example of the brain's plasticity—contributes to the development of *chronic* seizure activity via feedback excitation (Mathern et al., 1993). Such experimental results are consistent with recently accumulated data from the brains of adult temporal lobe epilepsy patients (undergoing surgery for intractable seizures) that suggest that mossy fiber sprouting is more pronounced in individuals in which seizures started at a very early age (Isokawa et al., 1993). Other structural abnormalities associated with seizures have also been found in the immature CNS (Walsh, Chapter 5). For example, regions of ectopic neurons, cell loss, or neuronal disorganization have been found in human neocortical and hippocampal tissues from individuals with seizures of very early onset (Chugani et al., 1990; Houser, 1990). Similar structural abnormalities have been identified in a number of animal model systems, inbred to produce abnormal neuronal discharge patterns (Farias et al., 1992; Ribak et al., 1993) or treated early in development to produce such pathoanatomic lesions (Rosen et al., 1992). Some of these animal models have spontaneous seizures or have low seizure thresholds (e.g., genetically epilepsy-prone rats, seizure-sensitive gerbils); in some cases, however, seizures are not characteristic. It remains unclear which, if any, of these early structural abnormalities are seizure-related—either for early-onset epilepsies or for later developing syndromes.

A variety of contrasting seizure-associated phenomena have been described in mature brain, but the relevance of these observations for the developing CNS is still unclear. For example, studies suggest that one of the more obvious changes associated with seizures in the mature brain involves an astrocytic reaction. Indeed, reactive gliosis has been identified in tissue from both experimental and human epileptic brain (Ward, 1978). Given the relatively slow glial development in the mammalian CNS, the reactive gliosis process may not play a significant role in immature seizures. However, the paucity of glia may itself be a key to the seizure susceptibility in immature brain. If glia do play an important role in ion buffering, transmitter uptake, and related processes (Dietzel et al., 1989; Walz, 1989) in normal mature CNS, then their relative absence in the immature brain leaves the system vulnerable to significant perturbations. This absence may be especially important given the apparently slower rate of neuronal ion exchanger mechanisms and general metabolic activity in the immature than the mature CNS (Holtzman and Olson, 1983). However, the immature brain appears to be well adapted to deal with traumatic challenges and to remain viable under conditions that would have devastating consequences in the adult (Jensen et al., 1993).

Another major effect of seizures reported in the literature is the loss of fine dendritic processes and dendritic spines (Isokawa et al., 1993). There is little evidence, however, that seizure activity in the immature mammalian brain leads to such loss. Experimental studies, particularly those from the alumina monkey focus, suggest that chronic seizures give rise to selective damage of GABAergic neurons (Ribak et al., 1986), a change that would certainly have dire consequences for mature as well as developing central nervous structures. However, the histopathology of human epileptic brain samples, especially as now detailed with various immunocytochemical methods, fails to support the idea of selective GABAergic neuron damage (Babb et al., 1989). There do appear to be identifiable cell populations that are more vulnerable than others to various types of epileptogenic insult, but the "generic" GABAergic interneuron—especially those cells colocalizing parvalbumin (Sloviter et al., 1991)—appears to be relatively spared. In the hippocampus, temporal lobe seizures have been associated with specific loss of mossy cells and somatostatin/NPY-containing neurons (which colocalize GABA), as well as CA_1 pyramidal cells (de Lanerolle et al., 1989). The hilar cell loss is mimicked by perforant path stimulation in animal models of epileptogenesis (Sloviter, 1987), suggesting that the cells are sensitive to high levels of synaptic input. The CA_1 cells also appear to be targeted in models of ischemic brain damage (Pulsinelli et al., 1982; Smith et al., 1984); their sensitivity in epileptic brain perhaps reflects unmet energy demands in these cells.

However, the patterns of epileptic (and ischemic) damage in immature brain are quite different; there is relative sparing of CA_1, and enhanced vulnerability of granule cells (Schwartz et al., 1992; see Chapter 10). It is interesting to note that cells in the hilus receive their major afferent input relatively late in development (Ribak et al., 1985) and that immature animals may therefore escape excitotoxic hilar cell damage due to a paucity of excitatory inputs to these neurons. Consistent with this theme, models of hypoxia/ischemia have generally shown considerably less damage in immature tissue than in the mature CNS. This relative "protection" of immature neurons seems somewhat paradoxical in light of current interest in the toxic effects of rises in intracellular calcium. If, as suggested, the enhanced plasticity of the immature system results at least in part from enhanced mechanisms for calcium influx (and/or intracellular release) and slower kinetics for intracellular calcium buffering, then one might expect greater vulnerability in the immature neurons in response to "excitotoxic" insult. Why these immature neurons are not exquisitely sensitive to damage-inducing stimuli remains to be determined. What *is* clear, given such different results from "identical" challenges in mature and immature CNS, is that there must be different processes underlying cell vulnerability and viability in the immature brain.

Early Intervention

Within the context of the mature CNS, there is now evidence for both seizure-induced damage and "plastic" alterations (whether they be appropriate repairs or aberrant responses) in reaction to that damage. If such changes occur in the immature brain, there are reasons to fear that the effects will be significant and long lasting. Thus an important clinical issue to be faced is whether seizure activity requires early intervention in the developing human brain. A variety of approaches—pharmacologic and surgical—have been proposed for early intervention.

Examples of, and rationales for, pharmacologic intervention in young children—for example, for absence seizure activity—have been discussed by other authors in this volume. There are a number of immature seizure types, however, that are particularly intriguing with respect to current treatments (see Chapter 1). Infantile spasms (or West syndrome) present at a very early stage of development and often involve generalized seizure activity covering large portions of the infant's brain. The underlying basis for the seizure activity is unclear, but investigators have empirically discovered one relatively effective treatment—the administration of ACTH (Aicardi, 1986; Baram, 1993; Hrachovy and Frost, 1989). Why this drug treatment should be effective, even in a subset of these young patients, is not clear. It is intriguing to note, however, that the adrenal steroid hormone–ACTH axis appears to be critically involved in modulation of normal cell structure in developing cortical regions (see above). Developmental effects of adrenal steroids, gonadal steroids, and thyroid hormone include support of cortical dendrites and spines (Gould et al., 1991; McEwen, Coirini et al., 1991) and of cell division and survival (particularly for the dentate granule cells) (Gould et al., 1992; Sloviter et al., 1992). One might conjecture that a naturally occurring developmental paucity (or overabundance, or imbalance) of such support factors could give rise to widespread regions of subtle structural abnormality.

Unfortunately, in many cases ACTH treatment is not effective. In such children, there may be no currently identified drug or modulatory agent that adequately controls these devastating seizures. Left unchecked, the seizures may spontaneously disappear, or they may lead to a CNS which is seriously compromised, for example, by severe mental retardation (Shields et al., 1992a). It is unclear whether the seizures themselves produce such devastating consequences or whether the underlying basis for the seizures is responsible for the behavioral or intellectual outcome. One glimpse into this issue is provided by the results of early surgical intervention, where removal of a significant portion of the infant's cortex results not only in seizure amelioration, but in a more normal developmental outcome (Shields et al., 1992b, 1993). These results suggest that under certain conditions, unchecked seizure activity in the young brain may have dire consequences, and that drastic measures are sometimes warranted to block ongoing seizures. The clinical—and basic science—challenge is to determine which cases are likely to recede spontaneously and/or produce no long-lasting behavioral or structural changes, and which are likely to remain and lead to abnormal developmental profiles. In many infantile seizure syndromes, the activity is apparently generalized and widespread. Although surgery cannot be restricted to discrete identifiable focal areas, new imaging technologies are able to provide lateralizing and regional guidance to identify the most abnormal brain regions (Chugani et al., 1990). That such surgical intervention is possible speaks to the great plasticity of the immature central nervous system. Indeed, surgical intervention for medically intractable seizures in children may have its best results (with respect to the behavior and psychosocial integration of the developing individual) when it is carried out in the very young child. Unfortunately, the optimal age for such interventions is still often unclear.

The surgeon now faces a considerable dilemma. On the one hand, there are conceptual and empirical bases for removing an offending epileptogenic region as quickly as possible. On the other hand, the evidence is relatively poor that immature seizure activity per se will lead to identifiable structural damage, although certain types of seizures may have severe consequences (Moshé and Shinnar, 1993). Since surgical resections have significantly better outcome when carried out on immature tissue, when "plasticity" can compensate for the effects of tissue removal, a decision about surgery often must be made before one can determine whether the syndrome will remit spontaneously. In severe cases surgical resection may be the only way to alleviate an ongoing and constant state of intolerable CNS activity. Given the absence of other effective treatments, the surgeries appear relatively attractive. Still to be evaluated, however, is the long-term effectiveness of such surgeries for reducing or preventing seizure activity in the nervous systems of such individuals. Given the dependence of these surgeries on the immature brain's innate plasticity, the possibility remains of abnormal reorganization following these gross resections.

References

Aicardi, J. (1986) *Epilepsy in Children.* New York: Raven Press, pp. 17–38.

Artola, A., Bröcher, S., and Singer, W. (1990) Different voltage-dependent thresholds for inducing long-term depression and long-term potentiation in slices of rat visual cortex. *Nature 347:69–72.*

Artola, A., and Singer, W. (1987) Long-term potentiation and NMDA receptors in rat visual cortex. *Nature 330:649–652.*

Attardi, D. G., and Sperry, R. W. (1963) Preferential selection of central pathways by regenerating optic fibers. *Exp. Neurol. 7:46–64.*

Babb, T. L. Pretorious, J. K., Kupfer, W. R., and Crandall, P. H. (1989) Glutamate decarboxylase–immunoreactive neurons are preserved in human epileptic hippocampus. *J. Neurosci. 9:2562–2574.*

Baram, T. Z. (1993) Pathophysiology of massive infantile spasms: Perspective on the putative role of brain adrenal axis. *Ann. Neurol. 33:231–236.*

Bashir, Z. I., Borolotto, Z. A., Davies, C. H., Beretta, N., Irving, A. J., Seal, A. J., Henley, J. M., Jane, D. E., Watkins, J. C., and Collingridge, G. L. (1993) Induction of LTP in the hippocampus needs synaptic activation of glutamate metabotropic receptors. *Nature 363:347–349.*

Baumbach, H. D., and Chow, K. L. (1981) Visuocortical epileptiform discharges in rabbits: Differential effects on neuronal development in the lateral geniculate nucleus and superior colliculus. *Brain Res. 209:61–76.*

Bear, M. F., and Singer, W. (1986) Modulation of visual cortical plasticity by acetylcholine and noradrenaline. *Nature 320:172–176.*

Ben-Ari, Y., Cherubini, E., Corradetti, R., and Gaiarsa, J.-L. (1989) Giant synaptic potentials in immature rat CA_3 hippocampal neurones. *J. Physiol. 416:303–325.*

Ben-Ari, Y., Cherubini, E., and Krnjevic, K. (1988) Changes in voltage dependence of NMDA currents during development. *Neurosci. Lett. 94:88–92.*

Bergey, G. K., Fitzgerald, S. C., Schrier, B. K., and Nelson, P. G. (1981) Neuronal maturation in mammalian cell culture is dependent on spontaneous electrical activity. *Brain Res. 207*:49–58.

Blakemore, C., and Cooper, G. F. (1970) Development of the brain depends on the visual environment. *Nature 228*:477–478.

Bliss, T. V. P., and Lømo, T. (1973) Long-lasting potentiation of synaptic transmission in the dentate area of the anesthetized rabbit following stimulation of the perforant path. *J. Physiol. 232*:331–356.

Borgens, R. B., Roederer, E., and Cohen, M. J. (1981) Enhanced spinal cord regeneration in lamprey by applied electric fields. *Science 213*:611–617.

Bowe, M. A., and Nadler, J. V. (1990) Developmental increase in the sensitivity to magnesium of NMDA receptors on CA_1 hippocampal pyramidal cells. *Dev. Brain Res. 56*:55–61.

Bröcher, S., Artola, A., and Singer, W. (1992a) Agonists of cholinergic and noradrenergic receptors facilitate synergistically the induction of long-term potentiation in slices of rat visual cortex. *Brain Res. 573*:27–36.

Bröcher, S., Artola, A., and Singer, W. (1992b) Intracellular injection of Ca^{2+} chelators blocks induction of long-term depression in rat visual cortex. *Proc. Natl. Acad. Sci. 89*:123–127.

Burgard, E. C., and Hablitz, J. J. (1993) Developmental changes in NMDA and non-NMDA receptor-mediated synaptic potentials in rat neocortex. *J. Neurophysiol. 69*:230–240.

Cain, D. P. (1989) Long-term potentiation and kindling: How similar are the mechanisms? *TINS 12*:6–10.

Cherubini, E., Gaiarsa, J. L., and Ben-Ari, Y. (1991) GABA: An excitatory neurotransmitter in early postnatal life. *TINS 14*:515–519.

Chugani, H. T., Shields, W. D., Shewmon, D. A., Sankar, R., Chen, B. C., and Phelps, M. E. (1990) Infantile spasms: I. PET identifies focal cortical dysgenesis in cryptogenic cases for surgical treatment. *Ann. Neurol. 27*:406–413.

Cline, H. T., and Constantine-Paton, M. (1990) NMDA receptor agonist and antagonists alter retinal ganglion cell arbor structure in the developing frog retinotectal projection. *J. Neurosci. 10*:1197–1216.

Collingridge, G. L., Kehl, S. J., and McLennan, H. (1983) Excitatory amino acids in synaptic transmission in the Schaffer collateral-commissural pathway of the rat hippocampus. *J. Physiol. 334*:33–46.

Connor, J. A., Tseng, H.-Y., and Hockberger, P. E. (1987) Depolarization- and transmitter-induced changes in intracellular Ca^{2+} of rat cerebellar granule cells in explant cultures. *J. Neurosci. 7*:1384–1400.

Connors, B. W., Benardo, L. S., and Prince, D. A. (1983) Coupling between neurons of the developing rat neocortex. *J. Neurosci. 3*:773–782.

Constantine-Paton, M., Cline, H. T., and Debski, E. (1990) Patterned activity, synaptic convergence, and the NMDA receptor in developing visual pathways. *Ann. Rev. Neurosci. 13*:129–154.

Cornell-Bell, A. H., Thomas, P. G., and Smith, S. J. (1990) The excitatory neurotransmitter glutamate causes filopodia formation in cultured hippocampal astrocytes. *Glia 3*:322–334.

Crabtree, J. W., Ostrach, L. H., Campbell, B. G., and Chow, K. L. (1983) Long-term effects of early cortical epileptiform activity on development of visuocortical receptive fields in the rabbit. *Dev. Brain Res. 8*:1–9.

Crepel, V., Hammond, C., Krnjevic, K., Chinestra, P., and Ben-Ari, Y. (1993) Anoxia-induced LTP of isolated NMDA receptor-mediated synaptic responses. *J. Neurophysiol. 69:*1774–1778.

De Lanerolle, N. C., Kim, J. H., Robbins, R. J., and Spencer, D. D. (1989) Hippocampal interneuron loss and plasticity in human temporal lobe epilepsy. *Brain Res. 495:*387–395.

Diamond, M. C. (1967) Extensive cortical depth measurements and neuron size increases in the cortex of environmentally enriched rats. *J. Comp. Neurol. 131:*357–364.

Dietzel, I., Heinemann, U., and Lux, H. D. (1989) Relations between slow extracellular potential changes, glial potassium buffering, and electrolyte and cellular volume changes during neuronal hyperactivity in cat brain. *Glia 2:*25–44.

Dingledine, R., Hume, R. I., and Heinemann, S. F. (1992) Structural determinants of barium permeation and rectification in non-NMDA glutamate receptor channels. *J. Neurosci. 12:*4080–4087.

Dodd, J., and Jessell, T. M. (1988) Axon guidance and the patterning of neuronal projections in vertebrates. *Science 242:*692–699.

Dudek, S. M., and Bear, M. F. (1992) Homosynaptic long-term depression in area CA_1 of hippocampus and effects of N-methyl-D-aspartate receptor blockade. *Proc. Natl. Acad. Sci. 89:*4363–4367.

Dugich-Djordjevic, M. M., Tocco, G., Willoughby, D. A., Najm, I., Pasinetti, G., Thompson, R. F., Baudry, M., Lapchak, P. A., and Hefti, F. (1992) BDNF mRNA expression in the developing rat brain following kainic acid-induced seizure activity. *Neuron 8:*1127–1138.

Ernfors, P., Merlio, J.-P., and Persson, H. (1993) Cells expressing mRNA for neurotrophins and their receptors during embryonic rat development. *Eur. J. Neurosci. 4:*1140–1158.

Farias, P. A., Low, S. Q., Peterson, G. M., and Ribak, C. E. (1992) Morphological evidence for altered synaptic organization and structure in the hippocampal formation of seizure-sensitive gerbils. *Hippocampus 2:*229–246.

Finger, S., and Stein, D. G. (eds.) (1982) *Brain Damage and Recovery.* London: Academic Press.

Gall, C., and Lauterborn, J. (1992) The dentate gyrus: A model system for studies of neurotrophin regulation. In C. E. Ribak, C. M. Gall, and I. Mody (eds.), *The Dentate Gyrus and Its Role in Seizures.* Amsterdam: Elsevier Science Publishers, pp. 171–185.

Goodman, C. S., and Shatz, C. J. (1993) Developmental mechanisms that generate precise patterns of neuronal connectivity. *Cell 72* (Suppl.):77–98.

Gould, E., Cameron, H. A., Daniels, D. C., Woolley, C. S., and McEwen, B. S. (1992) Adrenal hormones suppress cell division in the adult rat dentate gyrus. *J. Neurosci. 12:*3642–3650.

Gould, E., Woolley, C. S., and McEwen, B. (1991) The hippocampal formation: Morphological changes induced by thyroid, gonadal and adrenal hormones. *Psychoneuroendocrinology 16:*67–84.

Greenough, W. T. (1976) Enduring brain effects of differential experience and training. In M. R. Rosenzweig and E. L. Bennett (eds.), *Neural Mechanisms of Learning and Memory.* Cambridge, Mass.: MIT Press, pp. 255–278.

Grover, L. M., and Teyler, T. J. (1992) N-methyl-D-aspartate receptor-independent long-term potentiation in area CA_1 of rat hippocampus: Input-specific induction and preclusion in a non-tetanized pathway. *Neuroscience 49:*7–11.

Gutnick, M. J., Connors, B. W., and Prince, D. A. (1982) Mechanisms of neocortical epileptogenesis in vitro. *J. Neurophysiol. 48:*1321–1335.

Hallböök, F., Ibáñez, C. F., Ebendal, T., and Persson, H. (1993) Cellular localization of brain-derived neurotrophic factor and neurotrophin-3 mRNA expression in the early chicken embryo. *Eur. J. Neurosci. 5:*1–14.

Harris, A. B., and Lockard, J. S. (1981) Absence of seizures or mirror foci in experimental epilepsy after excision of alumina and astrogliotic scar. *Epilepsia 22:*107–122.

Harris, K. M., and Teyler, T. J. (1984) Developmental onset of long-term potentiation in area CA_1 of the rat hippocampus. *J. Physiol. 346:*27–48.

Henderson, T. A., Woolsey, T. A., and Joaquin, M. F. (1992) Infraorbital nerve blockade from birth does not disrupt central trigeminal pattern formation in the rat. *Dev. Brain Res. 66:*146–152.

Hesse, G. W., and Teyler, T. J. (1976) Reversible loss of hippocampal long-term potentiation following electroconvulsive seizures. *Nature 264:*562–564.

Hestrin, S. (1992) Developmental regulation of NMDA receptor-mediated synaptic currents at a central synapse. *Nature 357:*686–689.

Hockberger, P. E., Tseng, H.-Y., and Connor, J. A. (1989) Development of rat cerebellar Purkinje cells: Electrophysiological properties following acute isolation and in long-term culture. *J. Neurosci. 9:*2258–2271.

Holmes, G. L., and Thompson, J. L. (1988) Effects of kainic acid on seizure susceptibility in the developing brain. *Dev. Brain Res. 39:*51–59.

Holtzman, D., and Olson, J. (1983) Developmental changes in brain cellular energy metabolism in relation to seizures and their sequelae. In H. H. Jasper and N. M. Van Gelder (eds.), *Basic Mechanisms of Neuronal Hyperexcitability.* New York: Alan R. Liss, pp. 423–449.

Hopkins, W. F., and Johnston, D. (1984) Frequency-dependent noradrenergic modulation of long-term potentiation in hippocampus. *Science 226:*350–351.

Houser, C. R. (1990) Granule cell dispersion in the dentate gyrus of humans with temporal lobe epilepsy. *Brain Res. 535:*195–204.

Hrachovy, R. A., and Frost, J. D. (1989) Infantile spasms: A disorder of the developing nervous system. In P. Kellaway and J. L. Noebels (eds.), *Problems and Concepts in Developmental Neurophysiology.* Baltimore: Johns Hopkins University Press, pp. 131–147.

Hubel, D. H., and Wiesel, T. N. (1970) The period of susceptibility to the physiological effects of unilateral eye closure in kittens. *J. Physiol. 206:*419–436.

Isokawa, M., Levesque, M. F., Babb, T. L., and Engel, J., Jr. (1993) Single mossy fiber axonal systems of human dentate granule cells studied in hippocampal slices from patients with temporal lobe epilepsy. *J. Neurosci. 13:*1511–1522.

Jacobson, M., and Baker, R. E. (1969) Development of neuronal connections with skin grafts in frogs: Behavioral and electrophysiological studies. *J. Comp. Neurol. 137:*121–142.

Janigro, D., and Schwartzkroin, P. A. (1988) Effects of GABA and baclofen on pyramidal cells in the developing rabbit hippocampus: An "in vitro" study. *Dev. Brain Res. 41:*171–184.

Jensen, F., Tsuji, M., Offutt, M., Firkusny, I., and Holtzman, D. (1993) Profound, reversible energy loss in the hypoxic immature rat brain. *Dev. Brain Res. 73:*99–105.

Jensen, F. E., Applegate, C. D., Burchfield, J. L., and Lombroso, C. T. (1991) Dif-

ferential effects of perinatal hypoxia and anoxia on long term seizure susceptibility in the rat. *Life Sci. 49:*399–407.

Jessell, T. M. (1988) Adhesion molecules and the hierarchy of neural development.
*Neuron 1:*3–13.

Kamphuis, W., Monyer, H., De Rijk, T. C., and Lopes da Silva, F. H. (1992) Hippocampal kindling increases the expression of glutamate receptor-A Flip and
-B Flip mRNA in dentate granule cells. *Neurosci. Lett. 148:*51–54.

Kasamatsu, T., and Pettigrew, J. D. (1979) Preservation of binocularity after monocular deprivation in the striate cortex of kittens treated with 6-hydroxydopa-
mine. *J. Comp. Neurol. 185:*139–162.

Kasamatsu, T., Pettigrew, J. D., and Ary, M.-L. (1979) Restoration of visual cortical
plasticity by local microperfusion of norepinephrine. *J. Comp. Neurol.
185:*163–182.

Kato, N., Artola, A., and Singer, W. (1991) Developmental changes in the susceptibility to long-term potentiation of neurones in rate visual cortex slices. *Dev.
Brain Res. 60:*45–50.

Kennard, M. A. (1942) Cortical reorganization of motor function: Studies on a set of
monkeys of various ages from infancy to maturity. *Arch. Neurol. Psych.
48:*227–240.

Killisch, I., Dotti, C. G., Laurie, D. J., Luddens, H., and Seeburg, P. H. (1991)
Expression patterns of $GABA_A$ receptor subtypes in developing hippocampal
neurons. *Neuron 7:*927–936.

King, G. L., Dingledine, R., Giacchino, J. L., and McNamara, J. O. (1985) Abnormal
neuronal excitability in hippocampal slices from kindled rats. *J. Neurophysiol.
54:*1295–1304.

Köhler, M., Burnashev, N., Sakmann, B., and Seeburg, P. H. (1993) Determinants
of Ca^{2+} permeability in both TM1 and TM2 of high affinity kainate receptor
channels: Diversity by RNA editing. *Neuron 10:*491–500.

Kriegstein, A. R., Suppes, T., and Prince, D. A. (1987) Cellular and synaptic physiology and epileptogenesis of developing rat neocortical neurons in vitro. *Dev.
Brain Res. 34:*161–171.

Laurie, D. J., Wisden, W., and Seeburg, P. H. (1992) The distribution of 13 $GABA_A$
receptor subunit mRNAs in the rat brain: III. Embryonic and postnatal development. *J. Neurosci. 12:*4151–4172.

Lipton, S. A., and Kater, S. B. (1989) Neurotransmitter regulation of neuronal outgrowth, plasticity and survival. *TINS 12:*265–270.

Lo, Y.-J., and Poo, M.-M. (1991) Activity-dependent synaptic competition in vitro:
Heterosynaptic suppression of developing synapses. *Science 254:*1019–1022.

Lo Turco, J. J., and Kriegstein, A. R. (1991) Clusters of coupled neuroblasts in embryonic neocortex. *Science 252:*563–566.

Lohof, A. M., Ip, N. Y., and Poo, M.-M. (1993) Potentiation of developing neuromuscular synapses by the neurotrophins NT-3 and BDNF. *Nature 363:*350–
353.

Luhmann, H. J., and Prince, D. A. (1991) Postnatal maturation of the GABAergic
system in rat neocortex. *J. Neurophysiol. 65:*247–263.

Madison, D. V., Malenka, R. C., and Nicoll, R. A. (1991) Mechanisms underlying
long-term potentiation of synaptic transmission. *Ann. Rev. Neurosci. 14:*379–
397.

Maisonpierre, B. C., Belluscio, L., Friedman, B., Alderson, R. F., Wiegand, S. J.,
Furth, M. E., Lindsay, R. M., and Yancopoulous, G. D. (1990) NT-3, BDNF

and NGF in the developing rat nervous system: Parallel as well as reciprocal patterns of expression. *Neuron 5:*501–509.

Mathern, G. W., Cifuentes, F., Leite, J. P., Pretorious, J. K., and Babb, T. L. (1993) Hippocampal EEG excitability and chronic spontaneous seizures are associated with aberrant synaptic reorganization in the rat intrahippocampal kainate model. *Electroenceph. Clin. Neurophysiol. 87:*326–339.

Mattson, M. P., and Kater, S. B. (1989) Excitatory and inhibitory neurotransmitters in the generation and degeneration of hippocampal neuroarchitecture. *Brain Res. 478:*337–348.

Mattson, M. P., Lee, R. E., Adams, M. E., Guthrie, P. B., and Kater, S. B. (1988) Interactions between entorhinal axons and target hippocampal neurons: A role for glutamate in the development of hippocampal circuitry. *Neuron 1:*865–876.

Mattson, M. P., Murrain, M., Guthrie, P. B., and Kater, S. B. (1989) Fibroblast growth factor and glutamate: Opposing roles in the generation and degeneration of hippocampal neuroarchitecture. *J. Neurosci. 9:*3728–3740.

McEwen, B. S., Angulo, J., Cameron, H., Caho, H. M., Daniels, D., Gannon, M. N., Gould, E., Mendelson, S., Sakai, R., Spencer, R., and Woolley, C. (1991) Paradoxical effects of adrenal steroids on the brain: Protection versus degeneration. *Biol. Psychiatr. 31:*177–199.

McEwen, B. S., Coirini, H., Westlind-Danielsson, A., Frankfurt, M., Gould, E., Schumacher, M., and Woolley, C. (1991) Steroid hormones as mediators of neural plasticity. *J. Steroid Biochem. Molec. Biol. 39:*223–232.

Meister, M., Wong, R. O. L., Baylor, D. A., and Shatz, C. J. (1991) Synchronous bursts of action potentials in ganglion cells of the developing mammalian retina. *Science 252:*939–943.

Milner, B. (1974) Sparing of language functions after early unrelated brain damage. In E. Eidelberg and D. G. Stein (eds.), *Functional Recovery after Lesions of the Nervous System: Neuroscience Research Program Bulletin,* Vol 12. Cambridge, Mass: MIT Press, pp. 213–216.

Minakami, R., Hirose, E., Yoshioka, K., Yoshimura, R., Misumi, Y., Sakaki, Y., Tohyama, M., Kiyama, H., and Sugiyama, H. (1992) Postnatal development of mRNA specific for a metabotropic glutamate receptor in the rat brain. *Neurosci. Res. 15:*58–63.

Mody, I., Reynolds, J. N., Salter, M. W., Carlen, P. L., and MacDonald, J. F. (1990) Kindling-induced epilepsy alters calcium currents in granule cells of rat hippocampal slices. *Brain Res. 531:*88–94.

Mody, I., Stanton, P. K., and Heinemann, U. (1988) Activation of *N*-methyl-D-aspartate receptors parallels changes in cellular and synaptic properties of dentate gyrus granule cells after kindling. *J. Neurophysiol. 59:*1033–1054.

Monyer, H., Seeburg, P. H., and Wisden, W. (1991) Glutamate-operated channels: Developmentally early and mature forms arise by alternative splicing. *Neuron 6:*799–810.

Moore, S. D., Barr, D. S., and Wilson, W. A. (1993) Seizure-like activity disrupts LTP in vitro. *Neurosci. Lett. 163:*117–119.

Morrell, F. (1985) Secondary epileptogenesis in man. *Arch. Neurol. 42:*318–335.

Morrell, F., Tsuru, N., Hoeppner, T. J., Morgan, D., and Harrison, W. H. (1975) Secondary epileptogenesis in the frog forebrain: Effect of inhibition of protein synthesis. *Can. J. Neurol. Sci. 2:*407–416.

Moshé, S. L., and Ludvig, N. (1988) Kindling. In T. A. Pedley and B. S. Meldrum (eds.), *Recent Advances in Epilepsy*. New York: Churchill Livingstone, pp. 21–44.

Moshé, S. L., and Shinnar, S. (1993) Early intervention. In J. Engel, Jr. (ed.), *Surgical Treatment of the Epilepsies*. New York: Raven Press, pp. 123–132.

Moshé, S. L., Sperber, E. F., and Albala, B. J. (1991) Kindling as a model of epilepsy in developing animals. In F. Morrell (ed.), *Kindling and Synaptic Plasticity: The Legacy of Graham Goddard*. Boston: Birkhauser, pp. 177–194.

Mueller, A. L., Taube, J. S., and Schwartzkroin, P. A. (1984) Development of hyperpolarizing inhibitory postsynaptic potentials and hyperpolarizing response to gamma-aminobutyric acid in rabbit hippocampus studied in vitro. *J. Neurosci. 4:*860–867.

Mulkey, R. M., and Malenka, R. C. (1992) Mechanisms underlying induction of homosynaptic long-term depression in area CA_1 of the hippocampus. *Neuron 9:*967–975.

Müller, M., Gähwiler, B. H., Rietschin, L., and Thompson, S. L. (1993) Reversible loss of dendritic spines and altered excitability after chronic epilepsy in hippocampal slice cultures. *Proc. Natl. Acad. Sci. 90:*257–261.

Murakami, F., Song, W.-J., and Katsumaru, H. (1993) Plasticity of neuronal connections in developing brains of mammals. *Neurosci. Res. 15:*235–253.

Nelson, P. G., Yu, C., Fields, R. D., and Neale, E. A. (1989) Synaptic connections in vitro: Modulation of number and efficacy by electrical activity. *Science 244:*585–587.

Okada, R., Moshé, S. L., and Albala, B. J. (1984) Infantile status epilepticus and future seizure susceptibility in the rat. *Dev. Brain Res. 15:*177–183.

O'Leary, D. D. M., and Koester, S. E. (1993) Development of projection neuron types, axon pathways, and patterned connections of the mammalian cortex. *Neuron 10:*991–1006.

Oliver, M. W., and Miller, J. J. (1985) Alterations of inhibitory processes in the dentate gyrus following kindling-induced epilepsy. *Exp. Brain Res. 57:*443–447.

Patterson, P. H. (1988) On the importance of being inhibited, or saying no to growth cones. *Neuron 1:*263–267.

Patterson, S. L., Grover, L. M., Schwartzkroin, P. A., and Bothwell, M. (1992) Activity dependent neurotrophin expression in rat hippocampal slices: A stimulus paradigm inducing LTP in CA_1 evokes increases in BDNF and NT-3 mRNAs. *Neuron 9:*1081–1088.

Peinado, A., Yuste, R., and Katz, L. C. (1993) Extensive dye coupling between rat neocortical neurons during the period of circuit formation. *Neuron 10:*103–114.

Pellegrini-Giampietro, D. E., Bennett, M. V. L., and Zukin, R. S. (1991) Differential expression of three glutamate receptor genes in developing brain: An in situ hybridization study. *Proc. Natl. Acad. Sci. 88:*4157–4161.

Pellegrini-Giampietro, D. E., Bennett, M. V. L., and Zukin, R. S. (1992) Are Ca^{2+} permeable kainate/AMPA receptors more abundant in immature brain? *Neurosci. Lett. 144:*65–69.

Perkins, A. T., IV, and Teyler, T. J. (1988) A critical period for long-term potentiation in the developing rat visual cortex. *Brain Res. 439:*222–229.

Pulsinelli, W. A., Brierley, J. B., and Plum, F. (1982) Temporal profile of neuronal damage in a model of transient forebrain ischemia. *Ann. Neurol. 11:*491–498.

Purves, D., and Lichtman, J. W. (1985) *Principles of Neural Development*. Sunderland, Mass.: Sinauer Associates, pp. 251–267.

Qiao, X., and Noebels, J. L. (1993) Developmental analysis of hippocampal mossy fiber outgrowth in a mutant mouse with inherited spike-wave seizures. *J. Neurosci. 13:*4622–4635.

Racine, R. (1978) Kindling: The first decade. *Neurosurgery 3:*234–252.

Rami, A., Patel, A. J., and Rabié, A. (1986) Thyroid hormone and development of the rat hippocampus: Morphological alterations in granule and pyramidal cells. *Neuroscience 19:*1217–1226.

Reichardt, L. F., and Tomaselli, K. J. (1991) Extracellular matrix molecules and their receptors: Functions in neural development. *Ann. Rev. Neurosci. 14:*531–570.

Ribak, C. E., Hunt, C. A., Bakay, R. A. E., and Oertel, W. H. (1986) A decrease in the number of GABAergic somata is associated with the preferential loss of GABAergic terminals at epileptic foci. *Brain Res. 363:*78–90.

Ribak, C. E., Lauterborn, J. C., Navetta, M. S., and Gall, C. M. (1993) The inferior colliculus of GEPRs contains greater numbers of cells that express glutamate decarboxylase (GAD_{67}) mRNA. *Epilepsy Res. 14:*105–113.

Ribak, C. E., Seress, L., and Amaral, D. G. (1985) The development, ultrastructure and synaptic connections of the mossy cells of the dentate gyrus. *J. Neurocytol. 14:*835–857.

Rocamora, N., Garcia-Ladona, F. J., Palacios, J. M., and Mengod, G. (1993) Differential expression of brain-derived neurotrophic factor, neurotrophin-3, and low-affinity nerve growth factor receptor during the postnatal development of the rat cerebellar system. *Mol. Brain Res. 17:*1–8.

Rosen, G. D., Sherman, G. F., Richman, J. M., Stone, J. V., and Galaburda, A. M. (1992) Induction of molecular layer ectopias by puncture wounds in newborn rats and mice. *Dev. Brain Res. 67:*285–291.

Rovira, C., and Ben-Ari, Y. (1991) Benzodiazepines do not potentiate GABA responses in neonatal hippocampal neurons. *Neurosci. Lett. 130:*157–161.

Rubel, E. W., and Hyson, R. L. (1992) Afferent influences on brain stem auditory system development. *Brain Dysfunction 5:*65–93.

Rutishauser, U., and Jessell, T. M. (1988) Cell adhesion molecules in vertebrate neural development. *Physiol. Rev. 68:*819–857.

Sarvey, J. M. (1988) Protein synthesis in long-term potentiation and norepinephrine-induced long-lasting potentiation in hippocampus. In P. W. Landfield and S. A. Deadwyler (eds.), *Long-Term Potentiation: From Biophysics to Behavior.* New York: Alan R. Liss, pp. 329–353.

Schlaggar, B. L., Fox, K., and O'Leary, D. D. M. (1993) Postsynaptic control of plasticity in developing somatosensory cortex. *Nature 364:*623–626.

Schwab, M. E., and Caroni, P. (1988) Oligodendrocytes and CNS myelin are nonpermissive substrates for neurite growth and fibroblast spreading in vitro. *J. Neurosci. 8:*2381–2393.

Schwartz, P. H., Massarweh, W. F., Vinters, H. V., and Wasterlin, C. G. (1992) A rat model of severe neonatal hypoxic-ischemic brain injury. *Stroke 23:*539–546.

Schwartzkroin, P. A. (1982) Development of rabbit hippocampus: Physiology. *Dev. Brain Res. 2:*469–486.

Seeburg, P. H. (1993) The molecular biology of mammalian glutamate receptor channels. *TINS 16:*359–365.

Shatz, C. J., and Stryker, M. P. (1988) Prenatal tetrodotoxin infusion blocks segregation of retinogeniculate afferents. *Science 242:*87–89.

Shields, W. D., Duchowny, M. S., and Holmes, G. L. (1993) Surgically remediable syndromes of infancy and early childhood. In J. Engel, Jr. (ed.), *Surgical Treatment of the Epilepsies*. New York: Raven Press, pp. 35–48.

Shields, W. D., Shewmon, D. A., Chugani, H. T., and Peacock, W. J. (1992a) Treatment of infantile spasms: Medical or surgical? *Epilepsia 33* (Suppl.):26–31.

Shields, W. D., Shewmon, D. A., Chugani, H. T., and Peacock, W. J. (1992b) The role of surgery in the treatment of infantile spasms. *J. Epilepsy 3* (Suppl.):321–324.

Shoepp, D. D., and Conn, P. J. (1993) Metabotropic glutamate receptors in brain function and pathology. *TIPS 14:*13–20.

Sillito, A. M. (1975) The contribution of inhibitory mechanisms to the receptive field properties of neurones in the striate cortex of the cat. *J. Physiol. 250:*305–309.

Simon, D. K., Prusky, G. T., O'Leary, D. D. M., and Constantine-Paton, M. (1993) N-methyl-D-aspartate receptor antagonists disrupt the formation of a mammalian neural map. *Proc. Natl. Acad. Sci. 89:*10593–10597.

Sloviter, R. S. (1987) Decreased hippocampal inhibition and a selective loss of interneurons in experimental epilepsy. *Science 235:*73–76.

Sloviter, R. S., Sollas, A. L., Barbaro, N. M., and Laxer, K. D. (1991) Calcium-binding protein (Calbindin-D28K) and parvalbumin immunocytochemistry in the normal and epileptic human hippocampus. *J. Comp. Neurol. 308:*381–396.

Sloviter, R. S., Sollas, A. L., Dean, E., and Neubort, S. (1992) Adrenalectomy-induced granule cell degeneration in the rat hippocampal dentate gyrus: Characterization of an in vivo model of controlled neuronal death. *J. Comp. Neurol. 330:*324–336.

Smith, M.-L., Auer, R. N., and Siesjo, B. K. (1984) The density and distribution of ischemic brain injury in the rat following 2–10 minutes of forebrain ischemia. *Acta Neuropathol. 64:*319–332.

Sperber, E. F., Haas, K. Z., Stanton, P. K., and Moshé, S. L. (1991) Resistance of the immature hippocampus to seizure-induced synaptic reorganization. *Dev. Brain Res. 60:*89–93.

Sperry, R. W. (1963) Chemoaffinity in the orderly growth of nerve fiber pattern and connections. *Proc. Natl. Acad. Sci. 50:*703–710.

Sretavan, D. W., Shatz, C. J., and Stryker, M. P. (1988) Modification of retinal ganglion cell axon morphology by prenatal infusion of tetrodotoxin. *Nature 336:*468–471.

Stafstrom, C. E., Thompson, J. L., and Holmes, G. L. (1992) Kainic acid seizures in the developing brain: Status epilepticus and spontaneous recurrent seizures. *Dev. Brain Res. 65:*227–236.

Stryker, M. P., and Harris, W. A. (1986) Binocular impulse blockade prevents the formation of ocular dominance columns in cat visual cortex. *J. Neurosci. 6:*2117–2133.

Stryker, M. P., and Sherk, H. (1975) Modification of cortical orientation selectivity in the cat by restricted visual experience: A re-examination. *Science 190:*904–905.

Sutula, T., and Steward, O. (1986) Quantitative analysis of synaptic potentiation during kindling of the perforant path. *J. Neurophysiol. 56:*732–746.

Sutula, T., and Steward, O. (1987) Facilitation of kindling by prior induction of long-term potentiation in the perforant path. *Brain Res. 420:*109–117.

Taira, E., Takaha, N., and Miki, N. (1993) Extracellular matrix proteins with neurite promoting activity and their receptors. *Neurosci. Res. 17:*1–8.

Tremblay, E., Roisin, M. P., Represa, A., Charriaut-Marlangue, C., and Ben-Ari, Y. (1988) Transient increased density of NMDA binding sites in the developing rat hippocampus. *Brain Res. 461:*393–396.

Tsumoto, T. (1993) Long-term depression in cerebral cortex: A possible substrate of "forgetting" that should not be forgotten. *Neurosci. Res. 16:*263–270.

Velísek, L., Moshé, S. L., and Stanton, P. K. (1993) Age dependence of homosynaptic non-NMDA mediated long-term depression in field CA$_1$ of rat hippocampal slices. *Dev. Brain Res. 75:*253–260.

Walsh, C., and Cepko, C. L. (1992) Widespread dispersion of neuronal clones across functional regions of the cerebral cortex. *Science 255:*434–439.

Walz, W. (1989) Role of glial cells in the regulation of the brain ion microenvironment. *Progr. Neurobiol. 33:*309–333.

Ward, A. A. (1978) Glia and epilepsy. In E. Schoffeniels, G. Franck, L. Hertz, and D. B. Tower (eds.), *Dynamic Properties of Glial Cells.* New York: Pergamon, pp. 413–427.

White, C. A., Esguerra, M., and Sur, M. (1992) Electrophysiological properties of developing neurons recorded in slices of ferret LGN. *Neurosci. Abstr. 18:*923.

Wigstrom, H., and Gustafsson, B. (1985) Facilitation of hippocampal long-lasting potentiation by GABA antagonists. *Acta Physiol. Scand. 125:*159–172.

Williams, K., Russell, S. L., Shen, Y. M., and Molinoff, P. B. (1993) Developmental switch in the expression of NMDA receptors occurs in vivo and in vitro. *Neuron 10:*267–278.

Woolley, C. S., and McEwen, B. S. (1992) Estradiol mediates fluctuation in hippocampal synapse density during the estrous cycle in the adult rat. *J. Neurosci. 12:*2549–2554.

Xie, X., and Smart, T. G. (1991) A physiological role for endogenous zinc in rat hippocampal synaptic neurotransmission. *Nature 349:*521–524.

Yoon, M. G. (1973) Retention of the original topographic polarity by the 180° rotated tectal reimplant in young adult goldfish. *J. Physiol. 233:*575–588.

Yuste, R., and Katz, L. C. (1991) Control of postsynaptic Ca^{2+} influx in developing neocortex by excitatory and inhibitory neurotransmitters. *Neuron 6:*334–344.

Zhang, J.-H., Sato, M., Araki, T., and Tohyama, M. (1993) Postnatal ontogenesis of neurons containing GABA$_A$ α1 subunit mRNA in the rat forebrain. *Mol. Brain Res. 16:*193–203.

Zheng, F., and Gallagher, J. P. (1992) Metabotropic glutamate receptors are required for the induction of long-term potentiation. *Neuron 9:*163–172.

10

Seizure-Induced Changes in the Immature Brain

RAMAN SANKAR
CLAUDE G. WASTERLAIN
ELLEN S. SPERBER

Do seizures cause brain damage? Are seizures themselves an expression of brain damage, or are they an independent result of the illness that caused the damage? Studies in adult animals have shown that severe seizures can cause hippocampal damage (Bekenstein and Lothman, 1993; Nadler et al., 1978; Sloviter, 1987), which in turn results in chronic epilepsy (Lothman and Bertram, 1993; Mello et al., 1993; Shirasaka et al., 1994). A similar conclusion has been drawn from epidemiological studies on the outcome of status epilepticus in adult patients (Bone, 1993; Treiman, 1993). Regarding the immature brain, there is no such agreement among clinical researchers and basic scientists. Several studies in developing animals indicate that status epilepticus does not cause hippocampal damage in the immature brain (until the third or fourth week of life in the rat) (Albala et al., 1984; Holmes and Thompson, 1988; Nitecka et al., 1984; Sperber, 1992), although some extra-hippocampal damage may be seen. At the clinical level, early retrospective studies indicate that status epilepticus in children may have severe consequences (Aicardi and Chevrie, 1970) and that even mild seizures may produce small decreases in intellectual performance (Schiottz-Christensen and Bruhn, 1973). More recent clinical studies, performed in a prospective fashion, suggest that sequelae of status epilepticus may not be as devastating as previously thought (Dunn et al., 1988; Maytal et al., 1989). The differences in outcome may be due to wide divergences in the definition, diagnosis, and treatment for seizures, as documented in Wasterlain and Vert's (1990) survey of clinical practices in leading hospitals. Further, the study of seizure-induced damage in the immature brain is confounded by the fact that it is often difficult to distinguish the developmental disturbance or disease which caused the seizures from the deterioration in development caused by the epileptic condition itself. An additional complication is that patients are invariably treated with drugs that can themselves alter neural development (see Holmes, 1991, for review).

Despite these complications, it is reasonable to expect the impact of seizures on the developing brain to be a function of the type and severity of the seizures, as well as of the developmental stage of the brain when seizures (and/or epilepsy) occur. In this chapter we will discuss the often controversial data from both human and animal studies on the possible detrimental effects of seizures in the developing brain.

Human Studies

The available clinical data came from retrospective and prospective studies of neurological outcome following neonatal seizures and status epilepticus (SE) in children, as well as studies involving certain classic childhood syndromes such as febrile seizures, infantile spasms (ISs), and Lennox-Gastaut syndrome (LGS).

Neonatal Seizures

Outcome studies reveal a dramatic decline in the mortality rates for neonatal seizures, from 40 percent before 1969 to 15 percent for patients studied between 1969 and 1985 (Volpe, 1986). This change is presumably due to the increased aggressiveness with which such seizures are treated in modern neurologic facilities. In separate studies Bergman et al. (1983) and Lombroso (1983) found that approximately 50 percent of infants who experienced neonatal seizures had a normal outcome with only minor neurologic abnormalities. Bergman et al. found that although the seizure frequency and neonatal mortality associated with seizures were greatest in very premature infants, the outcome in premature infants who survived was similar to that of the term infants.

These studies indicated that the major prognostic factor for outcome is the underlying disease. This conclusion has been supported by the many studies attempting to correlate prognosis with EEG signs. In several of these studies (Holmes et al., 1982; Rose and Lombroso, 1970; Rowe et al., 1985; Watanabe et al., 1980) EEG background activity proved to be a much better predictor of outcome than the epileptiform abnormalities (e.g., focal spikes or sharp waves) per se. In general, poor prognosis was associated with an EEG background of electrocerebral inactivity, low voltage, or a burst suppression pattern. The correlation of poor neurologic outcome with certain seizure types (tonic, myoclonic, or subtle) in premature infants (Holden et al., 1982; Knauss and Marshall, 1977; Lombroso, 1983; Watanabe et al., 1982) is also consistent with the view that etiology of neonatal seizures may be the best predictor of outcome.

A number of other studies have supported this position (André et al., 1990). For example, seizures caused by isolated or transient metabolic abnormalities such as hypocalcemia or hypoglycemia have relatively favorable outcomes (Holmes, 1987) compared to those caused by developmental brain abnormalities or hypoxic-ischemic encephalopathy. The importance of the underlying etiology may also be reflected in recent studies which included only neonatal seizures confirmed by EEG. Those patients with severe neonatal insults had particularly bad outcomes. Of these patients only 30 percent developed normally in one study (Scher et al., 1989); other investigators found that 56 percent of the patients developed postnatal epilepsy (Clancy and Legido, 1991; Legido et al., 1991).

Status Epilepticus

The pioneering studies by Aicardi and Chevrie (1970) emphasized the poor outcome of patients who suffered status epilepticus early in life. Their retrospective study of 239 cases of SE in patients under 15 years of age showed that mental deterioration followed SE in 114 patients (48 percent). Since 78 of these 114 children had developed normally prior to the first bout of SE, their mental deterioration was attributed to the SE. This study was the first to suggest that prolonged convulsions appeared to be more devastating in babies than in older children. However, the higher incidence and severity of SE in young children may reflect the greater frequency of organic brain damage and symptomatic epilepsy in this age group (Lennox, 1960; Van den Berg and Yerushalmy, 1969). In their report, Aicardi and Chevrie emphasized that the number of cases of SE with unknown origin may have been inflated due to the limitations of the available methodology.

It is important to separate the acute sequelae following SE from those consequences that appear with longer latency. Acute sequelae, such as hippocampal damage (Corsellis and Bruton, 1983) and hemiatropha cerebri as a result of unilateral SE (Aicardi, 1986a; Aicardi and Baraton, 1971) may reflect an illness such as Rasmussen encephalitis. Concerning long-term outcomes, the recent studies of Dunn (1988) and Maytal et al. (1989) yielded virtually identical results. Both studies emphasized that outcome was related to SE etiology and that the age at the time of onset of SE was a minor factor. Both found neurologic sequelae mainly in symptomatic SE cases but not in idiopathic or febrile SE. Finally, both reports found (in partially prospective studies) that in the absence of an acute neurologic insult or a progressive neurologic disorder, the morbidity is low in children with aggressively treated SE.

There are important differences between the retrospective study of Ai-cardi and Chevrie (1970) and the study of Maytal et al. (1989). The former study was based on patients with SE examined between the years 1961 and 1968, several of whom were seen in small community hospitals where modern intensive care methods were unavailable; the latter study dealt with patients with SE seen between 1985 and 1987 in an urban, academic medical center, where modern treatment techniques were used. Further, the definition of SE used by Aicardi and Chevrie involved convulsions lasting more than 1 hour or a series of convulsions without return of consciousness for the same time; the more recent study by Maytal et al. used 30 minutes as the criterion duration, and only 26 percent of the patients had seizures lasting for more than 1 hour. It is likely, then, that the difference in SE outcome reported by the two studies reflects, at least in part, improvements in management strategies in recent years. Modern standards of aggressive treatment of SE probably shorten the duration of SE, and also better maintain perfusion, oxygenation, and euglycemia during and after the SE.

Dodrill and Wilensky (1990) summarized the 13 available studies of intellectual impairment as an outcome of SE. Their review reveals that SE is most common in the first 5 years of life, particularly before 2 years of age. They point out that all the studies that showed adverse consequences of SE on intellectual function were retrospective, whereas prospective studies (Dunn, 1988; Ellenberg and Nelson, 1978) did not show detrimental effects of SE on mental ability. However, Dodrill and Wilensky warned that few studies employed standardized psychological assessments (beyond an IQ test) and that the extent of the impairment resulting from SE may therefore be underestimated. Furthermore, they found that early studies tended to reveal greater mental deficits and morbidity than more recent studies, again reflecting the improvement resulting from more aggressive recent treatment of SE.

Febrile Seizures

The possibility of an etiologic connection between prolonged febrile seizures and subsequent development of complex partial seizures (CPSs) was first suggested by Falconer et al. (1964; Falconer, 1971), after reviewing patients who had undergone unilateral temporal lobectomy for intractable CPSs of temporal lobe origin. They found that a history of prolonged febrile seizures occurring between the ages of 6 months and 4 years occurred significantly more often in patients with CPS including mesial temporal sclerosis (MTS) than in CPS patients free of the MTS lesion. This result led to the hypothesis that febrile seizures result in selective neuronal damage leading to MTS. However, more recent studies (Hauser and Kurland, 1975; Lee et al., 1981) have not supported this hypothesis. Further, it appears that the types of epilepsy that develop in children after febrile seizures do not differ from those seen in children without a history of febrile seizures (Sofijanov et al., 1983;.Tsuboi, 1984).

The benign nature of simple febrile seizures is no longer in question; the preponderance of evidence does not support an etiologic role of febrile seizures in MTS. However, the prognosis of severe seizures triggered by fever, and the effect of such severe seizures on intellectual and brain development, is still disputed. The detrimental effect of febrile seizures on intellectual development appears controversial, however, only when data from retrospective studies are compared to data from prospective studies. Retrospective studies tend to be hindered by lack of information regarding neurologic functioning prior to the febrile seizure. Schiottz-Christensen and Bruhn (1973) evaluated behavior and scholastic achievement in twins discordant for febrile convulsions. They found a small deficit in psychologic functioning in those children who had seizures; among monozygous twins there was a significant difference in the Wechsler scale (performance IQ difference of 7 points). The National Institute of Neurological and Communicative Disorders and Stroke Collaborative Perinatal Project (NCPP) found no significant difference between the mean full-scale IQ of children who had experienced a febrile seizure and their normal siblings (Ellenberg and Nelson, 1978). Similar results had been reported by studies in Great Britain, where children with febrile convulsions did as well as the remainder of the population in school performance at 7 and 11 years of age (Ross et al., 1980). Another longitudinal study (Verity et al., 1985) examined the effect of febrile seizures on head circumference, intelligence, and behavior by following 303 children with febrile seizures until age 5. The children with febrile seizures were not found to differ from their peers in any of those parameters.

Infantile Spasms and Lennox-Gastaut Syndrome

These two distinctive childhood epileptic syndromes are considered to be catastrophic epilepsies of childhood. Both these syndromes are development-specific, and the seizures are the result of a wide variety of abnormalities. As in other seizure disorders, the prognosis appears to be related to the underlying etiology.

Long-term follow-up studies of children with infantile spasms have suggested that the prognosis is related to both the cause of seizures and the efficacy of seizure control (Fois et al., 1984; Riikonen, 1982). The neurologic sequelae may also be related to the seizures themselves. Investigators have argued that the progressive intellectual decline seen in association with infantile spasms results from the epileptic disturbance; their evidence is based on observations of dramatic developmental improvement following resective surgery of widespread, but lateralized, areas of cortical dysgenesis (Chugani et al., 1993; Shields, 1991). Initial results of such surgery indicated that in some cases there is cessation of seizures following surgery and resumption of a relatively normal developmental pattern. In Aicardi's (1986b) study of patients with the Lennox-Gastaut syndrome, mental retardation was present from the onset in 20–60 percent of the patients. The percentage of patients with mental retardation increased over time of illness, to 75–90 percent (Chevrie and Aicardi, 1972). This change is viewed as clinical evidence of marked deterioration in many children with this syndrome, including changes in children who had early periods of normal development. However, mental deterioration as a result of the syndrome is particularly difficult to define in this population, since these children tend to be treated with high doses of antiepileptic drugs.

Effect of Childhood Seizures on the Hippocampus

In an early study on brain damage associated with seizures, Norman (1964) described the hippocampi of a group of children, aged 1–6 years, who died during status epilepticus. All brains showed extensive cellular damage (pyknotic nuclei, eosinophilic cytoplasm) in CA_1 (Sommer sector) and most had changes in the end folium (CA_3 and dentate hilus); most showed, in addition, extrahippocampal damage (in thalamus, amygdala, striatum, and cerebellum). Corsellis and Bruton (1983) also found hippocampal lesions (and extrahippocampal damage) in the brains of patients who died in infancy during or shortly after status epilepticus. The acute changes differed from hippocampal sclerosis in the absence of scar tissue and atrophy. While the damage seen in such studies was clearly associated with the episodes of status epilepticus, no data are available to distinguish direct effects of seizures from effects of associated events such as hypoxia and hypotension. More recent retrospective clinical reports with histopathologic data suggest that there may be an association between seizures in early childhood and secondary hippocampal damage. Sagar and Oxbury (1987) found significantly lower than normal neuron counts in the hippocampal field CA_1, end folium, and the dentate gyrus (DG) of the resected temporal lobes of patients who had their first convulsion before the age of 3 years. Most of these patients had a first convulsion that was longer than 30 minutes or had experienced repetitive convulsions during the first day.

Represa et al. (1989) performed quantitative autoradiography to study high-affinity binding sites for kainate in the postmortem hippocampal specimens from epileptic children and from children who died without evidence of neurologic disease. The density of kainate binding sites was used as an estimate of the density of mossy fiber terminals in the stratum lucidum, and the pyramidal layers of CA_3, and in the supragranular layer of fascia dentata. Even though there was no evidence of hippocampal cell loss in this study, significantly increased binding was seen in the hippocampi of epileptic children, especially in the CA_3 field. This result provides evidence for the occurrence of neural "plasticity" in the human epileptic brain, even in the apparent absence of histologic lesions. The authors remarked on the possibility that the establishment of new connections may contribute to the hyperexcitability of the epileptic hippocampus.

Studies at UCLA on surgically resected hippocampi from children aged 5.5 months to 11.5 years with intractable seizures have revealed evidence of cell loss in the fascia dentate and aberrant mossy fiber sprouting into the inner molecular layer of the fascia dentata (Mathern et al., 1994). Mossy fiber sprouting was identified by neo-Timm staining, and postnatal granule cell development was studied by immunohistochemical localization of the embryonic form of neural cell adhesion molecule (NCAM-H). The greatest expression of NCAM-H was observed in the resected hippocampi of children under 2 years, suggesting that, as in other mammalian species, granule cells are produced postnatally in immature human brains.

These data point out potentially significant differences between mature and immature hippocampus; given such differences, it is possible that the expression of seizure-induced damage in the immature brain has a pattern that is distinct from that of the mature brain which develops MTS.

Animal Studies

The connection between seizures, which may or may not include one or several episodes of SE, and the development of MTS is difficult to discern from retrospective clinical studies. Certainly it is impossible to determine from such studies the actual age at which seizures produced the observed damage. Limitations of these clinical studies include problems of controlling for the age of onset of the initial seizure, number of subsequent seizures, the duration of seizures, and the presence of prior brain damage. Animal studies are therefore essential for understanding seizure consequences.

The paucity of animal models that mimic developmental epilepsies in the human has been a major limitation to our ability to gain clear understanding of the type and extent of risk posed by epilepsy to the developing brain. In general, most animal studies deal with SE, rather than with chronic epilepsies. It is safe to say that there is no animal model of hippocampal epilepsy that matches an epileptic syndrome of childhood in terms of pathologic damage produced by the seizures. Issues of comparative otogeny, discussed in detail in Chapter 2, impose some restrictions on development of chronic experimental models in animals (especially in rats), in part because of the shorter period of their brain maturation. It is estimated that a 7- to 10-day-old rat may be equivalent in some respects to a newborn human infant (Gottlieb et al., 1977; Moshé, 1987; Moshé et al., 1992). However, different aspects of biochemical and neurophysiologic maturity may be reached anywhere from 4 to 6 weeks of age. Thus the rate of maturation of different anatomic, biochemical, and neurophysiologic processes in a rodent may not demonstrate congruency with human brain development. These different patterns of maturation further complicate comparisons between animal models and human developmental epilepsy syndromes.

The animal experiments discussed in this section pertain for the most part to SE or limbic epilepsy.

Effects of Seizures on the Hippocampus

Kainic acid (KA), an excitatory neurotoxin, is known to produce severe seizures and a pattern of hippocampal damage in adult rats similar to Ammon's horn sclerosis (AHS). The damage is most severe in the pyramidal cells of CA_3 and the hilus, followed by some damage to CA_1; the CA_2 pyramidal cells, the granule cells of the dentate gyrus, and the fibers en passage are spared (Lothman and Collins, 1981; Nadler et al., 1978). However, SE induced by systemic KA injection in *immature* rats does not appear to produce hippocampal damage (Albala et al., 1984; Holmes and Thompson, 1988; Holmes et al., 1988; Nitecka et al., 1984; Sperber et al., 1991), even though the immature rat brain is more likely to undergo SE and have more severe seizures than adult rats (Moshé et al., 1983; Okada et al., 1984).

Seizures induced by KA, kindling, pentylenetetrazol (PTZ), and repetitive stimulation of the perforant path result in sprouting of the mossy fibers of dentate granule cells to the supragranular layer of the fascia dentate in mature rats (Cronin and Dudek, 1988; Golari et al., 1992; Nadler et al., 1980; Sloviter, 1992; Sperber et al., 1991; Sutula et al., 1988; Tauck and Nadler, 1985). However, such synaptic reorganization has not been seen in 15-day-old rat pups following KA-induced SE (Figure 10-1) or kindling (Sperber et al., 1991). These data suggest that hippocampal pathology akin to AHS is age-dependent (Moshé, 1987) and may be less likely to occur during the neonatal period and early infancy (Albala et al., 1984; Holmes and Thompson 1988). However, this conclusion is complicated by the fact that the dose of KA used in the pups is lower than that used in most adult experiments (the adult dose is lethal to immature animals). Although experiments in pups and adults are not strictly comparable in terms of convulsant dose, both age groups experience SE. In fact, SE is more severe in pups than in adults (Albala et al., 1984). As in the immature rat, systemic KA-induced seizures in immature rabbits spare CA_3 pyramidal cells but produce damage in the CA_1 region (Franck and Schwartzkroin, 1984). It is possible that this difference between rat and rabbit reflects the species-specific rates of regional hippocampal maturation and/or a difference in species sensitivity to hypoxic-ischemic damage.

In addition to determining structural damage, it is important for animal model studies to test for *functional* consequences of seizures in the immature hippocampus. The physiologic paradigm involving determination of the dentate granule cell response to paired-pulse stimulation of the perforant path has been used to estimate functional inhibition in hippocampal slices from adult and 15-day-old rats following KA-induced SE (Sperber, Haas, and Moshé, 1992; Sperber et al., 1991). In slices of adult rats following KA-induced SE, paired-pulse stimulation revealed a loss of facilitation (i.e., relatively more inhibition) at 25–100 ms interpulse interval compared to controls (Fig. 10-2). In 15-day-old rats, however, KA-induced SE produced no such change; the dentate responses from these rats were identical to controls. This physiologic measure parallels the absence of morphologic damage in developing rats with KA-induced SE.

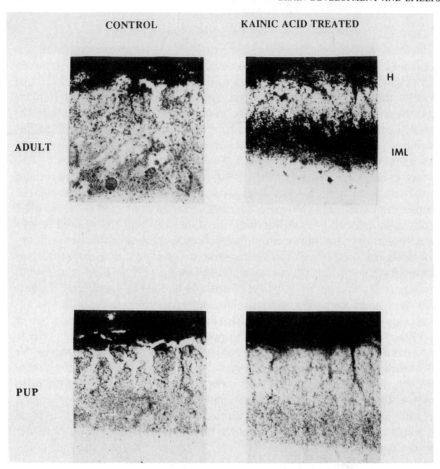

Figure 10-1. Kainic acid seizures produce age-related hippocampal damage. In adult rats, mossy fiber synaptic reorganization is extensive in the dentate gyrus following kainic acid seizures. Note the striking band of positive Timm staining in the inner molecular layer (IML) of the KA-treated adult rat as compared with the adult control animal, which shows Timm positivity only in the hilus (H). in contrast, 15-day-old rats that were exposed to kainic acid seizures show no mossy fiber synaptic reorganization in IML of the dentate gyrus (compared with age-matched control rats). (Reprinted with permission from Sperber et al., 1991.)

The explanation for this difference in response—and damage—between the mature and immature brain may be related to the late development of the kainic acid receptors (Campochiaro and Coyle, 1978). Although a recent study by Miller et al. (1990) examining both high- and low-affinity receptor sites demonstrated that KA receptors approximate adult density by 14 days of age in the dentate gyrus and CA_3, these data do not permit conclusions regarding structural and functional maturity of the receptors. Using in situ hybridization techniques, Pellegrini-Giampietro et al. (1991) showed unique

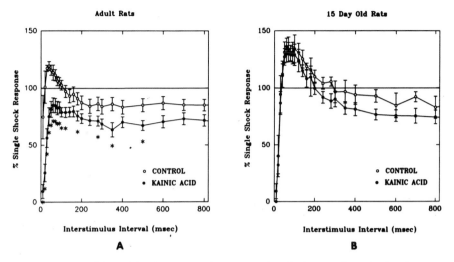

Figure 10-2. Kainic acid seizures produce age-related changes in paired-pulse per-forant path stimulation profiles. In adult control rats (A) an initial inhibition (0–20 ms) followed by excitation (25–200 ms) and then a late inhibition (200–800 ms) can be observed. Adult rats exposed to kainic acid seizures exhibit an enhancement of inhibition at all time intervals (25–500 ms). In contrast, 15-day-old rats (B) exposed to kainic acid had a triphasic profile that did not differ from controls. (Reproduced with permission from Sperber et al., 1991.)

developmental patterns in the mRNA expression of $GluR_1$, $GluR_2$, and $GluR_3$ subunits of the glutamate receptors in CA_1, CA_3, and dentate gyrus. Differences in receptor structure may be reflected in differences in receptor function, thus explaining (perhaps) the resistance of the immature hippocampus to damage.

It is noteworthy that age-related differences in the hippocampal response to seizures (e.g., cell loss, mossy fiber sprouting, and response of dentate granule cells to paired-pulse perforant path stimulation) occur in both KA-induced SE and kindling models (Sperber, Stanton, et al., 1992). Likewise, the hippocampal damage caused by pilocarpine-induced SE (Cavalheiro et al., 1987) and flurothyl-induced SE (Nevander et al., 1985; Sperber et al., 1991) appears to be age-dependent. These findings suggest that the lack of alterations in immature hippocampus after seizures is age-specific but not model-specific.

These results contrast with the lasting loss of inhibition in the paired-pulse stimulation paradigm seen in 14- to 16-day-old rats that have been sub-jected to sustained perforant path stimulation (Penix et al., 1994), a well-described model of SE in the adult rat (Sloviter, 1987, 1991). This loss of inhibition in young rats is associated with a histologic pattern that is quite different from that seen in the adult animals exposed to such stimulation. In the immature rat there is no damage to the pyramidal cells in the CA_3 field, but there is selective necrosis of some cells in the inner layers of stratum granulosum and of hilar neurons (Fig. 10-3). It has been hypothesized that the vulnerability of these cells in the inner layers of stratum granulosum is related to the ontogeny of the calcium binding protein calbindin D-28k (Goodman et al., 1993). Calbindin has been shown to protect CA_1 neurons in culture from glutamate-induced neurotoxicity (Baimbridge and Kao, 1988), and its expression in the dentate granule cells (Rami et al., 1987; Sloviter, 1992) coincides with the appearance of resistance to ischemia. The innermost layers of stratum granulosum are the last to show immunocytochemical evidence of calbindin presence; acquisition of calbindin-positivity in these cells coincides with a loss of their vulnerability to hypoxia-ischemia (Goodman et al., 1993).

The majority of the data from studies of seizure models in developing rats suggest that AHS is unlikely to result from seizures occurring during the perinatal period or very early in infancy. The experimental observations relevant to this issue are summarized in Table 10-1. Nevertheless, it is still quite possible that seizures in immature animals may have adverse effects on neurodevelopment.

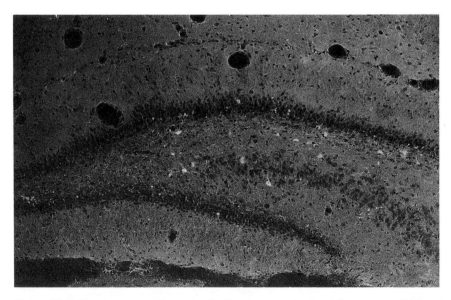

Figure 10-3. Dentate gyrus shows eosin fluorescence in necrotic neurons. This rat received 16 hours of ipsilateral perforant path stimulation under urethane anesthesia at the age of 15 days and was perfused-fixed with 4 percent paraformaldehyde 3 days later. Twenty-micrometer-thick cryostat sections were stained with hematoxylin-eosin. Under fluorescent light with a fluorescein filter, eosin in the cytoplasm of necrotic neurons fluoresced brightly. Most of the necrotic cells are hilar polymorphic or pyramidal-shaped neurons; a few are located in the granule cell layer. In this rat, the contralateral hippocampus showed no lesion.

TABLE 10-1. Summary of Animal Data on Seizures and Hippocampal Damage in the Developing Brain

Seizures Do Not Produce Damage	*Seizures Produce Damage*
KA → no hippocampal damage in rats (1–4)	KA → Damage to CA_1 in rabbits (5)
Flurothyl → no hippocampal damage (6)	Pilocarpine → extrahippocampal damage (7)
Pilocarpine → no hippocampal damage (7)	Prolonged perforant path stimulation → cell loss and loss of paired-pulse inhibition (9)
Kindling → no neuronal damage or mossy fiber sprouting (8)	
KA, kindling, flurothyl → no change in response to paired-pulse stimulation (3, 6, 8)	

Note: Numbers in parentheses indicate the following references:
1. Albala et al., 1984
2. Nitecka et al., 1984
3. Sperber et al., 1991
4. Holmes and Thompson, 1988
5. Franck and Schwartzkroin, 1984
6. Sperber, Haas, and Moshé, 1992
7. Cavalheiro et al., 1987
8. Sperber, Stanton, et al., 1992
9. Penix et al., 1994

Effect of Seizures on Behavior

In a study that subjected 10- and 25-day-old rats to KA-induced status epilepticus (de Feo et al., 1986) and followed them up to the age of 45 days, impairment of the ability to acquire conditioned avoidance responses in the shuttle-box situation was observed in both age groups. This long-term effect was interpreted as reflecting not SE but direct KA-induced damage to neocortical neurons, since PTZ-induced SE, equivalent in severity and duration, did not affect this learned behavior. Stafstrom et al. (1993) studied the effect of KA-induced SE in developing rats on their performance in three learning and memory tasks in adulthood. Their results showed that rats exposed to KA-induced SE at 5 and 10 days of age performed normally and did not have any hippocampal lesions; rats exposed to KA-induced SE at 20 days of age showed a deficit in one test and no hippocampal lesion; and older rats (30-day adults) had performance deficits in all three tests as well as hippocampal lesions. The data suggest that the detrimental effects of SE on performance are age-dependent; however, a correlation between behavioral deficit and seizure-induced cell loss is unclear. Indeed, these experiments also confirmed the results of previous studies (Holmes et al., 1988) showing that seizures in prepubescent animals (22–26 days) could produce behavioral deficits in the absence of obvious morphologic damage in hippocampus. On the basis of these studies, it remains unclear how to relate seizure-associated behavioral deficits with structural integrity in the brain.

Effect of Seizures on Brain Metabolism and Growth

The immature brain has unique metabolic adaptations to seizure activity. During epileptic seizures, the immature brain is protected by its lower metabolic rate, which in the newborn rat may be 10- to 20-fold lower than that of the adult (Vanucci and Duffy, 1975). The metabolic consequences of seizures in immature brain, although slower to develop, are similar to those associated with damage to the adult brain: depletion of energy reserves (Fujikawa et al., 1986); inhibition of protein synthesis (Dwyer and Wasterlain, 1984); and inhibition of DNA synthesis (Wasterlain, 1976). As a result, seizures may have to go on for hours in order to accumulate the same energy debt that might be reached within a fraction of that time in the adult. While starting from a lower baseline, cerebral energy use during seizures increases in the neonate as in the adult (Fujikawa et al., 1989). In some models of neonatal seizures, neocortical and hippocampal blood flow cannot keep up with metabolic demand (Fujikawa et al., 1986; Pereira et al., 1993). The immature blood–brain barrier has a limited capacity to transport glucose (Morin et al., 1988) and this capacity is severely taxed during seizures, which massively increase glycolytic rates (Dwyer and Wasterlain, 1985). Ketone bodies, which provide as much as one-third of the energy consumed by the brain of suckling mammals, cannot be utilized if seizures are accompanied by anoxia (Wasterlain et al., 1990). As a result, neonatal seizures can rapidly deplete cortical ATP (adenosine triphosphate) and cerebral energy reserves (Fujikawa et al., 1988).

The effect of hypoxia on the immature brain has been studied in vivo by ^{31}P NMR spectroscopy (Jensen et al., 1993). Hypoxia produced a severe but reversible reduction of phosphocreatine and nucleotide triphosphates during a particular developmental window (postnatal day 9–13). Thus during development there may be a specific period of vulnerability to relative hypoxia in terms of maintenance of energy stores. An earlier study by Jensen et al. (1992) demonstrated that hypoxia at this age resulted in a long-term increase in flurothyl seizure susceptibility. Although hypoxia was the primary insult in these studies, the results of these investigations highlight the possibility that seizure-induced hypoxia may be a mechanism by which seizures can injure the developing brain.

Neonatal seizures have been found to inhibit brain protein synthesis even if blood oxygenation is maintained (Dwyer and Wasterlain, 1984; Wasterlain, 1974). Such seizures also inhibit brain DNA synthesis (Wasterlain, 1976) and mitotic rates (Suga and Wasterlain, 1980). These effects are selective for brain regions that participate in seizure activity, while adjacent areas are unaffected (Dwyer and Wasterlain, 1984). In some experimental models severe seizures inhibit brain growth. Inhibition of protein and DNA synthesis could be expected to affect growth adversely, and indeed rats subjected to seizures at critical stages of development show evidence of reduced brain growth (Wasterlain, 1976) in the absence of any histologic lesions. If seizures are sufficiently prolonged or repetitive, these effects can be permanent (Wasterlain, 1976). These effects of seizures are age-specific in the rat; neonatal seizures reduce cell numbers, whereas later seizures reduce cell size, myelin markers, and synaptic markers (Wasterlain and Sankar, 1993). Some seizure types may alter the expression of the growth cone marker GAP-43 in immature rats (Fig. 10-4; Sankar et al., 1993), suggesting an effect on the plastic process important in the developing brain. There is no evidence to date that frequently repeated epileptiform discharges in children cause any of these more subtle effects.

Conclusion

In 1881 William Gowers stated that "seizures beget seizures." Recent studies of the adult brain suggest that Gowers was right. Experimental seizures can indeed induce hippocampal lesions, which in turn generate chronic epilepsy. In the immature brain, however, many types of experimental seizures fail to produce histologic lesions (or generate chronic epilepsy). We do not yet know whether the recent demonstration of neuronal necrosis in one

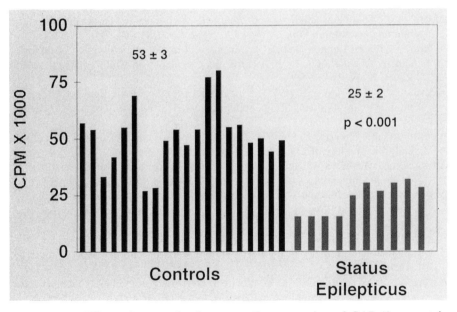

Figure 10-4. Effect of neonatal seizures on the expression of GAP-43, a protein marker of growth cones. Experimental rats were subjected to 2 hours of flurothyl seizures at the age of 4 days; littermate controls were handled the same way but received no flurothyl. Rats were sacrificed 2 days later, and proteins from the forebrain homogenates were separated by SDS-PAGE, transblotted onto nitrocellulose paper, incubated with a monoclonal antibody to GAP-43 then with a secondary antibody, and conjugated with ^{125}I-protein A. (Reproduced with permission from Sankar et al., 1993.)

model of SE in immature rats (Penix et al., 1994) represents a rare exception to that rule or an important clue to understanding when (and how) in development the rule applies. Deleterious effects of seizures on brain growth have been well-documented in young rodents but their relevance to human pathology remains unproven.

Although experimental data are compelling, there are several problems inherent in translating animal data into practical guidelines for the clinician. Critical seizure-sensitive periods of development have been identified in some animal models (see Chapter 2), but it is uncertain how these data apply to the developing human brain. It is perhaps fair to say that even if a preexisting lesion initiates seizures, recurrent or prolonged seizures may contribute to further deterioration. The value of Gowers's dictum appears to lie not so much in a simple and definitive answer to this important issue of seizure–damage interaction but rather in the enormous body of research it has generated. Our understanding of epilepsy, and of its impact on brain development, continues to increase as we focus on the complex relations between seizures and brain development.

References

Aicardi, J. (1986a) Consequences and prognosis of convulsive status epilepticus in infants and children. *Jpn. J. Psychol. Neurol. 40*:283–290.

Aicardi, J. (1986b) Lennox-Gastaut syndrome and myoclonic epilepsies of infancy and early childhood. In J. Aicardi (ed.), Epilepsy in Children. New York: Raven Press, pp. 39–65.

Aicardi, J., and Baraton, J. (1971) A pneumoencephalographic demonstration of brain atrophy following status epilepticus. *Dev. Med. Child. Neurol. 13*:660–667.

Aicardi, J., and Chevrie, J. J. (1970) Convulsive status epilepticus in infants and children: A study of 239 cases. *Epilepsia 11*:187–197.

Albala, B. J., Moshé, S. L., and Okada, R. (1984) Kainic acid-induced seizures: A developmental study. *Dev. Brain Res. 13*:139–148.

André, M., Matisse, N., and Vert, P. (1990) Prognosis of neonatal seizures. In C. G. Wasterlain and P. Vert (eds.), Neonatal Seizures. New York: Raven Press, pp. 61–67.

Baimbridge, K. G., and Kao, J. (1988) Calbindin D-28k protects against glutamate-induced neurotoxicity in rat CA1 pyramidal neuron cultures. *Soc. Neurosci. Abstr. 18*:1264.

Bekenstein, J. W., and Lothman, E. W. (1993) Dormancy of inhibitory interneurons in a model of temporal lobe epilepsy. *Science 259*:97–100.

Bergman, I., Painter, M. J., Hirsh, R. P., Crumrine, P. K., and David, R. (1983) Outcome in neonates with convulsions treated in an intensive care unit. *Ann. Neurol. 14*:642–647.

Bone, R. C. (1993) Treatment of status epilepticus: Epilepsy Foundation of America. *J. Am. Med. Assoc. 270*:854–859.

Campochiaro, P., and Coyle, J. T. (1978) Ontogenic development of kainate neurotoxicity: Correlates with glutamatergic innervation. *Proc. Natl. Acad. Sci. 75*:2025–2029.

Cavalheiro, L. A., Silva, D. F., Turski, W. A., Calderazzo-Filho, L. S., Bartolotto,

Z., and Turski, L. (1987) The susceptibility of rats to pilocarpine-induced seizures is age-dependent. *Dev. Brain Res. 37:*43–58.

Chevrie, J. J., and Aicardi, J. (1972) Childhood epileptic encephalopathy with slow spike-wave: A statistical study of 80 cases. *Epilepsia 13:*259–271.

Chugani, H. T., Shewmon, D. A., Shields, W. D., et al. (1993) Surgery for intractable infantile spasms: Neuroimaging perspectives. *Epilepsia 34:*764–771.

Clancy, R. R., and Legido, A. (1991) Postnatal epilepsy after EEG-confirmed neonatal seizures. *Epilepsia 32:*69–76.

Corsellis, J. A. N., and Bruton, C. J. (1983) Neuropathology of status epilepticus in humans. In A. V. Delgado-Escueta, C. G. Wasterlain, D. M. Treiman, R. J. Porter (eds.), Advances in Neurology, Vol. 34: Status Epilepticus. New York: Raven Press, pp. 129–139.

Cronin, J., and Dudek, F. E. (1988) Chronic seizures and collateral sprouting of dentate mossy fibers after kainic acid treatment in rats. *Brain Res. 474:*181–184.

De Feo, M. R., Mecarelli, O., Palladini, G., and Ricci, G. F. (1986) Long-term effects of early status epilepticus on the acquisition of conditioned avoidance behavior in rats. *Epilepsia 27:*476–482.

Dodrill, C. B., and Wilensky, A. J. (1990) Intellectual impairment as an outcome of status epilepticus. *Neurology 40* (Suppl. 2):23–27.

Dunn, D. W. (1988) Status epilepticus in children: Etiology, clinical features, and outcome. *J. Child. Neurol. 3:*167–173.

Dwyer, B. E., and Wasterlain, C. G. (1984) Selective focal inhibition of brain protein synthesis during generalized bicuculline seizures in newborn marmoset monkeys. *Brain Res. 308:*109–121.

Dwyer, B. E., and Wasterlain, C. G. (1985) Neonatal seizures in monkeys and rabbits: Brain glucose depletion in the face of normoglycemia, prevention by glucose loads. *Pediatr. Res. 19:*992–995.

Ellenberg, J. H., and Nelson, K. B. (1978) Febrile seizures and later intellectual performance. *Arch. Neurol. 35:*17–21.

Engel, J., Jr., and Shewmon, D. A. (1991) Impact of the kindling phenomenon on clinical epileptology. In F. Morrell (ed.), Kindling and Synaptic Plasticity. The Legacy of Graham Goddard. Boston: Birkhauser, pp. 195–210.

Falconer, M. A. (1971) Genetic and related aetiologic factors in temporal lobe epilepsy: A review. *Epilepsia 12:*13–31.

Falconer, M. A., Serafetindes, E. A., and Corsellis, J. A. N. (1964) Etiology and pathogenesis of temporal lobe epilepsy. *Arch. Neurol. 10:*233–248.

Fois, A., Malandrini, F., Balestri, P., and Giorgi, D. (1984) Infantile spasms: Long-term results of ACTH treatment. *Eur. J. Pediatr. 142:*51–55.

Franck, J. E., and Schwartzkroin, P. A. (1984) Immature rabbit hippocampus is damaged by systemic but not intraventricular kainic acid. *Dev. Brain Res. 13:*219–227.

Fujikawa, D. G., Dwyer, B. E., Lake, R. R., and Wasterlain, C. G. (1989) Local cerebral glucose utilization during status epilepticus in newborn primates. *Am. J. Physiol. 256 (Cell. Physiol. 25):*C1160–C1167.

Fujikawa, D. G., Dwyer, B. E., and Wasterlain, C. G. (1986) Preferential blood flow to brainstem during generalized seizures in the newborn marmoset monkey. *Brain Res. 397:*61–72.

Fujikawa, D. G., Vannucci, R. C., Dwyer, B. E., and Wasterlain, C. G. (1988) Generalized seizures deplete brain energy reserves in normoxemic newborn monkeys. *Brain Res. 454:*51–59.

Fujiwara, T., Ishida, S., Miyakoshi, M., et al. (1979) Status epilepticus in childhood: A retrospective study of initial convulsive status and subsequent epilepsies. *Folia Psychiatr. Neurol. Jpn. 33:*337–344.

Golari, G., Cavazos, G. E., and Sutula, T. P. (1992) Activation of dentate gyrus by pentylenetetrazol-evoked seizure-induced mossy fiber synaptic reorganization. *Brain Res. 593:*257–264.

Goodman, J. H., Wasterlain, C. G., Massarweh, W. F., Dean, E., Sollas, A. L., and Sloviter, R. S. (1993) Calbindin-D28k immunoreactivity and selective vulnerability to ischemia in the dentate gyrus of the developing rat. *Brain Res. 606:*309–314.

Gottlieb, A., Keydor, I., and Epstein, H. T. (1977) Rodent brain growth stages: An analytical review. *Biol. Neonate 32:*166–176.

Gowers, W. R. (1881) *Epilepsy and Other Chronic Convulsive Diseases.* London: J. A. Churchill.

Hauser, W. A., and Kurland, L. T. (1975) The epidemiology of epilepsy in Rochester, Minnesota, 1935 through 1967. *Epilepsia 16:*1–66.

Holden, K. R., Mellits, E. D., and Freeman, J. M. (1982) Neonatal seizures: 1. Correlation of prenatal and perinatal events with outcomes. *Pediatrics 70:*165–176.

Hollmann, M., Harley, M., and Heinnemann, S. (1991) Ca^{2+} permeability of KA-AMPA-gated glutamate receptor channels depends on subunit composition. *Science 252:*851–853.

Holmes, G. L. (1987) Diagnosis and Management of Seizures in Children. Philadelphia: W. B. Saunders, pp. 237–261.

Holmes, G. L. (1991) The long-term effects of seizures on the developing brain: Clinical and laboratory issues. *Brain Dev. 13:*393–409.

Holmes, G. L., Rowe, J., Hafford, J., Schmidt, R., Testa, M., and Zimmerman, A. (1982) Prognostic value of the electroencephalogram in neonatal asphyxia. *Electroenceph. Clin. Neurophysiol. 53:*60–72.

Holmes, G. L., and Thompson, J. L. (1988) Effects of kainic acid on seizure susceptibility in the developing brain. *Dev. Brain Res. 39:*51–59.

Holmes, G. L., Thompson, J. L., Marchi, T., and Feldman, D. S. (1988) Behavioral effects of kainic acid administration on the immature brain. *Epilepsia 29:*721–730.

Jensen, F., Holmes, G. L., Lombroso, C. T., Blume, H. K., and Firkunsy, I. R. (1992) Age-dependent changes in long-term seizure susceptibility and behavior after hypoxia in rats. *Epilepsia 33:*971–980.

Jensen, F., Tsuji, M., Offutt, M., Firkusny, I., and Holtzman, D. (1993) Profound reversible energy loss in the hypoxic immature rat brain. *Dev. Brain Res. 73:*99–105.

Jorgensen, O. S., Dwyer, B. E., and Wasterlain, C. G. (1980) Synaptic proteins after electroconvulsive seizures in immature rats. *J. Neurochem. 35:*1235–1237.

Knauss, T. A., and Marshall, R. E. (1977) Seizures in a neonatal intensive care unit. *Dev. Med. Child. Neurol. 19:*719–728.

Lee, K., Diaz, M., and Melchior, J. C. (1981) Temporal lobe epilepsy: Not a consequence of childhood febrile convulsions in Denmark. *Acta Neurol. Scand. 63:*231–236.

Legido, A., Clancy, R. R., and Berman, P. H. (1991) Neurologic outcome after electroencephalographically proven neonatal seizures. *Pediatrics 88:*583–596.

Lennox, W. G. (1960) Epilepsy and Related Disorders. Boston: Little, Brown.

Lombroso, C. T. (1983) Prognosis in neonatal seizures. In A. V. Delgado-Escueta, C. G. Wasterlain, D. M. Treiman, and R. J. Porter (eds.), Advances in Neurology: Vol. 34. Status Epilepticus. New York: Raven Press, pp. 101–113.

Lothman, E. W., and Bertram, E. H. (1993) Epileptogenic effects of status epilepticus. *Epilepsia 34:*S59–S70.

Lothman, E. W., and Collins, R. C. (1981) Kainic acid-induced limbic seizures: Metabolic, behavioral, electroencephalographic and neuropathological correlates. *Brain Res. 218:*299–318.

Mathern, G. W., Leite, J. P., Pretorius, J. K., Quinn, B., Peacock, W. J., and Babb, T. L. (1994) Children with severe epilepsy: Evidence of hippocampal neuron losses and aberrant mossy fiber sprouting during postnatal granule cell migration and differentiation. *Dev. Brain. Res. 78:*70–80.

Mathern, G. W., Leite, J. P., Pretorius, J. K., Quinn, B., Peacock, W. J., and Babb, T. L. (1994) Severe seizures in young children are associated with hippocampal neuron losses and aberrant mossy fiber sprouting during fascia dentata postnatal development. *Epilepsy Res. Suppl.* (in press).

Maytal, J., Shinnar, S., Moshé, S. L., and Alvarez, L. A. (1989) Low morbidity and mortality of status epilepticus in children. *Pediatrics 83:*323–331.

Mello, L. E., Cavalhiero, E. A., Tan, E. M., Kupfer, W. R., Pretorious, J. K., Babb, T. L., and Finch, D. M. (1993) Circuit mechanism of seizures in the pilocarpine model of chronic epilepsy: Cell loss and mossy fiber sprouting. *Epilepsia 34:*985–995.

Miller, L. P., Johnson, A. E., and Gelhard, R. E. (1990) The ontogeny of excitatory amino acid receptors in the rat forebrain: II. Kainic acid receptors. *Neuroscience 35:*45–51.

Morin, A. M., Dwyer, B. E., Fujikawa, D. G., and Wasterlain, C. G. (1988) Low [³H]-cytochalasin B binding in the cerebral cortex of newborn rat. *J. Neurochem. 51:*206–211.

Moshé, S. L. (1987) Epileptogenesis and the immature brain. *Epilepsia 28* (Suppl.):S3–S15.

Moshé, S. L., Albala, B. J., Ackermann, R. F., and Engel, J., Jr. (1983) Increased seizure susceptibility of the immature brain. *Dev. Brain Res. 7:*81–85.

Moshé, S. L., Sperber, E. F., Haas, K., Xu, S., and Shinnar, S. (1992) Effects of the maturational process on epileptogenesis. In H. Luders (ed.), Epilepsy Surgery. New York: Raven Press, pp. 741–748.

Nadler, J. V., Perry, B. W., and Cotman, C. W. (1978) Intraventricular kainic acid preferentially destroys hippocampal pyramidal cells. *Nature 271:*676–677.

Nadler, J. V., Perry, B. W., and Cotman, C. W. (1980) Selective reinnervation of hippocampal area CA1 and the fascia dentata after destruction of CA3-CA4 afferents. *Brain Res. 182:*1–9.

Nevander, G., Ingvar, M., Auer, R., and Siesjo, B. K. (1985) Status epilepticus in well-oxygenated rats causes neuronal necrosis. *Ann. Neurol. 19:*281–290.

Nitecka, L., Tremblay, E., Charton, G., Bouillot, J. P., Berger, M. L., and Ben-Ari, Y. (1984) Maturation of kainic acid seizure–brain damage syndrome in the rat: II. Histopathological sequelae. *Neuroscience 13:*1073–1094.

Norman, R. M. (1964) The neuropathology of status epilepticus. *Med. Sci. Law 4:* 46–51.

Okada, R., Moshé, S. L., and Albala, B. J. (1984) Infantile status epilepticus and future seizure susceptibility in the rat. *Dev. Brain Res. 15:*177–183.

Pellegrini-Giampietro, D. E., Bennett, M. V., and Zukin, R. S. (1991) Differential expression of three glutamate receptor genes in developing rat brain: An in situ hybridization study. *Proc. Natl. Acad. Sci. 88:*4157–4161.

Penix, L. P., Thompson, K., and Wasterlain, C. G. (1994) Selective vulnerability to perforant path stimulation: Role of NMDA and non-NMDA receptors. *Epilepsy Res.* (in press).

Pereira de Vasconcelos, A., Boyet, S., Koziel, V., and Nehlig, A. (1993) Effects of pentylenetetrazol-induced status epilepticus on local cerebral blood flow in the developing rat. *J. Cereb. Blood Flow Metabol. 13* (Suppl. 1):S412.

Rami, A., Brehier, A., Thomasset, M., and Rabie, A. (1987) The comparative immunocytochemical distribution of 28kDa cholecalcin (CaBP) in the hippocampus of rat, guinea pig and hedgehog. *Brain Res. 422:*149–153.

Represa, A., Robain, O., Tremblay, E., and Ben-Ari, Y. (1989) Hippocampal plasticity in childhood epilepsy. *Neurosci. Lett. 99:*351–355.

Reynolds, E. H. (1981) Biological factors in psychological disorders associated with epilepsy. In E. H. Reynolds and M. R. Trimble (eds.), Epilepsy and Psychiatry. Edinburgh: Churchill Livingston, pp. 264–290.

Riikonen, R. (1982) A long-term follow-up study of 214 children with the syndrome of infantile spasms. *Neuropediatrics 13:*14–23.

Rose, A. L., and Lombroso, C. T. (1970) Neonatal seizure states: A study of clinical, pathological, and electroencephalographic features in 137 full-term babies with a long-term follow-up. *Pediatrics 45:*404–425.

Ross, E. M., Peckham, C. S., West, P. B., et al. (1980) Epilepsy in childhood: Findings from the National Child Development Study. *Br. Med. J. 280:*207–210.

Rowe, J. C., Holmes, G. L., Hafford, J., Baboval, D., Robinson, S., Phillips, A., Rosenkrantz, T., and Raye, J. (1985) Prognostic value of the electroencephalogram in term and preterm infants following neonatal seizures. *Electroenceph. Clin. Neurophysiol. 60:*183–196.

Sagar, H. J., and Oxbury, J. M. (1987) Hippocampal neuron loss in temporal lobe epilepsy: Correlation with early childhood convulsions. *Ann. Neurol. 22:*334–340.

Sankar, R., Wallis, R. A., Thompson, K., Yang, C. X., Akira, T., and Wasterlain, C. G. (1993) Age-dependent changes in susceptibility to seizures and seizure-induced damage. In F. Andermann, A. Beaumanoir, L. Mira, J. Roger, and C. J. Tassinari (eds.), Occipital Seizures and Epilepsies in Children. London: John Libbey, pp. 15–29.

Scher, M. S., Painter, M. J., Bergman, I., Barmada, M. A., and Brunberg, J. (1989) EEG diagnoses of neonatal seizures: Clinical correlations and outcome. *Pediatr. Neurol. 5:*17–24.

Schiottz-Christensen, E., and Bruhn, P. (1973) Intelligence, behaviour and scholastic achievement subsequent to febrile convulsions: An analysis of discordant twin-pairs. *Develop. Med. Child. Neurol. 15:*565–575.

Shewmon, D. A., and Erwin, R. J. (1988) Focal spike–induced cerebral dysfunction is related to the after-coming slow wave. *Ann. Neurol. 23:*242–247.

Shields, W. D. (1991) Infantile spasms and developmental delay: Cause versus effect. *Epilepsia 32* (Suppl. 3):60.

Shirasaka, Y., and Wasterlain, C. G. (1994) Chronic epileptogenicity following focal status epilepticus. *Brain Res (in press)*.

Sloviter, R. S. (1987) Decreased hippocampal inhibition and a selective loss of interneurons in experimental epilepsy. *Science 235:*73–76.

Sloviter, R. S. (1991) Permanently altered hippocampal structure, excitability and inhibition after experimental status epilepticus in the rat: The "dormant basket cell" hypothesis and its possible relevance to temporal lobe epilepsy. *Hippocampus 1*:41–66.

Sloviter, R. S. (1992) Possible functional consequences of synaptic reorganization in the dentate gyrus of kainate-treated rats. *Neurosci. Lett. 137*:91–96.

Sofijanov, N., Sadikario, A., Dukovski, M., et al. (1983) Febrile convulsions and later development of epilepsy. *Am. J. Dis. Child. 137*:123–126.

Sperber, E. F. (1992) Developmental profile of seizure-induced hippocampal damage. *Epilepsia 33*:44.

Sperber, E. F., Haas, K. Z., and Moshé, S. L. (1992) Developmental aspects of status epilepticus. *Int. Pediatr. 7*:213–222.

Sperber, E. F., Haas, K. Z., Stanton, P. K., and Moshé, S. L. (1991) Resistance of the immature hippocampus to seizure-induced synaptic reorganization. *Dev. Brain Res. 60*:88–93.

Sperber, E. F., Stanton, P. K., Haas, K. Z., Ackermann, R. F., and Moshé, S. L. (1992) Developmental differences in the neurobiology of epileptic brain damage. In J. Engel, Jr., C. G. Wasterlain, E. A. Cavalheiro, U. Heinemann, and G. Avanzini (eds.), Molecular Neurobiology of Epilepsy. Amsterdam: Elsevier, pp. 67–81.

Stafstrom, C. E., Chronopoulos, A., Thurber, S., Thompson, J. L., and Holmes, G. L. (1993) Age-dependent cognitive and behavioral deficits after kainic acid seizures. *Epilepsia 34*:420–432.

Suga, S., and Wasterlain, C. G. (1980) Effects of neonatal seizures or anoxia on cerebellar mitotic activity in the rat. *Exp. Neurol. 67*:573–580.

Sutula, T., Xiao-Xian, H., Cavazos, J., and Scott, G. (1988) Synaptic reorganization in the hippocampus induced by abnormal functional activity. *Science 239*:1147–1150.

Tauck, D. L., and Nadler, J. V. (1985) Evidence of functional mossy fiber sprouting in hippocampal formation of kainic acid-treated rats. *J. Neurosci. 5*:1016–1022.

Till, K. (1967) Hemispherectomy for infantile hemiplegia. *Dev. Med. Child. Neurol. 9*:773–774.

Treiman, D. M. (1993) Generalized convulsive status epilepticus in the adult. *Epilepsia 34* (Suppl. 1):S2–S11.

Tsuboi, T. (1984) Epidemiology of febrile and afebrile convulsions in children in Japan. *Neurology 34*:175–181.

Van den Berg, B. J., and Yerushalmy, J. (1969) Studies on convulsive disorders in young children: 1. Incidence of febrile and non-febrile convulsions by age and other factors. *Pediatr. Res. 3*:298–304.

Vannucci, R. C., and Duffy, T. E. (1975) Oxidative and energy metabolism of fetal and neonatal rats during anoxia and during recovery. *Am. J. Physiol. 230*:1269–1275.

Verity, C. M., Butler, N. R., and Goldring, J. (1985) Febrile convulsions in a national cohort followed up from birth: II. Medical history and intellectual ability at 5 years of age. *Br. Med. J. 290*:1311–1315.

Volpe, J. J. (1986) Neonatal seizures. In J. J. Volpe (ed.), Neurology of the Newborn. Philadelphia: W. B. Saunders, pp. 129–157.

Wasterlain, C. G. (1974) Inhibition of protein synthesis by epileptic seizures without motor manifestations. *Neurology 24*:175–180.

Wasterlain, C. G. (1976) Effects of neonatal status epilepticus on rat brain development. *Neurology 26*:975–986.

Wasterlain, C. G., Hattori, H., Yang, C., Schwartz, P. H., Fujikawa, D. G., Morin,

A. M., and Dwyer, B. E. (1990) Selective vulnerability of neuronal subpopulations during ontogeny reflects discrete molecular events associated with normal brain development. In G. G. Wasterlain and P. Vert (eds.), Neonatal Seizures. New York: Raven Press, pp. 69–81.

Wasterlain, C. G., and Sankar, R. (1993) Excitotoxicity and the developing brain. In G. Avanzini, R. Fariello, U. Heinemann, and R. Mutani (eds.), Epileptogenic and Excitotoxic Mechanisms. London: John Libbey, pp. 135–151.

Wasterlain, C. G., and Vert, P. (eds.) (1990) Neonatal Seizures. New York: Raven Press.

Watanabe, K., Kuroyanagi, M., Hara, K., and Miyazaki, S. (1982) Neonatal seizures and subsequent epilepsy. *Brain Dev. 4:*341–346.

Watanabe, K., Miyazaki, S., Hara, K., and Hakamada, S. (1980) Behavioral state cycles, background EEGs and prognosis of newborns with perinatal hypoxia. *Electroencephalogr. Clin. Neurophysiol. 49:*618–625.

Woodruff, M. L. (1974) Subconvulsive epileptiform discharge and behavioral impairment. *Behav. Biol. 11:*431–458.

11

Age-Specific Antiepileptic Drug Treatment and Development of Age-Specific Antiepileptic Drugs

OLIVIER DULAC
ROBERT L. MACDONALD
KEVIN M. KELLY

The selection of optimal antiepileptic drug (AED) treatment is complicated by the great variety of etiologies and clinical phenotypes of epilepsy, by genetic background and age-dependent developmental features, and by the need to preserve normal cognitive function. Recognition of specific epilepsy syndromes is the most useful starting point for therapeutic decisions. Indeed, some types of epilepsy need no treatment. In other forms of epilepsy, intractability may be predicted from onset, and still other types may benefit from specific drug treatment or from early surgery. Since over one-quarter of infants and children with epilepsy are unsuccessfully treated by conventional antiepileptic drugs, there is a great need for new AEDs. However, both the design of new drugs and clinical trials need a rational basis that is still insufficiently developed. The Commission on Antiepileptic Drugs of the International League against Epilepsy (ILAE) has addressed specific aspects of AED trials in children (1989) and, following a workshop in Royaumont, France (1990), offered general proposals (1991).

Age- and Syndrome-Specific Drug Treatments

The development of age-specific AEDs must take into account specific age-related differences in pharmacokinetics, characteristics of epilepsy including age-specific epilepsy syndromes, tolerance, cognitive functions, formulation, and ethics.

Maturation of Metabolic Pathways and Drug Kinetics

Age-dependent maturation of metabolic pathways and drug kinetics have been discussed in detail by Morselli (1983) and White et al. (1983).

Absorption of AEDs

In the newborn, several factors may delay absorption of AEDs. First, there is a relative achlorhydria of the stomach, which improves during the first 20 to 30 months of life. Second, there is a prolonged and erratic gastric emptying time that persists until 6 to 8 months of age (Cavell, 1979). Third, and most important, the intestinal mucosa is functionally immature (Heiman, 1980). Thus bioavailability is very low for phenytoin (Jalling et al., 1970; Painter et al., 1978) and irregular for carbamazepine (Rey et al., 1979). Conversely, rectal absorption does not change with age (Dulac et al., 1978; Knudsen, 1977).

In contrast, in infants and children absorption is much faster than in adults, resulting in a higher peak drug concentration with an increased risk of adverse effects (Morselli et al., 1980). Carbamazepine syrup may produce somnolence 1 hour after its administration; it should therefore be given in three daily doses to prevent this side effect (Hoppner et al., 1980).

Distribution of AEDs

The distribution of AEDs is also modified because plasma protein binding is low in very young children due to low concentrations of albumin, globulins, and glycoproteins (Pacifici et al., 1984) and to a high level of free fatty acids and other substances capable of displacing the drug from its binding sites (Kurtz, Mauser-Granshorn, and Suckel, 1977; Kurtz, Michels, and Suckel, 1977). Plasma protein drug binding capacity becomes comparable to that of adults by 10 to 12 years of age.

Compared to adults, permeability of the blood–brain barrier to small molecules and extracellular fluid volume are increased in the newborn; cerebrospinal fluid (CSF) production, however, is diminished, thereby increasing the drug concentration in the brain extracellular fluid (White et al., 1983). Thus central nervous system drug concentrations can be quite variable, depending on the AED, acid–base equilibrium, and cerebral blood flow.

Metabolic Degradation of AEDs

The metabolic degradation of AEDs is reduced in the newborn. Metabolic pathways in the liver microsomes are influenced by exposure to inducing drugs (Aranda et al., 1974), particularly to phenobarbital (Boreus et al., 1975), phenytoin (Loughnan et al., 1977), and diazepam (Morselli et al.,

1973). Glucuronic acid conjugation activity is significantly reduced until 18 to 24 months of age. For instance, diazepam undergoes demethylation without glycuroconjugation, resulting in the accumulation of demethyldiazepam, which can be associated with severe and prolonged hypotonia.

The relative inefficiency of plasma clearance lasts until 2–3 weeks of life. By the end of the first month, there is a dramatic increase in the rate of drug metabolism from severalfold lower to severalfold higher than that of the adult (Morselli, 1983). Metabolic rate subsequently decreases to adult levels (Morselli, 1977).

Excretion of AEDs

Excretion of AEDs is mainly renal. Glomerular and, even more so, tubular function is immature in the newborn and reaches adult values in the middle of the first year of life. Phenobarbital clearance is thus 10 to 30 times lower in the newborn than in adults.

Drug Interactions

AED interactions have been widely studied in children (Levy et al., 1983). They are generally similar to those of adults with modifications due to the metabolic characteristics of this age range (Fig. 11-1). For example, with polytherapy, the concentration dosage ratio of carbamazepine is greatly influenced by age. It is higher in older patients because of the age-related changes in its half-life (Battino et al., 1980). In addition, the epoxy-10,11-carbamazepine blood levels are higher in polytherapy with increased side effects (Schoeman et al., 1984).

Brain Maturation

Brain maturation may affect response to drugs. Since available data on this issue are frequently drawn from animal studies, and since the maturational state of the newborn laboratory animal (e.g., the rat) is different from that of the human newborn, the relevance of these experimental data to clinical situations is unclear.

Astrocyte processes are poorly developed at birth, thereby precluding their normal buffering function at the synaptic cleft level (Rakic, 1981). Studies with strychnine and picrotoxin in rats have shown a rapid increase in the CD-50 (drug dose at which 50 percent of animals show convulsive behavior), thus indicating a rapid maturation of glycine and gamma aminobutyric acid (GABA) inhibitory pathways (Woodbury, 1967). N-methyl-D-aspartic acid (NMDA) binding sites are transiently increased in the newborn rat (Tremblay et al., 1988).

Rapid maturation of the brain in the first months of life results in changes such as establishment of connections between neurons, increasing density of neurotransmitter receptor channels, myelination and permeability of the blood–brain barrier. Kinetics of maturation vary with age and site in the

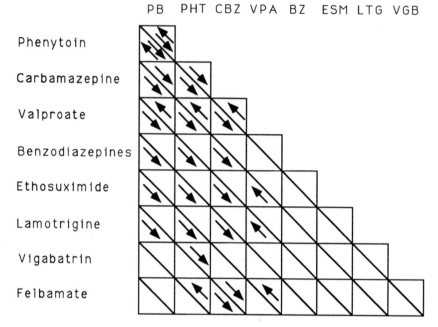

Figure 11-1. Metabolic interaction among antiepileptic drugs. For each pair of drugs, arrow in top/right part of box shows effect of interaction on blood level of the drug listed on the horizontal (top) axis; arrow in bottom/left part of box shows effect of interaction on blood level of the drug listed on the vertical (left) axis. Empty boxes indicate no interaction effect. For example, when valproate and carbamazepine are given together, the level of CBZ is increased and the level of VPA is decreased (relative to the blood level that would be achieved by the same drug dose if it were administered alone). Abbreviations: PB – phenobarbital; PHT – phenytoin; CBZ – carbamazepine; VPA – valproate; BZ – benzodiazepines; ESM – ethosuximide; LTG – lamotrigine; VGB – vigabatrin.

brain, as shown by quantified position emission tomography (Chugani et al., 1987) and single photon emission computed tomography with ^{133}Xe (Chiron et al., 1992). Perfusion and therefore metabolic activity maturation is rapid in early infancy and becomes slower as the child becomes older. Posterior areas of the brain exhibit early and rapid maturation that seems to be complete in the middle of the first year of life, whereas maturation of frontal areas is delayed, slower, and still ongoing at the end of the first year of life. The site of the epileptogenic focus is therefore likely to play a role in age of onset of focal epilepsy and response to drugs.

Difficulties Related to the Type of Epilepsy

AED Efficacy According to Seizure Types

All types of seizures observed in adults may also occur in children. Partial seizures are clearly recognized in infants (Duchowny, 1987; Luna, Dulac,

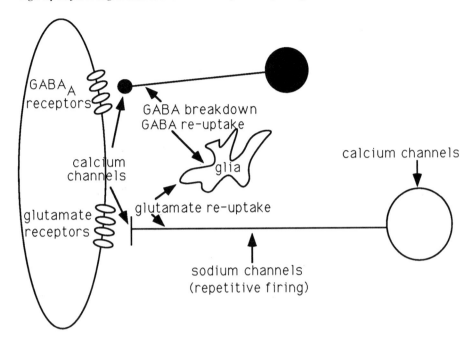

Figure 11-2. Possible targets for newly-developed antiepileptic drugs. Advances in molecular biology have revealed new information about the subunit composition of receptors and channels, and about the function and localization of uptake and degradative mechanisms. For example, a multitude of binding sites has been associated with different subunits of the GABA$_A$ receptor; drug interaction with such sites can produce specific modulation of the functional properties of the receptor. Since there is a change in subunit composition in many of these molecules during early development and maturation of the brain, it should be possible to identify drugs with specific effects on the immature CNS.

Pajot, and Beaumont, 1989; Luna, Dulac, and Plouin, 1989) (see Chapter 2). In addition, some types of seizures are specific to infancy. For example, clusters of spasms are rare after the first year of life. Many children exhibit more than one seizure type; one epidemiological study reported an average of more than 1.5 seizure types per patient (Luna et al., 1988).

Difficult-to-quantify seizures include myoclonus, spasms, and brief tonic seizures when falling asleep. For these seizures, even video-EEG monitoring may fail to reliably determine seizure frequency. Spontaneous seizure frequency may vary greatly, with seizure-free periods alternating with periods of increased seizure frequency, sometimes evolving into status epilepticus.

In a prospective study of adults, Mattson et al. (1985) demonstrated a specific spectrum of AED efficacy according to seizure type. Phenytoin and carbamazepine are more effective than phenobarbital and primidone against partial seizures, whereas the two latter drugs are more effective against secondarily generalized seizures. Penry and Dean (1988) showed that valproate is more effective against partial seizures with secondary generalization than those without. In children, as in adults, carbamazepine is more effective in partial than generalized seizures (Dulac et al., 1983), whereas the reverse is true for valproate (Dulac et al., 1986).

AEDs may modify the seizure pattern by controlling one of the several types of seizures exhibited by the patient, or by changing the type; for example, secondarily generalized seizures may evolve from complex partial or simple partial seizures. This response to therapy may be clinically relevant, since generalized seizures are much more disruptive to the patient than simple partial seizures. AED efficacy must therefore be assessed according to seizure type.

When starting a given AED, a new type of seizure may emerge. On the one hand, this change may reflect a toxic effect of the AED and worsen the condition of the patient. For instance, carbamazepine may produce myoclonic (Aguglia et al., 1987; Snead and Hosey, 1985), absence, and atonic seizures (Shields and Saslow, 1983), and benzodiazepines may trigger tonic seizures (Tassinari et al., 1972). On the other hand, the emergence of new types of seizures may be related to etiology and may represent a partial control of the epileptic process. Replacement of clusters of spasms by focal seizures in tuberous sclerosis treated with vigabatrin is one example (Chiron et al., 1991).

AED Efficacy According to Type of Epilepsy Syndrome

In addition to the type of seizures, other characteristics of the epilepsy should be taken into account (Table 11-1). A given type of seizure may result from several types of epilepsy syndromes, each of which may exhibit a different response to AEDs. More or less specific responses to AEDs thus characterize the various presently recognized epilepsy syndromes (Roger et al., 1985) classified by the Commission on Classification and Terminology of the International League against Epilepsy (1989). Partial seizures respond differently to drugs depending on whether they result from a brain lesion or from a benign partial epilepsy with centrotemporal spikes (BPECTS). Whereas phenytoin and carbamazepine are more efficient than valproate in symptomatic cases, all these drugs may be equally efficacious in the treatment of BPECTS (Chaigne and Dulac, 1989). A given AED may improve some epilepsy syndromes and worsen others. For instance, carbamazepine may worsen continuous spike waves in slow sleep (Marescaux et al., 1990). The overall result in a series of patients having different types of epilepsy syndromes may be an apparent lack of drug effect. This was the case in the Lunda, Dulac, Pajot, and Beaumont study of vigabatrin (1989). Patients with partial epilepsy responded best, whereas patients with myoclonic epilepsy exhibited impaired seizure control; the mean seizure frequency of the whole series was not significantly modified.

Several types of difficulties arise when taking into account the epilepsy syndromes:

1. At the onset of epilepsy, several clinical or EEG characteristics necessary for the syndromic diagnosis may be missing, and early diagnosis is

TABLE 11-1. First- and Second-Line AED According to Type of Epilepsy Syndrome

Syndrome	First Line	Second Line	Reference
Cryptogenic West	Steroids	Valproate	Snead et al., 1989
Symptomatic West	Steroids	Valproate	Siemes et al., 1988
	Vigabatrin		Chiron et al., 1991
		Benzodiazepines	Farrell, 1986
Benign myoclonic epilepsy of infancy	Valproate	Ethosuximide	Dravet et al., 1985
Severe myoclonic epilepsy of infancy	Valproate	Benzodiazepines	Dravet et al., 1985
Partial benign	Valproate		Chaigne and Dulac, 1989
		Carbamazepine	Lerman and Kivity-Ephraim, 1974
Lennox-Gastaut	Felbamate		Ritter et al., 1991
	Lamotrigine		Oller et al., 1991
		Benzodiazepines	Farrell, 1986
Myoclonic astatic	Valproate	Ethoxusimide	Doose, 1985
Infantile absences	Valproate		Sato et al., 1982
	Ethosuximide		Sato et al., 1982
		Lamotrigine	Schlumberger and Dulac, 1994
Continuous spike waves during slow sleep and Landau-Kleffner	Benzodiazepines		Marescaux et al., 1990
		Steroids	Lerman et al., 1991

295

often a challenge. BPECTS may lack centrotemporal spikes. Many cases of Doose syndrome (1985) are at first misdiagnosed as Lennox-Gastaut syndrome. Emergence of myoclonic jerks and spike waves is often delayed by several years in severe myoclonic epilepsy of infancy (Dravet et al., 1985).

2. A given syndrome may exhibit several stages, each one with a different response to AEDs. At the onset of severe myoclonic epilepsy in infancy, valproate and benzodiazepines are the most effective; 3 to 4 years later, phenytoin becomes the treatment of choice.

3. Each epilepsy syndrome comprises only a small number of patients. Thus in one epidemiological study of epilepsy in the first 10 years of life, not one epilepsy syndrome group comprised more than 10 percent of the cases, and most of them consisted of 0.5 to 2 percent of the cases. Multicenter studies with homogeneous diagnostic criteria are therefore necessary when dealing with the study of a given syndrome.

4. A consensus should be reached regarding the nosologic limits of various syndromes such as benign occipital epilepsy (Aicardi and Newton, 1983; Gastaut, 1985) and partial benign epilepsy with affective symptoms (Dalla Bernardina et al., 1985; Deonna et al., 1986).

5. There is growing evidence that some syndromes remain heterogeneous in terms of both clinical presentation and response to treatment. A given syndrome resulting from various etiologies may give different responses in different etiologies. This has been clearly shown in West syndrome, which is better controlled by steroids when it is cryptogenic than when it is symptomatic (Snead et al., 1989), and better controlled when it is due to periventricular leukomalacia than to tuberous sclerosis (Schlumberger and Dulac, 1994). In a recent study, patients with West syndrome had a better response to vigabatrin when there were radiologically demonstrable brain lesions (in particular, tuberous sclerosis and porencephaly) than in cryptogenic cases (Chiron et al., 1991). A clear etiologic diagnosis is therefore useful for an optimal therapeutic decision.

Response to AEDs is also variable within some idiopathic and cryptogenic epilepsy syndromes. The Doose syndrome (1985) includes the benign and severe myoclonic epilepsies of infancy (Roger et al., 1985) and also cases with onset in later childhood. Among the latter, some patients respond favorably to valproate and ethosuximide but are worsened by carbamazepine, whereas others are somewhat improved by carbamazepine (Chiron et al., 1987).

Difficulties Related to AED Toxicity in Children

Several AEDs have more side effects in children and adolescents than in adults. Fulminating hepatitis during valproate therapy is reported to be 30 to 100 times more frequent in infants than in adults (Dreifuss et al., 1989); the distinction between a toxic effect of the drug and an inborn error of metabolism (Egger et al., 1987) is often difficult to make (Dreifuss and Langer, 1987). Interaction between macrolides and carbamazepine has been reported in children (Mesdjian et al., 1980); hallucinations due to ethosuximide have been observed in adolescents (Roger et al., 1968).

Whether this heterogeneity in side effects corresponds to age-related specific metabolism of AEDs or to specific characteristics of the epilepsy syndrome remains unclear. For ethosuximide, drug-resistant cases of absence epilepsy are observed primarily in adolescents; in such cases, side effects may be seen as higher doses of ethosuximide are administered. Valproate is more likely to be used in polytherapy in infants than in adults; acetylsalicylic acid is often administered for fever in infants, and its combination with valproate in the presence of fever seems to be particularly prone to produce Reyes-like hepatic failure (Dreifuss and Langer, 1987). Thus the etiologic context seems to play a part in the occurrence of side effects of AEDs in children.

Difficulties Related to Cognitive Functions

Preexisting brain damage and psychological isolation contribute to altered cognitive function and behavior. Clinical seizures, electrographic spike-wave activity, and AEDs may further exacerbate these behaviors. Half the young epilepsy patients exhibit fluctuations of cognitive functions and behavior over periods of a few months (Bourgeois et al., 1983); some epilepsy syndromes are associated with rapid mental deterioration over a period of a few weeks.

Toxic drug blood levels may affect intellectual functioning. Cognitive disorders are easily overlooked, as shown in school-age children given phenobarbital (Vining et al., 1987) and carbamazepine (O'Dougherty et al., 1987). This point is of particular concern since children are in a period of rapid development of cognitive functions. However, after a few weeks of drug administration, the cognitive side effects may diminish. Drug combinations may modify cognitive tolerance compared to each drug administered alone. Very few data and standardized tests are available for testing cognitive functions in children under 6 years of age treated with AEDs. Behavioral disorders such as depression produced by phenobarbital may also be overlooked (Brent et al., 1987). Combination of drugs, as well as poor neuropsychological functioning due to an underlying condition, may increase the risk of behavioral side effects.

Surgery versus Use of New Drugs

After a long period with no development of new AEDs, the pharmaceutical industry is developing several new drugs. The clinician faced with a case of intractable epilepsy amenable to surgery may therefore prefer to try new AEDs before deciding on surgery. In fact, these approaches may not be mutually exclusive but rather complementary for several reasons:

1. Some patients have a clear focal lesion not involving functional areas, and surgery is therefore preferred, particularly if there is no clear etiological diagnosis.

2. Some patients have generalized epilepsies only amenable to callosotomy, and new drugs such as vigabatrin (Chiron et al., 1991), lamotrigine
(Schlumberger et al., 1992), and felbamate (Ritter et al., 1991) should have
priority.

3. Multifocal epilepsy with secondary generalization, such as West syndrome due to tuberous sclerosis, may be transformed by vigabatrin into
focal epilepsy (Chiron et al., 1991); thus patients with this condition may
become candidates for focal surgery.

4. Surgery should not be delayed too long since the potential for recovery
of brain function decreases with age, both for specific functions such as
speech and for interhemispheric connections. This factor applies to hemispherectomy, callosotomy (Lassonde et al., 1991), and subpial transection
involving functional areas such as speech in Landau-Kleffner syndrome
(Morrell et al., 1992), although this latter procedure remains controversial.

New Drugs and Drug Trials

Until the late 1980s AEDs were never licensed specifically for children, although childhood epileptic disorders are often clearly different from those
of adults. The situation has changed, but the development of a new AED for
children still faces a number of difficulties. As mentioned earlier, selective
action on specific epilepsy syndromes, potential adverse effects on cognitive
functions, and age-related side effects must be investigated early in the development of the drug.

Preclinical Difficulties Faced when Developing New AEDs

Evaluation of AEDs

Most new AEDs are initially tested for anticonvulsant action on animal seizure models—that is, pentylenetetrazol and maximal electroshock seizure
models—from which it is difficult to infer the type of human epilepsy for
which the drug would be effective. Indeed, there is evidence that such pre-
dictions may often be erroneous. For example, lamotrigine was predicted to
be effective against partial epilepsy but not absence epilepsy since (like phenytoin and carbamazepine) it was effective against maximal electroshock
and maximal pentylenetetrazol seizures but ineffective in threshold tests
(Miller et al., 1986). The reverse proved to be true in clinical practice.

The mechanism of action of AEDs has been studied extensively (Macdonald and Kelly, 1993, 1994). Current clinically used AEDs decrease membrane excitability by interacting with ion channels or neurotransmitter receptors. Currently approved AEDs appear to act on sodium channels,
$GABA_A$ receptors (GABARs), or T-type (transient-type) calcium channels
(Table 11-2). Phenytoin, carbamazepine, and possibly sodium valproate
decrease high-frequency repetitive firing of action potentials by enhancing
sodium channel inactivation. Benzodiazepines and barbiturates enhance

TABLE 11-2. Antiepileptic Drug Actions

Drug	Sodium Channels	GABA R Channels	T-Calcium Channels
Carbamazepine	+ +	−	−
Phenytoin	+ +	−	−
Primidone	+	−	?
Valproic acid	+ +	?/ +	?/ +
Barbiturates	+	+	−
Benzodiazepines	+	+ +	−
Ethosuximide	−	−	+ +

GABA$_A$-mediated inhibition. Ethosuximide and possibly sodium valproate reduce a low-threshold calcium current. The action of AEDs to reduce high-frequency repetitive firing of action potentials correlates well with activity against maximal electroshock seizures; enhancement of GABA$_A$ergic inhibition correlates well with activity against myoclonic seizures; and reduction of T-type calcium current correlates well with activity against generalized absence seizures. Unfortunately, use of the antimaximal electroshock and antipentylenetetrazol seizure tests selects for drugs with the same mechanisms of action, and therefore often excludes AEDs with novel mechanisms of action.

The Lack of Animal Models of Specific Epilepsy Syndromes

New animal models have been developed, including genetically determined absence epilepsy, which is considered to be a model of idiopathic generalized epilepsy (Hosford, 1992; Marescaux et al., 1984; Noebels, 1979); kainic acid (Ben Ari et al., 1979) and kindling (Goddard et al., 1969), which can be considered models of limbic epilepsy; and the alumina cream focus (Chauvel and Lamarche, 1975), which may be considered a model for neocortical focal epilepsy and epilepsia partialis continua. However, the predictive value of these models to determine the spectrum of activity of a new AED in humans remains to be determined. In addition, many childhood epilepsy syndromes—West syndrome, Lennox-Gastaut syndrome, cryptogenic myoclonic epilepsies, partial benign epilepsy, continuous spike waves in slow sleep, Landau-Kleffner syndrome, and Rasmussen's encephalitis—still lack reliable animal models. Until specific animal models of the epilepsies of childhood are developed and their pathophysiology is understood, it will be difficult to develop AEDs that will have specific actions on the childhood seizures.

Novel Approaches to Development of AEDs

Advances in the understanding of central nervous system neurotransmitter receptor channels and voltage-gated ion channels have presented opportunities for the development of AEDs that may have specific actions in the childhood epilepsies—without first understanding the specific pathophysiology of the childhood epilepsies. Many of the important excitatory and inhibitory neurotransmitter receptor channels and the voltage-gated ion channels that are essential for membrane excitability and synaptic transmission in the central nervous system have been cloned, and their amino acid sequences have been identified. Techniques have been developed to express human recombinant neurotransmitter receptor channels and voltage-gated ion channels in heterologous expression systems, that is, in nonneuronal cells which do not normally express these transmitter receptors or channels. These techniques allow the evaluation of potential AEDs on human neurotransmitter receptors or ion channels directly (Fig. 11-2).

Another important discovery has been the identification of multiple subtypes of specific neurotransmitter receptor channels or voltage-gated ion channels. For example, GABARs appear to be composed of combinations of different subtypes ($\alpha_1-\alpha_6$, $\beta_1-\beta_4$, $\gamma_1-\gamma_3$, δ, and $\rho_1-\rho_2$) of polypeptide subunits (Cutting et al., 1991; Pritchett, Luddens, and Seeburg, 1989; Schofield et al., 1987; Shivers et al., 1989). There is a differential regional expression in the central nervous system and spinal cord of various subunit subtype mRNAs (Laurie, Seeburg, and Wisden, 1992; Wisden et al., 1992), and the distribution of mRNAs for these receptor subtypes changes during development (Laurie, Wisden, and Seeburg, 1992). Thus differential expression and assembly of various subunit subtypes could produce a multitude of GABAR isoforms which may differ during development.

Differences in expression of specific GABAR isoforms may be of considerable significance for the effectiveness of specific AEDs. For example, GABARs formed from α_1 and β_1 subunits are insensitive to benzodiazepines (Moss et al., 1990; Pritchett, Sontheimer, and Shivers, 1989). The basis for this insensitivity was determined when two forms of a third GABAR subunit, the γ_1 and γ_2 subunits, where transiently coexpressed with α_1 and β_1 subunits in human embryonic kidney (HEK) cells and shown to form fully functional GABARs that were sensitive to benzodiazepines, β carbolines, barbiturates, and picrotoxin (Pritchett, Sontheimer, and Shivers, 1989). Analysis of binding of various benzodiazepines to purified GABARs from brain regions revealed the existence of two subclasses of benzodiazepine binding sites, type I and type II benzodiazepine sites (Braestrup and Nielsen, 1981; Eichinger and Sieghart, 1986; Garret and Tabakoff, 1985; Klepner et al., 1978; Lipa et al., 1981). The molecular basis for type I and II benzodiazepine binding sites was determined using transient expression of $\alpha_{x(x=1-6)}\beta_1\gamma_{2s}$ subunit combinations in HEK293 cells (Pritchett, Luddens, and Seeburg, 1989; Pritchett and Seeberg, 1990). The combination of $\alpha_1\beta_1\gamma_{2s}$ GABAR subtypes produced type I benzodiazepine binding sites and expression of $\alpha_2\beta_1\gamma_{2s}$, $\alpha_3\beta_1\gamma_{2s}$ or $\alpha_5\beta_1\gamma_{2s}$ GABAR subtype combinations produced type II benzodiazepine binding sites. Expression of the α_4 or α_6 subtype with β_1 and γ_{2s} subtypes produced benzodiazepine binding sites that did not bind the prototypical benzodiazepines, diazepam and flunitrazepam, or β carbolines, but did bind the benzodiazepine receptor inverse agonist Ro15-4513 and the benzodiazepine receptor antagonist flumazenil (Ro15-1788) (Sieghart et al., 1987; Wisden et al., 1991). Benzodiazepine receptor pharmacology was not altered by substituting other β subtypes. Thus, despite the finding that the γ subunit conferred benzodiazepine sensitivity to GABARs, the α subunit appeared to determine the type of benzodiazepine receptor expressed. Clearly, GABAR isoforms composed of different GABAR subunit subtypes have different pharmacologic properties, and it is therefore possible that enhancement of current through specific GABAR isoforms may produce different antiepileptic actions (see also Chapter 2).

Calcium channels have also been shown to be heterogeneous (Hui et al., 1991; Mori et al., 1991; Snutch et al., 1990, 1991; Starr et al., 1991; Williams et al., 1992). At least four different types of voltage-dependent calcium channels have been described: L-type, T-type, N-type, and P-type channels (Mintz et al., 1992; Nowycky et al., 1985). These four types of calcium channel have different voltage ranges for activation and inactivation and different rates of activation and inactivation. Each channel type has been cloned and shown to be composed of several subunits (L-type channel: Campbell et al., 1988; Catterall, 1988; N-type channel: Williams et al., 1992; P-type channel: Mori et al., 1991; and T-type channel: Soong et al., 1993). In additional, many subtypes of channels have been identified. With the finding that neurons express multiple calcium channels, it may be that AEDs act upon specific types of channels in specific regions of the central nervous system.

It is thus possible that specific neurotransmitter receptor channels or voltage-gated ion channels that appear early in development and then become less prominent later in development may be excellent molecular targets for age-specific AEDs. For example, a GABAR that is present early in development in areas such as hippocampus or thalamus or substantia nigra, but which is less significant or disappears later in life, would be an excellent target for a new selective childhood AED. Similarly, a calcium channel present in thalamus early in development might also be an excellent molecular target for a novel childhood AED.

Clinical Difficulties Faced When Developing New AEDs

Difficulties Related to Etiology and Prognosis

Newly-appearing seizures may be either the first expression of epilepsy or occasional, and prognosis varies accordingly. More than half the cases of childhood epilepsy are benign, but nearly one-fourth are intractable. Improvement in AED treatment of benign cases would mainly concern drug tolerance, whereas for intractable cases it should also concern efficacy. In all three conditions, drug trials are faced with several difficulties.

Etiological Considerations. Epilepsy is a chronic disorder, and it contrasts with reactive (provoked) seizures triggered by fever, transient metabolic disorders, or acute brain damage. The relative frequency of reactive seizures compared to epilepsy decreases with age; reactive seizures are relatively frequent in the newborn period and may consist of status epilepticus with poor prognosis. However, there is growing evidence that in the infant (Maytal et al., 1989), and to a greater degree in the newborn, neurological sequelae are more likely to result from the underlying acute disorder than from the status epilepticus it has triggered. Evaluation of new AED efficacy in the newborn is therefore particularly difficult.

Patients with Benign Childhood Epilepsy. Prospective controlled monotherapy may be advisable when dealing with cases of benign childhood epilepsy. The new drug needs to be compared with a reference drug in a randomized parallel study. Unfortunately, since the interictal EEG often shows focal spikes in these patients, there is a great temptation for the general practitioner or pediatrician to start drug therapy from the very first seizure. Patients so treated are poorly suited for prospective studies. The benign epilepsy syndrome may need treatment only in rare cases with frequent seizures (Ambrosetto et al., 1987); most patients recover spontaneously without treatment (Beaussart and Faou, 1978). Even in the case when no treatment is given after the first seizure, less than 40 percent of the patients will exhibit a second seizure within 2 years (Boulloche et al., 1989). For a controlled study of such a group, it would be necessary to include at least three times more patients than would otherwise be needed to obtain significant results. An alternative sample is patients with frequent seizures from onset; however, they may in fact constitute a particular group of their own.

Patients with Intractable Cases of Epilepsy. Patients with intractable epilepsy are often treated with two or more drugs. In some cases reduction of polytherapy has a favorable effect on seizure frequency, particularly when there is a metabolic drug interaction. An add-on design in the case of polytherapy may lead to complex metabolic interactions. However, reduction to monotherapy or even dual therapy may be difficult to obtain in other patients because of an increase in seizure frequency, risk of status epilepticus, and risk of epilepsy that can no longer be brought under control. Although the majority of AEDs are more efficient when used in monotherapy, others may gain efficacy in combination with another drug.

In addition, many patients have fluctuations in seizure frequency over a period of months (Dravet et al., 1985). In a recent study, an add-on placebo period of 1 month proved useful since it was possible to study regression toward the median seizure frequency between baseline and placebo period. The regression plot presented a slope of 0.985, thus demonstrating a very small "oscillation" during the baseline period (Luna, Dulac, Pajot, and Beaumont, 1989). In some patients, seizure frequency was reduced dramatically each time a new AED was introduced, but the improvement was only transient and was followed by a progressive increase in seizure frequency after a few weeks or months. A long-term follow-up study should therefore be part of the initial design. It is not clear, however, whether the increase in seizure frequency represents a worsening of the epileptic process or the development of tolerance.

Difficulties Related to Caretaking, Seizure Quantification, and Definition of Endpoints

Most children share their daytime among several caretakers, parents, teachers, and others, who may not have the same definition of seizure types and quality of observation. Special training based on video recording thus may be warranted. Certain types of seizures, such as myoclonus, absences, and brief atonic seizures, are particularly difficult to quantify. Some investigators have proposed quantification of seizures on video EEG, since the frequency based on video monitoring has been found to differ dramatically from the frequency reported by caretakers. Video-EEG quantification has several drawbacks, however, including hospital admission, which modifies the daily living conditions and seizure frequency. Consecutive recording sessions are not absolutely comparable, since the child grows accustomed to conditions of the recording session. A decrease of 50 percent in seizure frequency for this type of epilepsy may not be clinically relevant if the seizures still occur several times a day. Therefore, it may be more appropriate to determine, for example, the proportion of patients who become seizure-free, those who have less than one seizure a day, and those who have less than one a week. The number of seizure-free days may also be relevant. The value of intensive parental observation in prescheduled periods remains to be demonstrated. In childhood and juvenile absence epilepsy, ictal events can be identified and therefore quantified on EEG. Prolonged ambulatory recordings while lacking video correlation can also be helpful since recordings can be obtained in the patient's normal environment.

Cognitive Functions

Half the children with epilepsy exhibit fluctuations of cognitive functions over a period of months (Bourgeois et al., 1983). Some epilepsy syndromes are associated with rapid mental deterioration over a period of a few weeks. In other cases the effect on cognition may be insidious, detected only by standardized tests (Vining et al., 1987). In addition, drug effects in combination may modify cognition differently from effects of a single monotherapy. Few data and standardized tests are available for testing cognitive functions in children under 6 years treated with AEDs. Although studies of cognitive functions early in life are difficult to perform, they are necessary to determine the risk of drug toxicity on intellectual functioning and other behaviors.

Ethical Issues

Two types of ethical problems are faced by the clinical investigator. To what extent can parents give informed consent for the child? When should studies in children be started?

The Problems of Informed Consent. In most developed countries, the investigator is obliged by law to obtain approval of the local ethical committee and a written informed consent for each patient prior to any drug trial. For pediatric drug trials, only the parents are able to give such a consent. Whenever possible, the child is also required to give consent. To what extent is the parents' acceptance sufficient? Whereas for "therapeutic" research there is no doubt, for "nontherapeutic" research there are significant reservations. Double-blind placebo-controlled trials are acceptable only if they concern a type of seizure or a type of epilepsy syndrome specific to children (or with onset in early childhood), and provided the design is likely to permit evaluation of the risk-to-benefit ratio for each patient. A prospective study of untreated patients comparing a new AED to an effective reference drug would not be acceptable if it required frequent visits and blood samples which would otherwise not be indicated during treatment with the effective reference drug, unless there is a good reason to suspect that the new drug may be better tolerated than the reference.

When Should Therapeutic Research in Children Be Initiated? Morselli and Regnier (1983) disagreed with the FDA and with several medical societies that had previously developed guidelines suggesting that a drug should be tested in children only after safety and efficacy had been proven in adult patients. These authors argued that it would delay by 2 to 5 years the evaluation of AEDs in children, and that it is not acceptable to refuse to offer the same benefits to children as to adults. In addition, there are several historic examples of drugs being registered for adults but not studied for children. The ILAE commission (Commission on Antiepileptic Drugs, 1989) and a recent workshop sponsored by the Epilepsy Branch of the NINDS (1994) reached the same conclusion as Morselli and Regnier. Studies in children need a well-equipped institution with medical staff experienced in this type of research to obtain rapid and wide knowledge on both efficacy and tolerance in children. Trials without direct benefit to a child can be performed only if there is no potential for serious risk, if collection of the data is necessary to treat other children, and if it is impossible to obtain the data by any other means (Fagot-Largeault, 1985).

Objectives and Strategy for Drug Trial Design

For ethical reasons, early studies on normal volunteers are restricted to adults. However, since syndromes, tolerance, and pharmacokinetics differ in adults and children, there is no scientific or ethical reason to delay the clinical development of effective treatments in children with epilepsy compared to adults with epilepsy. When studies in animal models suggest specific drug action on a type of epilepsy syndrome restricted to childhood, studies in children could even precede studies in adults.

An initial open trial is important to determine drug effectiveness, side effects, and tolerance (based on biochemical, hematologic, and cognitive functions). Such studies may also include analysis of pharmacokinetics according to age as well as interaction with other medication. If possible, the trial should be stratified by epilepsy syndromes. Worsening of specific types of seizures and/or syndromes should also be determined. In patients with partial improvement, a randomized withdrawal trial could complete the study. However, the reliability of such a study remains to be determined; withdrawal seizures may complicate evaluation of the antiepileptic effect of the drug.

Controlled studies in selected syndromes could then be designed based on the findings of the open study. They should mainly involve syndromes that are specific to children (Commission on Antiepileptic Drugs of the International League against Epilepsy, 1994). Such controlled studies may have to be very restricted in terms of patient selection—for example, patients with only one etiologic condition of West syndrome. Inclusion criteria should comprise precise diagnostic criteria. Factors should be determined according to type and frequency of seizures, risk of rapid deterioration of cognitive functions by the epilepsy, the eventual existence of a standard drug registered for this indication, and the likely time lag for the effect of the drug based on data drawn from open studies. Thus parallel versus crossover design, duration of the baseline and study periods, placebo or reference drug as the control group, and endpoints are major issues to address for the study design.

The practical design of a controlled study should determine:

1. Operational diagnostic criteria, based on clinical (age of occurrence, types of seizures) and EEG characteristics and on etiology (depending on the type of syndrome mainly in West and Lennox-Gastaut syndromes); differential diagnosis should be detailed in the exclusion criteria.

2. The rationale, depending on the type of seizures, including the risk of status epilepticus, variability of seizure type and frequency over time and their clinical consequences, difficulties in seizure quantification, cognitive impairment, and the existence of a reference drug.

3. The aim of the study based on the rationale.

4. The endpoints: clinical seizure quantification, EEG ictal (absences) or interictal spike (continuous spike waves in slow sleep) quantification, and/or cognitive functions.

Given the susceptibility to withdrawal seizures in children with convulsive seizures (including the risk of status epilepticus), a parallel design is always preferred to a crossover design. Parents and caretakers should be trained to recognize seizure types, using video-recorded typical seizures of each type. Indeed, seizure types may change during the trial. The use of a placebo is ethically acceptable when no registered standard and well-tolerated drug is available for this indication. For the design of parallel add-on trials, metabolic interaction of study and reference drugs with comedication must be taken into account.

The open and controlled studies should avoid prolonged baseline and study periods to prevent selection of the most intractable cases. In addition, they should be completed by long-term follow-up studies of responders to determine the frequency, time lag, and conditions of occurrence of relapse, and whether reduction of comedication is possible.

Registration of the drug is not the end of the drug development process. The value of the drug in everyday clinical practice may differ from the conclusions drawn from trials designed to demonstrate its antiepilepsy efficacy for registration. Postmarketing studies are therefore necessary.

Current Controlled AED Trials

Few double-blind controlled AED trials have been performed in infants and children. Two trials involved patients with infantile spasms, comparing ACTH to nitrazepam (Dreifuss et al., 1986) or prednisone (Hrachovy et al., 1983), and both studies failed to show any difference. However, the etiology was not taken into account even though the syndrome is very heterogeneous. A single controlled drug trial for absence epilepsy compared valproate to ethosuximide (Sato et al., 1982), also finding no difference.

The only double-blind placebo-controlled trials in children with epilepsy involved patients with Lennox-Gastaut syndrome treated with cinromide (Group for the Evaluation of Cinromide in the Lennox-Gastaut Syndrome, 1989) and felbamate (Ritter et al., 1991). The first trial found no significant difference, but the second trial showed a significant reduction of seizure frequency.

Mechanisms of Action of AEDs Currently under Clinical Investigation or Recently Licensed

Vigabatrin

Vigabatrin (γ-vinyl-GABA; VGB), 4-amino-hex-5-enoic acid, is licensed in most western European countries. Open studies with add-on design suggest that the drug is mainly effective in cryptogenic and symptomatic partial epilepsy and in symptomatic West syndrome, particularly when due to tuberous sclerosis and porencephaly (Chiron et al., 1991; Dulac et al., 1991; Livingston et al., 1989). VGB is effective in the treatment of human partial seizures with or without secondary generalization. The only controlled study performed in children was a withdrawal study that demonstrated a significant increase in seizure frequency (Chiron et al., unpublished).

VGB has been shown to be an effective anticonvulsant in a variety of animal models of epilepsy. In studies with rodents, VGB inhibited strychnine-induced and audiogenic seizures (Schechter et al., 1979). Other studies showed that only the active $S(+)$-enantiomer of VGB was effective in inhibiting audiogenic seizures in mice (Meldrum and Murugaiah, 1983). VGB inhibited epileptic responses in photosensitive baboons (Meldrum and Horton, 1978) and inhibited the development of kindling (Loscher et al., 1987; Shin et al., 1986) as well as fully developed generalized seizures in the amygdala-kindled rat (Kalichman et al., 1982). VGB was less effective in inhibiting seizures caused by bicuculline and picrotoxin (Schechter and Tranier, 1977).

VGB is a synthetic derivative and structural analogue of GABA and was developed to be an enzyme-activated, irreversible inhibitor of GABA-transaminase (GABA-T), the primary presynaptic degradative enzyme of GABA. VGB's selective inhibition of GABA-T was intended to have potential therapeutic value by increasing GABA levels in the brain and thereby enhancing GABAergic transmission (Table 11-3; Jung et al., 1977; Schecter et al., 1979). Enhancement of GABA concentrations has been shown in all brain areas assayed; quantitative differences reflect the relative regional distribution of GABAergic neurons (Chapman et al., 1982). VGB markedly increased the synaptosomal GABA pool in rat cortex compared with nonsynaptosomal GABA (Sarhan and Seiler, 1979), suggesting a greater effect of VGB on neuronal GABA-T rather than glial GABA-T. This effect is consistent with the finding that neurons have a high-affinity GABA uptake system, whereas astrocytes have a low-affinity system (Schousboe et al., 1986).

In human studies, VGB dose-dependently increased cerebrospinal fluid levels of free and total GABA (Ben-Menachem, 1989; Grove et al., 1981; Schechter et al., 1984) but did not significantly affect other neurotransmitter systems (Riekkinen et al., 1989; Schechter et al., 1984). In recent studies with healthy subjects, nuclear magnetic resonance spectroscopy showed that occipital lobe GABA concentrations were elevated after administration of VGB (Petroff et al., 1993).

In summary, VGB is a selective irreversible inhibitor of GABA-T, the main degradative enzyme of GABA. Inhibition of GABA-T may produce greater available pools of presynaptic GABA for release in central nervous system synapses, resulting in increased inhibition of neurons important in controlling the abnormal electrical activity of seizures. These actions likely account for the clinical antiepileptic effects of VGB.

Lamotrigine

Open studies with add-on design suggest that lamotrigine (LTG), 3,5,-diamino-6-(2,3-dichlorophenyl)-1,2,4-triazine, is mainly effective in absence epilepsy, in Lennox-Gastaut syndrome (Oller et al., 1991), and in cryptogenic partial epilepsy with secondary generalization. LTG has been effective as add-on therapy in the treatment of human partial and generalized tonic-clonic seizures (Matsuo et al., 1993). Controversial data have been reported

TABLE 11-3. New Antiepileptic Drug Actions

Drug	Sodium Channels	GABA R Channels	T-Calcium Channels	NMDAR Channels
Felbamate	+/?	+/?	?	+/?
Gabapentin	+/?	−	−	−
Lamotrigine	+ +	−/?	−/?	?
Oxcarbazepine	+/?	?	?	?
Vigabatrin	?	+	?	?

regarding myoclonic epilepsy (Schlumberger et al., 1992; Wallace, 1989). No controlled study has been reported in children.

LTG has anticonvulsant activity in several animal seizure models including hindlimb extension in maximal electroshock and maximal pentylenetetrazol seizures in rodents (Miller et al., 1986).

LTG is a phenyltriazine with weak antifolate activity. It was developed following the observations that use of phenobarbital, primidone, and phenytoin resulted in reduced folate levels and that folates could induce seizures in experimental animals (Reynolds et al., 1966). It was proposed that antifolate activity may be related to anticonvulsant activity; however, this has not been demonstrated by structure-activity studies (Rogawski and Porter, 1990).

The action of LTG on the release of endogenous amino acids from rat cerebral cortex slices in vitro has been studied. LTG potently inhibited release of glutamate and aspartate evoked by the sodium channel activator veratrine and was much less effective in the inhibition of release of acetylcholine or GABA. At high concentrations LTG had no effect on spontaneous or potassium-evoked amino acid release. These studies suggested that LTG acted at voltage-dependent sodium channels resulting in decreased presynaptic release of glutamate (Table 11-3; Leach et al., 1986). In radioligand studies, the binding of ^{3}H-batrachotoxinin A 20-α-benzoate, a neurotoxin that binds to receptor site 2 on voltage-dependent sodium channels, was inhibited by LTG in rat brain synaptosomes (Cheung et al., 1992). Several electrophysiologic studies have tested the effects of LTG on voltage-dependent sodium channels. LTG blocked sustained repetitive firing in cultured mouse spinal cord neurons in a dose-dependent manner at concentrations therapeutic in the treatment of human seizures (Cheung et al., 1992). In cultured rat cortical neurons LTG reduced burst firing induced by glutamate or potassium, but not unitary sodium action potentials evoked at low frequencies (Lees and Leach, 1993). In cultured hippocampal neurons LTG reduced sodium currents in a voltage-dependent manner, and at depolarized potentials it showed a small frequency-dependent inhibition (Mutoh and Dichter, 1993). LTG increased steady-state inactivation of rat brain type IIA sodium channel α subunit currents expressed in Chinese hamster ovary cells (Taylor, 1993) and produced both tonic and frequency-dependent inhibition of voltage-dependent sodium channels in clonal N4TG1 mouse neuroblastoma cells, but it had no effect on cationic currents induced by stimulation of glutamatergic receptors in embryonic rat hippocampal neurons (Wang et al., 1993).

In cultured rat cortical neurons LTG at high concentrations was able to inhibit peak high threshold calcium currents and appeared to shift the threshold for inward currents to more depolarized potentials (Lees and Leach, 1993). In clonal rat pituitary GH3 cells LTG at the same concentration did not inhibit high threshold calcium currents, caused only slight inhibition of low threshold calcium currents, reduced rapidly inactivating voltage-dependent potassium currents, and had no significant effect on calcium-activated potassium currents (Lang and Wang, 1991). In cultured rat cortical neurons LTG did not appear to mimic the effect of diazepam when tested on GABA-evoked chloride currents (Lees and Leach, 1993).

These results suggest that the antiepileptic effect of LTG is due to a specific interaction at the voltage-dependent sodium channel that results in voltage- and frequency-dependent inhibition of the channel. These results are similar to those found for phenytoin and carbamazepine. It remains to be determined whether this action results in a significant preferential decreased release of presynaptic glutamate.

Oxcarbazepine

Oxcarbazepine (OCBZ), 10,11-dihydro-10-oxo-carbamazepine, is licensed in a few countries of Europe and Latin America. In an open study, 55 children were switched from carbamazepine to oxcarbazepine with excellent tolerance (Schobben and Willemse, 1985). No efficacy trial is available.

OCBZ is a derivative of the dibenzazepine series and is structurally very similar to carbamazepine. OCBZ differs from carbamazepine by a keto substitution at the 10,11 position of the dibenzazepine nucleus. The keto substitution causes a different biotransformation and greater tolerability in humans compared to carbamazepine. OCBZ is rapidly and nearly completely metabolized to 10,11-dihydro-10-hydroxy carbamazepine (GP 47779; HCBZ), the active metabolite responsible for the antiepileptic activity of OCBZ (Jensen et al., 1991). Metabolism of OCBZ does not result in the formation of 10,11-epoxy carbamazepine. OCBZ and HCBZ are effective in inhibiting hindlimb extension in rats and mice elicited by maximal electroshock but are approximately two to three times less effective against pentylenetetrazol-induced seizures in mice (Baltzer and Schmutz, 1978). In studies using rats at different developmental ages, OCBZ, HCBZ, and carbamazepine dose-dependently reduced the tonic phase of generalized seizures induced by pentylenetetrazol and appeared to have identical anticonvulsant profiles in this model (Kubova and Mares, 1993). OCBZ and HCBZ have relatively poor anticonvulsant efficacy against picrotoxin- and strychnine-induced seizures in mice (Baltzer and Schmutz, 1978). OCBZ was able to completely suppress seizures in rhesus monkeys in a chronic aluminum focus model of partial seizures; at comparable doses, HCBZ was less effective in suppressing seizures in this model (Jensen et al., 1991). OCBZ is effective in the treatment of human generalized tonic-clonic seizures and partial seizures with and without secondary generalization (Dam and Jensen, 1989).

In electrophysiologic studies of rat hippocampal slices, OCBZ and HCBZ enantiomers dose-dependently decreased paroxysmal discharges induced by penicillin. Additionally, the drugs' ability to suppress discharges was decreased by 4-amino-pyridine, a potassium channel blocker (Schmutz et al., 1993). Because OCBZ and HCBZ are similar to carbamazepine in both structure and clinical efficacy, it is likely that their mechanism of action may be similar to that of carbamazepine, namely, inhibition of sustained high-frequency repetitive firing of voltage-dependent sodium action potentials (Table 11-3). However, this has not been demonstrated by electrophysiological testing, and the mechanism of action of OCBZ remains unknown.

Felbamate

Felbamate (FBM), 2-phenyl-1,3-propanediol dicarbamate, has been shown to be significantly effective in Lennox-Gastaut syndrome defined as the combination of several types of generalized seizures, slow spike waves, and fast rhythms in sleep (Ritter et al., 1991). The favorable effect was maintained over the long term (Espe-Lillo and Ritter, 1992). Two small, open studies suggested an effect on absence seizures (Devinski et al., 1992) and on juvenile myoclonic epilepsy (Sachdeo et al., 1992). Felbamate was recently approved for use in the United States. However, early experience with the drug was associated with an unacceptably high incidence of aplastic anemia (Pennell et al., in press) and in August of 1994 the manufacturer and the FDA recommended that patients be withdrawn from felbamate if clinically possible.

In experimental animals, FBM was effective in blocking seizures induced by maximal electroshock, pentylenetetrazol, and picrotoxin (Swinyard et al., 1986). FBM inhibited bicuculline-induced seizures at high concentrations but was ineffective against strychnine-induced seizures (Sofia et al., 1991). In subprotective doses, FBM enhanced the protective effects of diazepam against seizures induced by maximal electroshock, pentylenetetrazol, and isoniazid, but not bicuculline, suggesting that felbamate may have indirect effects on the $GABA_A$ receptor complex or be involved in other mechanisms of action (Gordon et al., 1991).

Felbamate is a dicarbamate that has a structure similar to meprobamate, an antianxiety agent. FBM has been tested for interaction with the $GABA_A$ receptor complex as a possible mechanism of its antiepileptic activity. In rat brain cortical membranes, FBM did not affect ligand binding to the GABA, benzodiazepine, or picrotoxin binding sites of the $GABA_A$ receptor complex; in radiolabeled Cl^- influx studies in cultured mouse spinal cord neurons, FBM did not affect GABA-induced ^{36}Cl influx (Ticku et al., 1991). However, in cultured rat hippocampal neurons, FBM produced an increase in GABA-evoked Cl^- currents, which was not blocked by the benzodiazepine receptor antagonist flumazenil, suggesting that FBM was active at the $GABA_A$ receptor complex but not as an agonist at the benzodiazepine recognition site (Rho et al., 1994). In other studies using mouse spinal cord neurons, FBM reduced sustained repetitive firing of action potentials of voltage-dependent sodium channels (IC_{50} of 67 mg/ml when compared with a control population of neurons of which 72 percent responded with sustained repetitive firing) (White et al., 1992). It remains to be determined whether these results indicate a direct interaction of FBM with voltage-dependent sodium channels.

FBM has also been tested for a possible effect on excitatory amino acid receptors. FBM inhibited NMDA- and quisqualate-induced seizures in mice but did not significantly inhibit MK-801 binding (Sofia et al., 1991). FBM has been shown to inhibit the binding of [^{3}H]5,7-dichlorokynurenic acid, a competitive antagonist, at the strychnine-insensitive glycine site of the NMDA receptor (McCabe et al, 1993). FBM also reduced the ability of glycine to enhance NMDA-induced calcium currents in cerebellar granule cells measured by the fluorescent probe indo-1. In other studies, D-serine, a glycine site agonist, was administered intracerebroventricularly in audiogenic seizure-susceptible mice and produced a parallel right shift in FBM's anticonvulsant dose-response curve (Harmsworth et al., 1993). The results of these different studies suggest that FBM has activity at the glycine site of the NMDA receptor that may be related to its antiepileptic mechanism of action. However, studies in cultured rat hippocampal neurons showed that FBM's inhibition of NMDA receptor currents could not be overcome by increasing the concentration of NMDA or glycine, suggesting that FBM's activity was more consistent with open channel block than with antagonism at the glycine site of the NMDA receptor (Rho et al., 1994).

Further experiments are required to more fully characterize the potential antiepileptic mechanisms of action of FBM. These mechanisms of action may include enhancement of GABA$_A$ receptor-mediated inhibition, inhibition of high-frequency repetitive firing of sodium channels, and inhibition at the NMDA receptor ion channel complex (Table 11-3). Diverse mechanisms of action of FBM may underlie its unique anticonvulsant profile and clinical effectiveness.

Gabapentin

Gabapentin (GBP), 1-(aminomethyl)cyclohexane-acetic acid, is most effective in the treatment of human partial and generalized tonic-clonic seizures. GBP's effect on absence seizures has also been studied in both animal models of absence seizures and as add-on therapy in patients with epilepsy who are drug-resistant. In animal studies using pentylenetetrazol-induced clonic seizures, GBP protected mice from clonic convulsions in both the subcutaneous metrazol test and the intravenous threshold test (Bartoszyk et al., 1986). However, in a rat genetic model of absence epilepsy GBP increased electroencephalographic spike-and-wave bursts in a dose-dependent manner (Foot and Wallace, 1991). In human studies GBP reduced more than 50 percent of absence seizures in half the patients in one study (Bauer et al., 1989), and GBP reduced absence seizures and generalized spike-and-wave complexes in patients undergoing 24-hour electroencephalogram monitoring in another study (Rowan et al., 1989).

GBP is a cyclic GABA analogue originally designed to mimic the steric conformation of GABA (Schmidt, 1989), to have high lipid solubility to penetrate the blood–brain barrier, and to be a centrally active GABA agonist with potential therapeutic value (Rogawski and Porter, 1990). Early work with GBP also suggested that it may act on GABAergic neurotransmitter systems since it protected mice from tonic extension in chemical convulsion models using inhibitors of GABA synthesis (3-mercaptopropionic acid, isonicotinic acid, semicarbazide) or antagonists acting at the GABA$_A$ receptor complex (bicuculline, picrotoxin) (Bartoszyk et al., 1983; Bartoszyk and Reimann, 1985). However, subsequent work has not clearly demonstrated a specific effect of GBP on GABAergic neurotransmitter systems. Inhibition of monoamine release by GBP in electrically stimulated rabbit caudate nucleus (Reimann, 1983) and rat cortex (Schlicker et al., 1985) was not modified by GABA, baclofen, or bicuculline, suggesting that GBP did not act at GABA$_A$ or GABA$_B$ receptors. Binding experiments in rat brain and spinal cord have shown that GBP has no significant affinity for the GABA$_A$ or GABA$_B$ binding sites measured by ^{3}H-muscimol and ^{3}H-baclofen displacement, respectively. GBP did not significantly inhibit the binding of ^{3}H-diazepam, had only a weak inhibitory effect on the GABA-degrading enzyme GABA-aminotransferase, did not elevate GABA content in nerve terminals, and did not affect the GABA uptake system (Bartoszyk et al., 1986). However, GBP has been shown to increase GABA turnover in several regions of rat brain (Loscher et al., 1991) and to increase release of GABA from rat striatal slices (Gotz et al., 1993). Recent work has shown that GBP binds to a novel high-affinity site in the central nervous system (Hill et al., 1993; Suman-Chauhan et al., 1993) and was potently displaced by the anticonvulsant 3-isobutyl GABA (Taylor et al., 1993), but the identity of this binding site remains uncertain. Additionally, GBP has been shown to be a substrate for a saturable L-amino acid transport system in rat gut tissues (Stewart et al., 1993), and GBP appeared to be concentrated from brain interstitial fluid into brain tissue by an active process (Welty et al., 1993). The results of these studies raise the possibility of a specific binding site of GBP for active transport across neuronal membranes. This hypothesis remains to be tested. In electrophysiologic studies, GBP did not affect depolarizations elicited by iontophoretic application of GABA on cultured mouse spinal cord neurons (Rock et al., 1993; Taylor et al., 1988). Additionally, GBP appeared to act by GABA receptor–independent mechanisms in studies with rat hippocampal slices (Haas and Wieser, 1986) and the feline trigeminal nucleus (Kondo et al., 1991). GBP has been shown to decrease inhibition evoked by paired-pulse orthodromic stimulation of pyramidal neurons in the hippocampal slice preparation (Dooley et al., 1985; Taylor et al., 1988); however, the specific effect of GBP in this paradigm is not known.

GBP protected mice from convulsions caused by strychnine, a glycine receptor antagonist, but was unable to displace ^{3}H-strychnine in binding studies at the highest concentrations tested (Bartoszyk et al., 1986). Electrophysiologic studies showed no effect of GBP on the response of spinal cord neurons to iontophoretically applied glycine (Rock et al., 1993).

GBP has been tested in animal seizure models where seizures are induced by administration of excitatory amino acids. GBP prolonged the onset latency of clonic convulsions and tonic extension and death in mice following intraperitoneal injections of NMDA but not kainic acid or quinolinic acid. GBP did not have a clear effect on convulsions when these compounds or glutamate was injected into the lateral ventricle of rats (Bartoszyk, 1983). Intraperitoneal injections in mice of GBP or the NMDA receptor competitive antagonist 3-((±)-2-carboxypiperazin-4-yl)-propyl-1-phosphonic acid (CPP) antagonized tonic seizures. The effect of GBP, but not CPP, was dose-dependently antagonized by the administration of serine, an agonist at the glycine receptor on the NMDA receptor complex, suggesting an involvement of the strychnine-insensitive glycine site of the NMDA receptor in the anticonvulsant activity of GBP (Oles et al., 1990). In unpublished studies, GBP reportedly antagonized NMDA-induced, but not kainate-induced, depolarizations in thalamic and hippocampal slice preparations and antagonized NMDA-induced currents in the presence of glycine in cultured striatal neurons, an effect that was reversed by the addition of serine or increased glycine (Chadwick, 1992). Other studies did not show a significant effect of GBP on neuronal responses to iontophoretic application of glutamate or on membrane depolarizations and single channel currents evoked by NMDA with or without coapplication of glycine (Rock et al., 1993). These results are similar to the findings that GBP had no effect on spinal cord neuron depolarizations elicited by iontophoretically applied glutamate (Taylor et al., 1988) or pressure-ejected NMDA (Wamil et al., 1991). Additionally, in extracellular recordings from rat hippocampal slice preparations GBP had no effect on long-term potentiation, making it unlike NMDA receptor antagonists (Taylor et al., 1988).

GBP had no effect on sustained repetitive firing of action potentials in mouse spinal cord neurons (Rock et al., 1993; Taylor et al., 1988). In other experiments using the same neuronal preparation, prolonged times of exposure (12–48 hours) and/or application of GBP resulted in a voltage- and frequency-dependent limitation of sustained repetitive firing of sodium action potentials at therapeutically relevant concentrations (Wamil et al., 1994). However, GBP had no effect on rat brain type IIA sodium channel α subunit currents expressed in Chinese hamster ovary cells following 24-hour bath application of GBP or when GBP was delivered by blunt pipette or the recording electrode (Taylor, 1993). The results of these different studies suggest that the antiepileptic activity of GBP is not due to a direct interaction with voltage-dependent sodium channels limiting sustained repetitive firing of action potentials.

In studies of mouse spinal cord neurons, GBP blocked responses to Bay K 8644, an agonist at the dihydropyridine binding site of the L-type calcium channel (Wamil et al., 1991). In other electrophysiologic studies, however, GBP did not significantly affect any calcium channel current subtype (T, N, or L), suggesting that its basic mechanism of action was not on voltage-dependent calcium channels (Rock et al., 1993).

In summary, the results of several studies have not demonstrated a major effect of GBP on ligand- or voltage-gated channels (Table 11-3). Further work on the high-affinity binding site of GBP and the possibility of active transport of GBP across neuronal membranes should contribute significantly to understanding its mechanism of action.

Conclusion

Multiple AEDs are available for treatment of childhood epilepsies, and several AEDs have recently been approved for treatment of epilepsies in adults and for some childhood epilepsies. Furthermore, many other promising AEDs are currently under development or in clinical trials. While many of these new AEDs may be effective in treating the childhood epilepsies, few controlled clinical trials have been carried out with pediatric patients. In addition, during preclinical development of the AEDs, few studies on seizures in immature animals have been reported. It is clear that the developing nervous system has an organization different from that of the adult; it may have different isoforms of neurotransmitter receptors and ion channels—the presumed molecular targets of the AEDs. It is essential, therefore, that preclinical studies include evaluation of the AED actions on seizures in immature animals, studies of AED mechanisms of action on immature nervous system preparations, and clinical trials which include pediatric patients when appropriate and ethically possible.

Acknowledgments

Data and ideas have been shared with the participants in the Royaumont meeting (1990); the members of the Commission on Drugs of ILAE, L. Gram, A. Perret, I. Leppik, A. Gonzalez-Astiazaran, P. Loiseau, and H. Frey; the chairperson of the Commission on Pediatric Epileptology of ILAE, J. Roger; and C. Dravet, W. Renier, J. Mumford, and K. Farrell.

References

Aguglia, U., Zappia, M., and Quattrone, A. (1987) Carbamazepine-induced nonepileptic myoclonus in a child with benign epilepsy. *Epilepsia 28:*515–518.

Aicardi, J., and Newton, R. (1983) Clinical findings in children with occipital spike wave complexes suppressed by eye-opening. *Neurology (Cleveland) 33:*1526–1529.

Ambrosetto, G., Rossi, P. G., and Tassinara, L. A. (1987) Predictive factors of seizure frequency and duration of antiepileptic treatment in rolandic epilepsy: A retrospective study. *Brain Dev. 6:*300–304.

Aranda, J. V., MacLeod, S. M., Renton, K. W., and Eade, N. R. (1974) Hepatic microsomal drug oxidation and electron transport in newborn infants. *J. Pediatr. 85:*534–542.

Baltzer, V., and Schmutz, M. (1978) Experimental anticonvulsive properties of GP 47 680 and of GP 47 779, its main human metabolite: Compounds related to carbamazepine. In H. Meinardi and A. J. Rowan (eds.), *Advances in Epileptology, 1977.* Amsterdam/Lisse: Swets and Zeitlinger, pp. 295–299.

Bartoszyk, G. D. (1983) Gabapentin and convulsions provoked by excitatory amino acids. *Naunyn-Schmiedeberg's Arch. Pharmacol. 324:*R24.

Bartoszyk, G. D., Fritschi, E., Herrmann, M., and Satzinger, G. (1983) Indications for an involvement of the GABA-system in the mechanism of action of gabapentin. *Naunyn-Schmiedeberg's Arch. Pharmacol. 322:*R94.

Bartoszyk, G. D., Meyerson, N., Reimann, W., Satzinger, G., and Von Hodenberg, A. (1986) Gabapentin. In B. S. Meldrum and R. J. Porter (eds.), *Current Problems in Epilepsy: New Anticonvulsant Drugs.* London: John Libbey, pp. 147–164.

Bartoszyk, G. D., and Reimann, W. (1985) Preclinical characterization of the anticonvulsant gabapentin. *16th Epilepsy International Congress, Hamburg (Abstracts).*

Battino, D., Bossi, L., Croci, D., Franceschetti, S., Gomenti, C., Moise, A., and Vitali, A. Carbamazepine plasma levels in children and adults: Influence of age, dose, and associated therapy. *Ther. Drug Monit. 2:*315–322.

Bauer, G., Bechinger, D., Castell, M., et al. (1989) Gabapentin in the treatment of drug-resistant epileptic patients. *Adv. Epileptol. 17:*219–221.

Beaussart, M., and Faou, M. (1978) Evolution of epilepsy with rolandic paroxysmal foci: A study of 324 cases. *Epilepsia 19:*337–342.

Ben Ari, Y., Tremblay, E., Ottersen, O. P., and Naquet, R. (1979) Evidence suggesting secondary epileptogenic lesions afer kainic acid: Pretreatment with diazepam reduces distant but not local brain damage. *Brain Res. 165:*362–365.

Ben-Menachem, E. (1989) Pharmacokinetic effects of vigabatrin on cerebrospinal fluid amino acids in humans. *Epilepsia 30* (Suppl. 3):S12–S14.

Boreus, L. O., Jalling, B., and Kallberg, N. (1975) Clinical pharmacology of phenobarbital in the neonatal period. In P. L. Morseli, S. Garattini, and F. Serini (eds.), *Basic and Therapeutic Aspects of Perinatal Pharmacology.* New York: Raven Press, pp. 331–340.

Boulloche, J., Leloup, P., Mallet, E., Parrain, D. and Tron, P. (1989) Risk of recurrence after a single, unprovoked, generalized tonic-clonic seizure. *Dev. Med. Child. Neurol. 31:*626–632.

Bourgeois, B. F. D., Prensky, A. L., Palkes, H. S., Talent, B. K., and Busch, S. G. (1983) Intelligence in epilepsy: A prospective study in children. *Ann. Neurol. 14:*438–444.

Braestrup, C., and Nielsen, M. J. (1981) [^{3}H]-propyl-*b*-carboline-3-carboxylate as a selective radioligand for the BZI benzodiazepine receptor subclass. *J. Neurochem. 7:*333–341.

Brent, D. A., Crumrine, P. K., Varma, R. R., Allan, M., and Callman, C. (1987) Phenobarbital treatment and major depressive disorder in children with epilepsy. *Pediatrics 80:*909–917.

Campbell, K. P., Leung, A. T., and Sharp, A. H. (1988) The biochemistry and molecular biology of the dihydropydrine-sensitive calcium channel. *Trends Neurosci. 11:*425–430.

Catterall, W. A. (1988) Structure and function of voltage-sensitive ion channels. *Science 242:*50–61.

Cavell, B. (1979) Gastric emptying in preterm infants. *Acta Paediatr. Scand. 68:*725–730.

Chadwick, D. (1992) Gabapentin. In T. A. Pedley and B. S. Meldrum (eds.), *Recent Advances in Epilepsy.* New York: Churchill Livingstone, pp. 211–221.

Chaigne, D. and Dulac, O. (1989) Carbamazepine versus valproate in partial epilepsies of childhood. *Adv. Epilepsy 17:*198–200.

Chapman, A. G., Riley, K., Evans, M. C., and Meldrum, B. S. (1982) Acute effects of sodium valproate and δ-vinyl GABA on regional amino acid metabolism in the rat brain: Incorporation of 2[^{14}C]glucose into amino acids. *Neurochem. Res. 7*:1089–1105.

Chauvel, P., and Lamarche, M. (1975) Analyse d'une "Épilepsie du movement" chez un singe porteur d'un foyer rolandique. *Neurochirurgie 21*:121–127.

Cheung, H., Kamp, D., and Harris, E. (1992) An in vitro investigation of the action of lamotrigine on neuronal voltage-activated sodium channels. *Epilepsy Res. 13*:107–112.

Chiron, C., Dulac, O., Beaumont, D., Palacios, L., Pajot, N., and Mumford, J. (1991) Therapeutic trials of vigabatrin in refractory infantile spasms. *J. Child. Neurol. 6* (Suppl.):2S52–2S59.

Chiron, C., Dulac, O., and Plouin, P. (1987) Cryptogenic myoclonic epilepsy of childhood: To give or not to give carbamazepine? Presented at the 17th Epilepsy International Symposium, Jerusalem, September 6–11.

Chiron, C., Raynaud, C., Maziere, B., Zilbovicius, M., LaFlaunne, L., Mazure, M. C., Dulac, O., Bourguignon, M., and Syrota, A. (1992) Changes in regional cerebral blood flow during brain maturation in children and adolescents. *J. Nucl. Med. 33*:697–703.

Chugani, H., Phelps, M. E., and Mazziota, J. C. (1987) Positron emission tomography of human brain functional development. *Ann. Neurol. 22*:487–497.

Commission on Antiepileptic Drugs in the International League against Epilepsy. (1989) Guidelines for clinical evaluation of antiepileptic drugs. *Epilepsia 30*:400–408.

Commission on Antiepileptic Drugs of the International League against Epilepsy. (1991) Workshop on antiepileptic drug trials in children. *Epilepsia 32:* 284–285.

Commission on Antiepileptic Drugs of the International League against Epilepsy. (1994) Guidelines for antiepileptic drug trials in children. *Epilepsia 35*:94–100.

Commission on Classification and Terminology of the International League against Epilepsy. (1989) Proposal for revised classification of epilepsies and epileptic syndromes. *Epilepsia 30*:389–399.

Cutting, G. R., Lu, L., O'Hara, B. F., et al. (1991) Cloning of the γ-aminobutyric acid (GABA) p_1 cDNA: A GABA receptor subunit highly expressed in the retina. *Proc. Natl. Acad. Sci. 88*:2673–2677.

Dalla Bernardina, B., Chiamenti, C., Capovilla, G., Trevisan, E., and Tassinari, C. A. (1985) Benign partial epilepsy with affective symptoms. In J. Roger, C. Dravet, M. Bureau, F. E. Dreifuss, and P. Wolf (eds.), *Epileptic Syndromes in Infancy, Childhood and Adolescence.* London: Libbey Eurotext, pp. 171–175.

Dam, M., and Jensen, P. K. (1989) Potential antiepileptic drugs: Oxcarbazepine. In R. H. Levy, F. E. Dreifuss, R. H. Mattson, B. S. Meldrum, and J. K. Penry (eds.), *Antiepileptic Drugs,* 3rd ed. New York: Raven Press, pp. 913–924.

Deonna, T., Ziegler, A. L., Despland, P. A., Van Melle, G. (1986) Partial epilepsy in neurologically normal children: clinical syndromes and prognosis. *Epilepsia 27*:241–247.

Devinski, O., Kothari, M., Rubin, R., Marcandetti, R., and Luciano, D. (1992) Felbamate in absence epilepsy. *Epilepsia 33* (Suppl. 3):84.

Dooley, D. J., Bartoszyk, G. D., Rock, D. M., and Satzinger, G. (1985) Preclinical characterization of the anticonvulsant gabapentin. *16th Epilepsy International Congress, Hamburg.* (Abstracts)

Doose, H. (1985) Myoclonic astatic epilepsy of early childhood. In J. Roger, C. Dravet, M. Bureau, F. E. Dreifuss, and P. Wolf (eds.), *Epileptic Syndromes in Infancy, Childhood and Adolescence*. London: Libbey Eurotext, pp. 78–88.

Dravet, C., Natale, O., Magaudda, A., Larrieu, J. L., Bureau, M., Roger, J., and Tassinari, C. A. (1985) Les États de mal dans le syndrome de Lennox-Gastaut. *Rev. EEG Neurophysiol. Clin. 15:*361–368.

Dravet, C., Roger, J., and Bureau, M. (1985) Severe myoclonic epilepsy in infancy. In J. Roger, C. Dravet, M. Bureau, F. E. Dreifuss, and P. Wolf (eds.), *Epileptic Syndromes in Infancy, Childhood and Adolescence*. London: Libbey Eurotext, pp. 58–67.

Dreifuss, F., Farwell, J., Holmes, G., Joseph, C., Lockman, L., Masden, J. A., Minarcik, C. J., Rothnen, A. D., and Shewmon, A. D. (1986) Infantile spasms, comparative trial of nitrazepam and corticotropin. *Arch. Neurol. 43:*1107–1110.

Dreifuss, F. E., and Langer, D. H. (1987) Hepatic considerations in the use of antiepileptic drugs. *Epilepsia 28* (Suppl. 2):S23–S29.

Dreifuss, F. E., Langer, D. H., Moline, K. A., and Maxwell, J. E. (1989) Valproic acid hepatic fatalities. II. U.S. experience since 1984. *Neurology 69:*201–207.

Duchowny, M. S. (1987) Complex partial seizures in infancy. *Arch. Neurol. 44:*911–914.

Dulac, O., Aicardi, J., Rey, E., and Olive, G. (1978) Blood levels of diazepam after single rectal administration in infants and children. *J. Pediatr. 93:*1039–1041.

Dulac, O., Bouguerra, L., Rey, E., De Lauture, D., and Arthuis, M. (1983) Monotherapie par la carbamazepine dans les épilepsies de l'enfant. *Arch. Fr. Pediatr. 40:*415–419.

Dulac, O., Chiron, C., Luna, D., Cusmai, R., Pajot, N., Beaumont, D., Mondragon, S. (1991) Vigabatrin in childhood epilepsy. *J. Child. Neurol. 6* (Suppl):2S30–2S37.

Dulac, O., Steru, D., Rey, E., Perret, A., and Arthuis, M. (1986) Sodium valproate monotherapy in childhood epilepsy. *Brain Dev. 8:*47–52.

Egger, J., Harding, B. N., Boyd, S. G., Wilson, J., and Erdohazi, M. (1987) Progressive neuronal degeneration of childhood with liver disease. *Clin. Pediatr. 26:*167–173.

Eichinger, A., and Sieghart, W. (1986) Postnatal development of proteins associated with different benzodiazepine receptors. *J. Neurochem. 46:*173–180.

Espe-Lillo, J., and Ritter, F. J. (1992) Long term follow-up of felbamate treatment in children with Lennox-Gastaut syndrome. *Epilepsia 33* (Suppl. 3):118. (Abstract)

Fagot-Largeault, A. (1985) *L'Homme bioéthique*. Paris: Maloine.

Farrell, K. (1986) Benzodiazepines in the treatment of children with epilepsy. *Epilepsia 27* (Suppl. 1):S45–S51.

Foot, M., and Wallace, J. (1991) Gabapentin. In F. Pisani, E. Peruxxa, G. Avazini, and A. Richens (eds.), *New Antiepileptic Drugs*. Amsterdam: Elsevier, pp. 109–114.

Fujita, Y., Mynlieff, M., Kirksen, R. T., Kim, M. S., Niidome, T., Nakai, J., Friedrich, T., Iwabe, N., Miyata, T., Furuichi, T., Furutama, D., Mikoshiba, K., Mori, Y., and Beam, K. G. (1993) Primary structure and functional expression of the w-contotoxin-sensitive *N*-type calcium channel from rabbit brain. *Neuron 10:*585–598.

Garret, K. M., and Tabakoff, B. (1985) The development of type I and type II benzodizepine receptors in the mouse cortex and cerebellum. *Pharmacol. Biochem. Behav. 22:*985–992.

Gastaut, H. (1985) Benign epilepsy of childhood with occipital paraoxysms. In J. Roger, C. Dravet, M. Bureau, F. E. Dreifuss, and P. Wolf (eds.), *Epileptic Syndromes in Infancy, Childhood and Adolescence.* London: Libbey Eurotext, pp. 159–170.

Goddard, G. V., McIntyre, D. C., and Leech, C. K. (1969) A permanent change in brain function resulting from daily electrical stimulation. *Exp. Neurol. 25:*295–330.

Gordon, R., Gels, M., Diamantis, W., and Sofia, R. D. (1991) Interaction of felbamate and diazepam against maximal electroshock seizures and chemoconvulsants in mice. *Pharmacol. Biochem. Behav. 40:*109–113.

Gotz, E., Feuerstein, T. L., Lais, A., and Meyer, D. K. (1993) Effects of gabapentin on release of γ-aminobutyric acid from slices of rat neostriatum. *Arzneim.-Forsch./Drug Res. 43:*636–638.

Group for the Evaluation of Cinromide in the Lennox-Gastaut Syndrome. (1989) Double-blind placebo-controlled evaluation of cinromide in patients with Lennox-Gastaut syndrome. *Epilepsia 30:*422–430.

Grove, J., Schechter, P. J., Tell, G., Koch-Weser, J., Sjoerdsma, A., Warter, J. M., Marescaux, C., and Rumbach, L (1981) Increased gamma-aminobutyric acid (GABA), homocarnosine and β-alanine in cerebrospinal fluid of patients treated with gamma-vinyl GABA (4-amino-hex-5-enoic acid). *Life Sci 28:* 2431–2439.

Haas, H. L., and Wieser, H. G. (1986) Gabapentin: Action on hippocampal slices of the rat and effects in human epileptics. *Northern European Epilepsy Meeting, York.* (Abstracts)

Harmsworth, W. L., Wolf, H. H., Swinyard, E. A., and White, H. S. (1993) Felbamate modulates glycine receptor function. *Epilepsia 34* (Suppl. 2):92–93.

Heiman, G. (1980) Enteral absorption and bioavailability in children in relation to age. *Eur. J. Clin. Pharmacol. 18:*43–50.

Hill, D. R., Suman-Chauhan, N., and Woodruff, G. N. (1993) Localisation of [^{3}H]gabapentin to a novel site in rat brain: Autoradiographic studies. *Eur. J. Pharmacol. Mol. Pharmacol. 244:*303–309.

Hoppner, R. J., Kuger, A., Meijer, J. N. A., and Hulsman, J. (1980) Correlation between daily fluctuations of carbamazepine serum levels and intermittent side-effects. *Epilepsia 21:*341–350.

Hosford, D. A., Clark, S., Cao, B., Wilson, W. A., Jr., Lin, F. H., Morrisett, R. A., and Huin, A. (1992) The role of $GABA_B$ receptor activation in absence of lethargic (1h/1h) mice. *Science 257:*398–401.

Hrachovy, R. A., Frost, J. D., Kellaway, P., and Zion, T. E. (1983) Double blind study of ACTH vs prednisone therapy in infantile spasms. *J. Pediatr. 103:*641–645.

Hui, A., Ellinor, P. T., Krizanova, O., Wang, J. J., Diebold, R. J., and Schwartz, A. (1991) Molecular cloning of multiple subtypes of a novel rat brain isoform of the α_1 subunit of the voltage-dependent calcium channel. *Neuron 7:*35–44.

Jalling, B., Boreus, L. O., Rane, A., Sjaqvist, F. (1970) Plasma concentration of diphenylhydantoin in young infants. *Pharmacol. Clin. 2:*200–202.

Jensen, P. K., Gram, L., and Schmutz, M. (1991) Oxcarbazepine. In F. Pisani, E. Perucca, G. Avanzini, and A. Richens (eds.), *New Antiepileptic Drugs.* Amsterdam: Elsevier, pp. 135–140.

Jung, M. J., Lippert, B., Metcalf, B., Bohlen, P., and Schechter, P. J. (1977) γ-Vinyl GABA (4-amino-hex-5-enoic acid), a new irreversible inhibitor of GABA-T: Effects on brain GABA metabolism in mice. *J. Neurochem. 29:*797–802.

Kalichman, M. W., Burnham, W. M., and Livingstone, K. E. (1982) Pharmacological investigation of gamma-aminobutyric acid (GABA) and fully developed generalized seizures in the amygdala-kindled rat. *Neuropharmacology 21:*127–131.

Klepner, C. A., Lippa, A. S., Benson, D. I., Sano, M. C., and Beer, B. (1978) Resolution of two biochemically and pharmacologically distinct benzodiazepine receptors. *Pharmacol. Biochem. Behav. 11:*457–462.

Knudsen, F. V. (1977) Plasma diazepam in infants after rectal administration in solution and by suppositories. *Acta Paediatr. Scand. 67:*699–704.

Kondo, T., Fromm, G. H., and Schmidt, B. (1991) Comparison of gabapentin with other antiepileptic and GABAergic drugs. *Epilepsy Res. 8:*226–231.

Kubova, H., and Mares, P. (1993) Anticonvulsant action of oxcarbazepine, hydroxycarbamazepine, and carbamazepine against metrazol-induced motor seizures in developing rats. *Epilepsia 34:*188–192.

Kurtz, H., Mauser-Granshorn, A., and Suckel, H. H. (1977) Differences in the binding of drugs to plasma proteins from newborn and adult man. *Eur. J. Clin. Pharmacol. 11:*463–467.

Kurtz, H., Michels, H., and Suckel, H. H. (1977) Differences in the binding of drugs to plasma proteins from the newborn and adult man. *Eur. J. Clin. Pharmacol. 11:*469–472.

Lang, D. G., and Wang, C. M. (1991) Lamotrigine and phenytoin interactions on ionic currents present in N4TG1 and GH3 clonal cells. *Soc. Neurosci. Abstr. 17:*1256.

Lassonde, M., Sauerwein, H., Chicoine, A. J., and Geoffroy, G. (1991) Absence of disconnexion syndrome in callosal agenesis and early callosotomy: Brain reorganization or lack of structural specificity during ontogeny. *Neuropsychologia 29:*480–495.

Laurie, D. J., Seeburg, P. H., and Wisden, W. (1992) The distribution of 13-GABA$_A$ receptor subunit messenger RNAs in the rat brain. II. Olfactory bulb and cerebellum. *J. Neurosci. 12:*1063–1076.

Laurie, D. J., Wisden, W., and Seeburg, P. H. (1992) The distribution of 13-GABA$_A$ receptor subunit messenger RNAs in the rat brain. III. Embryonic and early postnatal development. *J. Neurosci. 12:*4151–4172.

Leach, M. J., Marden, C. M., and Miller, A. A. (1986) Pharmacological studies on lamotrigine, a novel potential antiepileptic drug: II. Neurochemical studies on the mechanism of action. *Epilepsia 27:*490–497.

Lees, G., and Leach, M. J. (1993) Studies on the mechanism of action of the novel anticonvulsant lamotrigine (Lamictal) using primary neuroglial cultures from rat cortex. *Brain Res. 612:*190–199.

Lerman, P., and Kivity-Ephraim, S. (1974) Carbamazepine sole anticonvulsant for focal epilepsy of childhood. *Epilepsia 15:*229–234.

Lerman, P., Lerman-Sagie, T., and Kivity, S. (1991) Effect of early corticosteroid therapy for Landau-Kleffner syndrome. *Dev. Med. Child. Neurol. 33:*257–266.

Levy, R. H., Moreland, T. A., and Farwell, J. R. (1983) Drug interactions in epileptic children. In P. L. Morselli, C. E. Pippenger, and J. Penry (eds.), *Antiepileptic Drug Therapy in Paediatrics.* New York: Raven Press, pp. 75–84.

Lipa, A. S., Beer, B., Sano, M. C., Vogel, R. A., and Myerson, L. R. (1981) Differential ontogeny of type I and type II benzodiazepine receptors. *Life Sci.* *28*:2343–2347.

Livingston, J. H., Beaumont, D., Arzimangolou, A., Aicardi, J. (1989) Vigabatrin in the treatment of epilepsy in children. *Br. J. Clin. Pharmacol.* *27* (Suppl. 1):109–112.

Loscher, W., Czuczwar, S. J., Jackel, R., and Schwarz, M. (1987) Effect of microinjections of gamma-vinyl GABA or isoniazid into substantia nigra on the development of amygdala kindling in rats. *Exp. Neurol.* *95*:622–638.

Loscher, W., Honack, D., and Taylor, C. P. (1991) Gabapentin increases aminooxyacetic acid-induced GABA accumulation in several regions of rat brain. *Neurosci. Lett.* *128*:150–154.

Loughnan, P. M., Greenwald, A., Purton, W. N., Aranda, J. V., Watters, G., and Neims, A. H. (1977) Pharmacokinetic observations of phenytoin disposition in the newborn and young infant. *Arch. Dis. Child.* *52*:302–309.

Luna, D., Chiron, C., Pajot, N., Dulac, O., and Jallon, P. (1988) *Epidémiologie des épilepsies de l'enfant dans le d'épartement de l'Oise* (France). London: John Libbey, Eurotext, pp. 41–53.

Luna, D., Dulac, O., Pajot, N., and Beaumont, D. (1989) Vigabatrin in the treatment of childhood epilepsies: A single blind placebo-controlled study. *Epilepsia* *30*:430–437.

Luna, D., Dulac, O., and Plouin, P. (1989) Ictal characteristics of cryptogenic partial epilepsies in infancy. *Epilepsia* *30*:827–832.

Macdonald, R. L., and Kelly, K. M. (1993) Antiepileptic drug mechanisms of action. *Epilepsia 34* (Suppl. 5):S1–S8.

Macdonald, R. L., and Kelly, K. M. (1994) Mechanisms of action of currently prescribed and newly developed antiepileptic drugs. *Epilepsia 35* (Suppl. 4):S41–S50.

Marescaux, C., Hirsh, E., Finck, S., Maquet, P., Schlumberger, E., Sellal, F., Metz-Lutz, M. N., Alembik, Y., Salmon, E., Franck, G., and Kurtz, D. (1990) Landau-Kleffner syndrome: A pharmacologic study of five cases. *Epilepsia* *31*:768–777.

Marescaux, C., Micheletti, G., Vergnes, M., Depaulis, A., Rumbach, L., and Warter, J. M. (1984) A model of chronic spontaneous petit mal-like seizures in the rat: Comparison with pentylenetetrazol induced seizures. *Epilepsia* *25*:326–331.

Matsuo, F., Bergen, E., Faught, E., Messenheimer, J. A., Dran, A. T., Rudd, G. D., and Lineberry, C. G. (1993) Placebo-controlled study of the efficacy and safety of lamotrigine in patients with partial seizures. *Neurology 43*:2284–2291.

Mattson, R. H., Cramer, C., Collins, J., Smith, D., Delgado-Escueta, A., Brown, E. T., Williamson, T., Treiman, D., McNamara, J., McKutchen, C., Homan, R., Crill, W., Lubozynski, M., Rosenthal, N., and Mayersdorf, A. (1985) Comparison of carbamazepine, phenobarbital, phenytoin and primidone in partial and secondarily generalized tonic-clonic seizures. *New Engl. J. Med.* *313*:145–151.

Maytal, J., Shinnar, S., Moshé, S. L., and Alvarez, L. A. (1989) Low morbidity and mortality of status epilepticus in children. *Pediatrics 83*:323–331.

McCabe, R. T., Wasterlain, C. G., Kucharczyk, N., Sofia, R. D., and Vogel, J. R. (1993) Evidence of anticonvulsant and neuroprotectant action of felbamate mediated by strychnine-insensitive glycine receptors. *J. Pharmacol. Exp. Ther. 264:*248–252.

Meldrum, B. S., and Horton, R. (1978) Blockade of epileptic responses in photosensitive baboon *Papio papio* by two irreversible inhibitors of GABA-transaminase, gamma-acetylenic GABA (4-amino-hex-5-ynoic acid) and gamma-vinyl GABA (4-amino-hex-5-enoic acid). *Psychopharmacologia 59:*47–50.

Meldrum, B. S., and Murugaiah, K. (1983) Anticonvulsant action in mice with sound-induced seizures of the optical isomers of gamma-vinyl GABA. *Eur. J. Pharmacol. 89:*149–152.

Mesdjian, E., Dravet, C., Cenraud, B., and Roger, J. (1980) Carbamazepine intoxication due to triacetyloleandomycin administration in epileptic patients. *Epilepsia 21:*489–496.

Miller, A. A., Wheatley, P., Swayer, D. A., Baxter, M. G., and Roth, B. (1986) Pharmacological studies on lamotrigine, a novel potential antiepileptic drug: I. Anticonvulsant profile in mice and rats. *Epilepsia 27:*483–489.

Mintz, I. M., Adams, M. E., and Bean, B. P. (1992) P-Type calcium channels in rat central and peripheral neurons. *Neuron 9:*85–95.

Mori, Y., Friedrich, T., Man-Suk, K., Mikami, A., Nakai, J., Ruth, P., Bosse, E., Hofmann, F., Flockerzi, V., Furuichi, T., Mikoshiba, K., Imoto, K., Tanabe, T., and Numa, S. (1991) Primary structure and functional expression from complementary DNA of a brain calcium channel. *Nature 350:*398–402.

Morrell, F., Whisler, W. W., Smith, S., Pierre-Louis, J. C., Hoeppner, T. J., Chez, M. G., and Hasegawa, H. (1992) Clinical outcome in Landau-Kleffner syndrome treated by multiple subpial transection. *Epilepsia 33* (Suppl. 3):100. (Abstract)

Morselli, P. L. (1977) *Drug Disposition during Development.* New York: Spectrum.

Morselli, P. L. (1983) Development and physiological variables important for drug kinetics. In P. L. Morselli, C. E. Pippenger, and J. Penry (eds.), *Antiepileptic Drug Therapy in Paediatrics* New York: Raven Press. pp. 1–12.

Morselli, P. L., Franco-Morselli, R., and Bossi, L. (1980) Clinical pharmacokinetics in newborns and infants: Age-related differences and therapeutic implications. *Clin. Pharmacokinet. 5:*485–527.

Morselli, P. L., Principi, N., Togoni, G., Reali, F., Belvedere, G., Standen, S. M., and Sereni, F. (1973) Diazepam elimination in premature and fullterm infants and children. *J. Perinat. Med. 1:*133–141.

Morselli, P. L., and Regnier, F. (1983) Ethics in pediatric research for new antiepileptic drugs. In P. L. Morselli, C. E. Pippenger, and J. Penry (eds.), *Antiepileptic Drug Therapy in Paediatrics.* New York: Raven Press, pp. 309–314.

Moss, S. J., Smart, T. A., Porter, N. M., et al. (1990) Cloned GABA receptors are maintained in a stable cell line: Allosteric and channel properties. *Eur. J. Pharmacol. 189:*77–88.

Mutoh, K., and Dichter, M. A. (1993) Lamotrigine blocks voltage-dependent Na currents in a voltage-dependent manner with a small use-dependent component. *Epilepsia 34* (Suppl. 6):87.

Noebels, J. (1979) Analysis of inherited epilepsy using single locus mutations in mice. *Fed. Proc. 38:*2405–2410.

Nowycky, M. C., Fox, A. P., and Tsien, R. W. (1985) Three types of neuronal calcium channels with different agonist sensitivity. *Nature 316:*440–443.

O'Dougherty, M., Wright, F. S., Cox, S., and Walson, P. (1987) Carbamazepine plasma concentration: Relationship to cognitive impairment. *Arch. Neurol.* *44*:863–877.

Oles, R. J., Singh, L., Hughes, J., and Woodruff, G. N. (1990) The anticonvulsant action of gabapentin involves the glycine/NMDA receptor. *Soc. Neurosci. Abstr. 16*:783.

Oller, L. F. V., Russi, A., and Oller-Daurella, L. (1991) Lamotrigine in the Lennox-Gastaut syndrome *Epilepsia 32* (Suppl. 3):58. (Abstract)

Pacifici, G. M., Taddeuci-Brunlli, G., and Rane, A. (1984) Clonazepam serum protein banding during development. *Clin. Pharmacol. Ther. 35*:354–359.

Painter, M. J., Pippenger, C., McDonald, H., and Pitlick, W. (1978) Phenobarbital and diphenylhydantoin levels in neonates with seizures. *J. Pediatr. 92*:315–319.

Pennell, P. B., Ogaily, M. S., and Macdonald, R. L. (1994) Aplastic anemia in a patient receiving felbamate for partial complex seizures. *Neurology* (in press).

Penry, J. K., and Dean, J. C. (1988) Valproate monotherapy in partial seizures. *Am. J. Med. 84* (Suppl. 1A):14–16.

Petroff, O. A. C., Rothman, D. L., Behar, K. L., and Mattson, R. H. (1993) Effect of vigabatrin on GABA levels in human brain measured in vivo with [^{1}H] NMR spectroscopy. *Epilepsia 34* (Suppl. 6):68.

Pritchett, D. B., Luddens, H., and Seeburg, P. H. (1989) Type I and type II GABA$_A$-benzodiazepine receptors produced in transfected cells. *Science 245*:1389–1392.

Pritchett, D. B., and Seeburg, P. H. (1990) Gamma-aminobutyric acid$_A$ receptor α5-subunit creates novel type II benzodiazepine receptor pharmacology. *J. Neurochem. 54*:1802–1804.

Pritchett, D. B., Sontheimer, H., Shivers, B. D., et al. (1989) Importance of a novel GABA$_A$ receptor subunit for benzodiazepine pharmacology. *Nature 338*:582–584.

Rakic, P. (1981) Neuronal–glial interaction during brain development. *Trends Neurosci. 4*:184–187.

Reimann, W. (1983) Inhibition by GABA, baclofen, and gabapentin of dopamine release from rabbit caudate nucleus: Are there common or different sites of action? *Eur. J. Pharmacol. 94*:341–344.

Rey, E., D'Athis, P., De Lauture, D., Dulac, O., Aicardi, J., and Olive, G. (1979) Pharmacokinetics of carbamazepine in the neonate and in the child. *Int. J. Clin. Pharmacol. Biopharm. 17*:90–96.

Reynolds, E. H., Milner, G., Matthews, D. M., and Chanarin, I. (1966) Anticonvulsant therapy, megaloblastic haemopoiesis and folic acid metabolism. *Q. J. Med. 35*:521–537.

Rho, J. M., Donevan, S. D., and Rogawski, M. A. (1994) Mechanism of action of the anticonvulsant drug Felbumate: Opposing effects on N-Methyl-D-Aspartate and γ-Aminobutyric Acid$_A$. *Ann. Neurology 35*:229–233.

Riekkinen, P. J., Pitkanen, A., Ylinen, A., Sivenius, J., and Halonen, T. (1989) Specificity of vigabatrin for the GABAergic system in human epilepsy. *Epilepsia 30* (Suppl. 3):S18–S22.

Ritter, F., Dreifuss, F. E., Sackallares, J. C., Shields, D., French, J., Dodson, W. E., Kramer, L. D., and Rosenberg, A. (1991) Double-blind trial of felbamate in Lennox-Gastaut syndrome. *Epilepsia 32* (Suppl. 3):13. (Abstract)

Rock, D. M., Kelly, K. M., and Macdonald, R. L. (1993) Gabapentin actions on ligand- and voltage-gated responses in cultured rodent neurons. *Epilepsy Res.* *16*:89–98.

Rogawski, M. A., and Porter, R. J. (1990) Antiepileptic drugs: Pharmacological mechanisms and clinical efficacy with consideration of promising developmental stage compounds. *Pharmacol. Rev. 42*:223–286.

Roger, J., Dravet, C., Bureau, M., Dreifuss, F. E., and Wolf, P. (1985) *Epileptic Syndromes in Infancy, Childhood and Adolescence.* London: Libbey Eurotext.

Roger, J., Grandgeon, H., Guey, J., and Lob, H. (1968) Psychiatric and psychological complications of ethosuximide treatment in epileptics. *Encéphale 57*:407–438.

Rowan, A. J., Schear, M. J., Wiener, J. A., and Luciano, D. (1989) Intensive monitoring and pharmacokinetic studies of gabapentin in patients with generalized spike-wave discharges. *Epilepsia 30*:30.

Sachdeo, R. C., Murphy, J. V., and Kamin, M. (1992) Felbamate in juvenile myoclonic epilepsy. *Epilepsia 33* (Suppl. 3):118 (Abstract)

Sarhan, S., and Seiler, N. (1979) Metabolic inhibitors and subcellular distribution of GABA. *J. Neurosci. Res. 4*:399–421.

Sato, S., White, B. G., Penry, J. K., Dreifuss, F. E., Sackellares, J. C., and Kupferberg, H. J. (1982) Valproic acid versus ethosuximide in the treatment of absence seizures. *Neurology 32*:157–163.

Schechter, P. J., Hanke, N. F. J., Grove, J., Huebert, N., and Sjoerdsma, A. (1984) Biochemical and clinical effects of gamma-vinyl GABA in patients with epilepsy. *Neurology 34*:182–186.

Schechter, P. J., and Tranier Y. (1977) Effects of elevated brain GABA concentrations on the action of bicuculline and picrotoxin in mice. *Psychopharmacology 54*:145–148.

Schechter, P. J., Tranier, Y., and Grove, J. (1979) Attempts to correlate alterations in brain GABA metabolism by GABA-T inhibitors with their anticonvulsant effect. In P. Mandel and F. V. DeFeudis (eds.), *GABA-Biochemistry and CNS Function.* New York: Plenum, pp. 43–57.

Schlicker, E., Reimann, W., and Gothert, M. (1985) Gabapentin decreases monoamine release without affecting acetylcholine release in the brain. *Arzneim.-Forsch./Drug Res. 35*:1347–1349.

Schlumberger, E., Chavez, F., Dulac, O., and Moszkowski, J. (1992) Open study with lamotrigine (LTG) in child epilepsy. *Seizure 1* (Suppl. A):P9/21. (Abstract)

Schlumberger, E., and Dulac, O. (1994) A simple, effective, well-tolerated treatment regime for West syndrome. *Dev. Med. Child Neurol.* (in press).

Schmidt, B. (1989) Potential antiepileptic drugs: Gabapentin. In R. H. Levy, F. E. Dreifuss, R. H. Mattson, B. S. Meldrum, and J. K. Penry (eds.), *Antiepileptic Drugs,* 3rd ed. New York: Raven Press, pp. 925–935.

Schmutz, M., Ferret, T., Heckendorn, R., Jeker, A., Portet, C. H., and Olpe, H. R. (1993) GP 47779, the main human metabolite of oxcarbazepine (Trileptal), and both enantiomers have equal anticonvulsant activity. *Epilepsia 34* (Suppl. 2):122.

Schobben, F., and Willemse, J. (1985) Substitution of carbamazepine by oxcarbazepine in epileptic children. Poster presented at the 16th Epilepsy International Congress, Hamburg.

Schoeman, J. F., Elyas, A. D., Brett, E. M., and Lascelles, P. T. (1984) Altered ratio of carbamazepine-10,11-epoxide in plasma of children: Evidence of anticonvulsant drug interaction. *Dev. Med. Child. Neurol. 26:*749–755.

Schofield, P. R., Darlison, M. G., Fujita, M., et al. (1987) Sequence and functional expression of the GABA$_A$ receptor shows a ligand-gated receptor super-family. *Nature 328:*221–227.

Schousboe, A., Larsson, O. M., and Seiler, N. (1986) Stereoselective uptake of the GABA-transaminase inhibitors gamma-vinyl GABA and gamma-acetylenic GABA into neurons and astrocytes. *Neurochem. Res. 11:*1497–1505.

Shields, W. D., and Saslow, E. (1983) Myoclonic, atonic and absence seizures following the institution of carbamazepine therapy in children. *Neurology 33:*1487–1489.

Shin, C., Rigsbee, L. C., and McNamara, J. O. (1986) Anti-seizure and anti-epileptogenic effect of gamma-vinyl gamma-aminobutyric acid in amygdaloid kindling. *Brain Res. 398:*370–374.

Shivers, B. D., Killisch, I., Sprengel, R., et al. (1989) Two novel GABA$_A$ receptor subunits exist in distinct neuronal subpopulations. *Neuron 3:*327–337.

Sieghart, W., Eichinger, A., Richards, J. G., and Mohler, H. (1987) Photoaffinity labelling of benzodiazepine receptor proteins with the partial inverse agonist [^{3}H]Ro15-4513: A biochemical and autoradiographic study. *J. Neurochem. 48:*46–52.

Siemes, H., Spohr, H. L., Michael, T., and Nau, T. (1988) Therapy of infantile spasms with valproate: Results of a prospective study. *Epilepsia 29:*553–560.

Snead, O. C., Benton, L. W., Hosey, L. C., Swann, L. W., Spink, D., Martin, D., and Rej, R. (1989) Treatment of infantile spasms with high-doses ACTH: Efficacy and plasma levels of ACTH and cortisol. *Neurology 39:*1027–1031.

Snead, O. C., and Hosey, L. C. (1985) Exacerbation of seizures in children by carbamazepine. *New Engl. J. Med. 313:*916–922.

Snutch, T. P., Leonard, J. P., Gilbert, M. M., Lester, H. A., and Davidson, N. (1990) Rat brain expresses a heterogeneous family of calcium channels. *Proc. Natl. Acad. Sci. 87:*3391–3395.

Snutch, T. P., Tomlinson, W. J., Leonard, J. P., and Gilbert, M. M. (1991) Distinct calcium channels are generated by alternative splicing and are differentially expressed in the mammalian CNS. *Neuron 7:*45–57.

Sofia, R. D., Kramer, L., Perhach, J. L., and Rosenberg, A. (1991) Felbamate. In F. Pisani, E. Perucca, G. Avanzini, and A. Richens (eds.), *New Antiepileptic Drugs.* Amsterdam: Elsevier, pp. 103–108.

Soong, T. W., Stea, A., Hodson, C. D., Dubel, S. J., Vincent, S. R., and Snutch, T. P. (1993) Structure and functional expression of a member of the low voltage-activated calcium channel family. *Science 260:*1133–1136.

Starr, T. V. B., Prystay, W., and Snutch, T. P. (1991) Primary structure of a calcium channel that is highly expressed in the rat cerebellum. *Proc. Natl. Acad. Sci. 88:*5621–5625.

Stewart, B. H., Kugler, A. R., Thompson, P. R., and Bockbrader, H. N. (1993) A saturable transport mechanism in the intestinal absorption of gabapentin is the underlying cause of the lack of proportionality between increasing dose and drug levels in plasma. *Pharm. Res. 10:*276–281.

Suman-Chauhan, N., Webdale, L., Hill, D. R., and Woodruff, G. N. (1993) Characterisation of [^{3}H]gabapentin binding to a novel site in rat brain: Homogenate binding studies. *Eur. J. Pharmacol. Mol. Pharmacol. 244:*293–301.

Swinyard, E. A., Sofia, R. D., and Kupferberg, H. J. (1986) Comparative anticonvulsant activity and neurotoxicity of felbamate and four prototype antiepileptic drugs in mice and rats. *Epilepsia 27:*27–34.

Tassinari, C. A., Draver, C., Roger, J., Cano, J. P., and Gastaut, H. (1972) Tonic status epilepticus precipitated by intravenous benzodiazepine in five patients with Lennox-Gastaut syndrome. *Epilepsia 13:*421–435.

Taylor, C. P. (1993) The anticonvulsant lamotrigine blocks sodium currents from cloned alpha-subunits of rat brain Na$^+$ channels in a voltage-dependent manner but gabapentin does not. *Soc. Neurosci. Abstr. 19:*1631.

Taylor, C. P., Rock, D. M., Weinkauf, R. J., and Ganong, A. H. (1988) In vitro and in vivo electrophysiology effects of the anticonvulsant gabapentin. *Soc. Neurosci. Abstr. 14:*866.

Taylor, C. P., Vartanian, M. G., Yuen, P. W., and Bigge, C. (1993) Potent and stereospecific anticonvulsant activity of 3-isobutyl GABA relates to in vitro binding at a novel site labeled by tritiated gabapentin. *Epilepsy Res. 14:* 11–15.

Ticku, M. K., Kamatchi, G. L., and Sofia, R. D. (1991) Effect of anticonvulsant felbamate on GABA$_A$ receptor system. *Epilepsia 32:*389–391.

Tremblay, E., Roisin, M. P., Represa, A., Charriaut-Marlangue, C., and Benari, Y. (1988) Transient increased density of NMDA binding sites in the developing rat hippocampus. *Brain Res. 46:*393–396.

Vining, E. P. G., Mellits, E. D., Dorsen, M. M., Cataldo, M. F., Quaskey, S. A., Spielberg, S. P., and Freeman, J. M., (1987) Psychologic and behavioural effects of antiepileptic drugs in children: A double-blind comparison between phenobarbital and valproic acid. *Pediatrics 80:*165–174.

Wallace, S. J. (1989) Lamotrigine in resistant childhood epilepsy. *Neuropediatrics 20:*116. (Abstract)

Wamil, A. W., and McLean, M. J. (1994) Limitation by gabapentin of high frequency action potential firing by mouse central neurons in cell culture. *Epilepsy Res. 17:*1–11.

Wamil, A. W., McLean, M. J., and Taylor, C. P. (1991) Multiple cellular actions of gabapentin. *Neurology 41* (Suppl. 1):140.

Wang, C. M., Lang, D. G., and Cooper, B. R. (1993) Lamotrigine effects on ion channels in cultured neuronal cells. *Epilepsia 34* (Suppl. 6):117–118.

Welty, D. F., Schielke, G. P., Vartanian, M. G., and Taylor, C. P. (1993) Gabapentin anticonvulsant action in rats: Disequilibrium with peak drug concentrations in plasma and brain microdialysate. *Epilepsy Res. 16:*175–181.

White, H. S., Kemp, J. W., and Woodbury, D. M. (1983) Effects of central nervous system maturation on drug metabolism. In P. L. Morselli, C. E. Pippenger, and J. Penry (eds.), *Antiepileptic Drug Therapy in Paediatrics*. New York: Raven Press, pp. 13–35.

White, H. S., Wolf, H. H., Swinyard, E. A., Skeen, G. A., and Sofia, R. D. (1992) A neuropharmacological evaluation of felbamate as a novel anticonvulsant. *Epilepsia 33:*564–572.

Williams, M. E., Feldman, D. H., McCue, A. F., Brenner, R., Velicelebi, G., Ellis, S. B., and Harpold, M. M. (1992) Structure and functional expression of α_1 subunits of a novel human neuronal calcium channel subtype. *Neuron 8:*71–84.

Wisden, W., Herb, A., Wieland, H., Keinanen, K., Luddens, H., and Seeburg,

P. H. (1991) Cloning, pharmacological characteristics and expression pattern of the rat GABA$_A$ receptor α4 subunit. *FEBS Lett. 289:*227–230.

Wisden, W., Laurie, D. J., Monyer, H., and Seeburg, P. H. (1992) The distribution of 13-GABA$_A$ receptor subunit messenger RNAs in the rat brain: 1. Telencephalon, diencephalon, mesencephalon. *J. Neurosci. 12:*1040–1062.

Woodbury, D. M. (1967) Effects of drugs on various parameters of the developing nervous system. *Drugs Poison 297:*227–244.

Epilogue

DOMINICK P. PURPURA

The frequent occurrence of seizure disorders in infancy and childhood, while long recognized, remains poorly understood. Developmental perturbations are likely candidates but we know little about them and even less about their impact on the mature brain. Understanding the principles of brain development is one of the central issues of biology. Fortunately, much progress has been made recently in defining these principles as evidenced by the present volume. If the picture of brain development is incomplete, it is not for the lack of effort. Consider the magnitude of the problem!

Brain development begins with the commitment of over 100 billion neurons and a half a trillion glial cells to formation of the most complex structure in the universe. For the most part neurons are generated in a zone surrounding the central cavity of the neural tube and its cephalic enlargements. Post-mitotic bipolar neurons leave this germinative zone and find their way to populate different structures (cerebral cortex, basal ganglia, thalamus, etc.). In the case of the cerebral cortex, the vast proportion of neurons utilize close application to radial fibers of specialized astroglia as guidelines to attain their correct address in the cortex. Some primitive neurons utilize other cell surface contacts as they migrate in orthogonal trajectories. How these elements navigate over relatively great distances is a subject of hot pursuit. Most likely, cytoskeletal components that induce cell mobility are activated by surface-to-surface macromolecular interactions. A point of some importance is that neurons destined for different positions in the cerebral cortex are born and migrate at different times. But this is not always the case as revealed by findings of early generated subcortical plate neurons that transiently serve important directional and facilitating functions for incoming afferent pathways. When their job is done these neurons disappear, which emphasizes the significant contribution that programmed cell death (apoptosis) makes to the developmental process.

When primitive neurons have attained their correct position, they undergo extensive differentiation of dendritic and axonal arbors. Then afferent pathways are fine tuned to appropriate targets through a process that is activity-dependent. The process of synaptogenesis that ensues will produce specified interconnected systems of neurons with about 10^{15} synapses. All of this occurs under the influence of several dozen growth factors and trophic agents, many of which will acquire other duties as neurotransmitters and neuromodulatory agents. Finally, at a stage when functionally validated connections have been effected and intrinsic neuronal circuitry completed, myelination of rapidly conducting pathways occurs to ensure high-fidelity communication between and among related neuronal organizations.

This brief description of brain development embarrasses reality. For nothing has been said about developmentally regulated genetic mechanisms expressed at each stage of the temporally overlapping sequence of maturational events. Nor has the important contribution of epigenetic and environmental factors been considered. We now know that profound alterations in receptor families occur during ontogenesis that significantly modify the effects which neurotransmitters have on developing neuronal systems. Additionally, receptors and related ionic channels undergo structural changes during development that modify ligand and voltage sensitivity and activation of coupled G-protein related intracellular events. Changes in the variety and distribution of cytosolic and membrane bound kinases, so critical for driving the machinery of protein phosphorylation, are also demonstrable in the developing brain. Information is accumulating rapidly on these molecular and genetic processes as the complexity of brain development unfolds.

What does this wealth of information tell us about seizure disorders in the immature brain? The question provokes remembrances of things past. Before the present revolution in developmental neuroscience, candidate hypotheses relating to seizure susceptibility and brain development suffered the burden of "yin-yang" theories based on excitatory-inhibitory interactions. I first utilized intracellular recording from hippocampal and neocortical neurons in neonatal and young kittens to demonstrate that excitatory postsynaptic potentials (EPSPs) appeared earlier in development than inhibitory postsynaptic potentials (IPSPs). A morphological correlate of these observations was seen in the relatively late appearance of axosomatic as opposed to axodendritic synapses, the former presumably reflecting inhibitory processes. Other peculiarities of immature cortical neurons were observed in the tendency for immature neurons to exhibit partial and full impulse initiation in dendrites, a rare finding in mature neocortical neurons. The relative imbalance of excitatory and inhibitory processes in cortical networks and the capacity of dendrites of immature neurons for impulse generation were thus viewed as contributory factors in epileptogenesis in the developing brain. Looking back over the three decades since these studies were reported provides perspect and prospect.

Based on what we now know about brain development, the range of potential perturbations likely to impact on the excitability characteristics of the immature nervous system seems boundless. While some factors will be found to be more critical than others, ease of detection provides no clue to importance. Thirty years ago the essence of parsimony was to attribute seizures to overexcitation, underinhibition, and membrane instabilities. We now recognize these phenomena as reflections of a spectrum of causal factors. Some have only recently come to light, most were not even dreamt of in earlier philosophies. "Developmental epileptology" has come of age.

In the awakening, many problems and questions leap to mind. A few bear mention. For example, we don't know what the normal ratio of inhibitory to excitatory neurons ought to be in the cerebral cortex for optimal functioning, to say nothing about total numbers of both. Immunocytochemical studies of GABA-ergic neurons disclose large numbers in different lamina, with altered distributions in epileptogenic areas. Could neurogenetic processes play a role in producing an imbalance of excitatory and inhibitory neurons? What role might target elements play in determining neuronal phenotype in cerebral cortex? What can be said about factors in migration that lead to disorganization of normal cortical columnar and inter-columnar connectivity? Activity-dependent mechanisms are at play in sorting out functional domains of neuronal networks. These might be susceptible to modification and alter the valence of excitation and inhibition in particular pathways. "Yinyang" hypotheses wax eternal.

Immature neurons undergo sequential synapse formation. Earliest contacts are effected on the shafts of dendrites of cortical neurons, later on spines and cell bodies. Dendritic spine, neck, and shaft alterations as well as changes in presynaptic terminal contact area occur during development. If everything we now know about glutaminergic (NMDA and non-NMDA) spine synapses is correct regarding their essential role in learning and memory on the one hand, and seizure mechanisms on the other, the importance of dendritic spine synapses in epileptology takes on ever greater significance.

A decade ago studies by my colleagues and me demonstrated that changes in dendrites and dendritic spines of cortical neurons in biopsy tissue obtained from infants and children with intractable seizure disorders were associated with a profound disarray of intradendritic microtubules. In view of the role of microtubules in dendritic morphology and in somatodendritic transport of macromolecules and other elements, it is evident that studies of seizure related structural alterations in dendritic morphology must take into account cellular processes that regulate the integrity and function of the cytoskeleton.

Reference was made above to observations indicating that many closely related families of receptors undergo developmentally regulated changes in subunit structure. The future holds great promise for assessing how such alterations influence related short and long term changes in neuronal excitability through calcium, inositol triphosphate, and other secondary messenger systems. Indeed, as evidence accumulates on immediate early gene transcription in relation to changes in neuronal activity, neuroscience is well on the way to evolving a "grand unified theory" that links experientially driven long-term alterations in neuronal activity to genetically regulated changes in neuronal structure and metabolism as well as to transporter, receptor, and ion channel properties. Neurons make synapses and synapses make behavior. This was the central dogma of neuroscience *before* it was realized that activity (behavior) could modify synapses and so modify neurons! The implications of this dynamic relationship between activity and persistent excitability change, involving genetic mechanisms for developmental epileptology, is a problem of no little consequence considering current interests in "kindling" and its presumed relation to long-term potentiation.

Epilepsy does not exist in a culture dish or a brain slice. It is an emergent manifestation of abnormal neuronal activity and the behavioral states this engenders. Clinical inquiry may reveal more about epilepsy than we can currently translate into bench science. But this is no reason to avoid the issue. The developing brain works in strange ways, its secrets to unfold in seizure. One of the missions of developmental epileptology will be to identify those features of seizure disorders in infancy and childhood that translate into productive basic research. It must not be forgotten that before the dawning of the "age of brain imaging," clinical studies of epilepsy provided much of what we now know about cerebral functional localization. Nor should history treat lightly the contributions to the brain sciences derived from studies of seizure mechanisms. New age imaging and computer-assisted electrophysiological methods will increase, not diminish, the importance of close coupling of clinical and basic science collaborative research in developmental epilepsy.

Clinical and basic scientists interested in seizure mechanisms have an opportunity to effect dramatic improvements in the management of childhood epilepsy by facilitating the identification of effective anticonvulsant agents derived from new principles of neuronal operations. As the knowledge base of developmental processes increases along with an understanding of their relationship to seizure manifestations in the maturing brain, it can be anticipated that new medications will come to the fore.

For example, the current plethora of studies of the NMDA-receptor channel complex are likely to yield new pharmacological insights that could revolutionize antiepileptic drug therapies in the years ahead. These drugs will be all the more relevant to childhood seizure disorders as the changing properties of receptor complexes during maturation become more firmly established. It bears noting that the most effective antiepileptic drug in history, phenytoin, was discovered by two clinicians with extraordinary insight into the workings of the human brain in health and disease. We've come a long way since then in our appreciation of both brain development and epilepsy, and we hope that clinical insights will continue to be a driving force in energizing the new discipline of developmental epileptology in this the *decade of the brain.*

Index